BRAIN TUMORS

Their Biology and Pathology

AMERICAN EDITION
based on the Second German Edition

Translated by **ALAN B. ROTHBALLER, M.D., M.Sc.**
Assistant Professor of Anatomy (Neuroanatomy) and Surgery (Neurosurgery), Albert Einstein College of Medicine, and Assistant Attending Neurosurgeon, Bronx Municipal Medical Center, New York, N. Y. Formerly Research Fellow, Montreal Neurological Institute

and **JERZY OLSZEWSKI, M.D., Ph.D.**
Associate Professor of Pathology (Neuropathology), College of Medicine, University of Saskatchewan, and Medical Research Associate, Canadian National Research Council Formerly Assistant Professor of Neuroanatomy and Neuropathology, McGill University and the Montreal Neurological Institute

BRAIN TUMORS

THEIR BIOLOGY AND PATHOLOGY

By **K. J. ZÜLCH, M. D.**

Professor of Neurology, University of Cologne,
and Head, Department of General Neurology,
Max Planck Institute for Brain Research

 SPRINGER SCIENCE+BUSINESS MEDIA, LLC

ISBN 978-1-4899-6264-5   ISBN 978-1-4899-6571-4 (eBook)
DOI 10.1007/978-1-4899-6571-4

Library of Congress Catalog Card Number: 57-14807

FOREWORD

When I began, in 1922, the study of Cushing's collection of tumors of the nervous system, it was my hope and intention to publish with him a comprehensive treatise correlating their biological behavior with their pathology. This ambitious project I was unable to complete because, in 1928, I left his clinic to create one of my own at the University of Chicago. Although I found time there to publish an account of the astroblastomas and, with Bucy, another of the oligodendrogliomas, I was soon forced by the pressure of clinical responsibilities to abandon the project.

Yet such a treatise was greatly needed and I am happy that the need has been so brilliantly satisfied by the exhaustive study of Dr. Zülch that has appeared in the Handbuch der Neurochirurgie. This study, profusely illustrated, is an inexhaustible mine of information concerning tumors of the brain. It is, however, too long and involved to be of everyday use to the busy neurosurgeon and neurologist. For this reason Dr. Zülch has put the essence of his vast experience into the present smaller volume which is equally authoritative but more manageable. Its translation into English makes it more readily utilizable to the American clinician.

Dr. Zülch discusses the origin of brain tumors, their frequency, their age-distribution and other biological characteristics according to a classification that has the purpose of being useful to the clinician without doing violence to our knowledge of tumor pathology. This procedure leaves room for argument, and the author gives his reasons for his own decisions.

Since the present book is addressed to the neurologist and neurosurgeon, I might point out that some diagnoses—the medulloepitheliomas and neuroepitheliomas—would have to be discussed at more length were the book intended for ophthalmologists, whereas pinealomas and papillomas would drop out. In other words, tumors with the structure described under these names exist and may be included or excluded from a classification depending upon its purpose. It should be pointed out also that any classification is somewhat artificial. This is true in general pathology as well as in neuropathology. The pathologist may be forced, in a particular case, to diagnose osteo-fibro-chondro-sarcoma, but this does not invalidate the isolation of groups with fairly typical and uniform structure so that it is possible to describe helpfully and individually fibromas, osteomas, chondromas and sarcomas.

To come now to the author's classification as used in this book, I think that it is very reasonable. I should perhaps differ only in including the astroblastomas, rather than with the astrocytomas, with the glioblastomas which they resemble more in their clinical behavior; the author is correct in including the pineoblastomas with the medulloblastomas, the site of the tumor being easily identified by an adjective—medulloblastoma pinealis.

In introducing this admirably concise treatment of an important subject to the American medical public, I am reminded of a statement of Robert Louis Stevenson to the effect that to live deliberately through one's ages is to get the best from a liberal education. One of the things that is learned with advancing age is that one is not going to be able to fulfill all of the dreams of one's youth. I am happy that one of mine has been so admirably realized by Dr. Zülch and that Drs. Rothballer and Olszewski have been willing to undertake the difficult task of translation.

Percival Bailey

PREFACE

Ever since the appearance of Bailey and Cushing's monograph in 1930, their new classification of brain tumors has gradually gained acceptance everywhere, including Germany and other German-speaking countries. When the first German edition of this book appeared in 1951, it was intended as an aid in the classification of brain tumors and as a means of dispelling some of the obscurity which seems to surround the subject. Through accurate macroscopic and microscopic examination and especially through a precise differential diagnosis, the classification of these tumors may become a real science, and one readily accessible to anyone prepared to make the necessary effort. The first edition, I may hope, made some progress in this direction. Beyond the mere classification however, the data thus acquired needed to be compiled and analyzed. Figures on preferential site, age incidence, sex predilection, and general incidence are therefore included. Moreover, the form of the tumor, its manner of growth, and type of spread, as well as such reactions of the surrounding brain as alterations in its shape or shifts in its position have been considered. All of the foregoing data—and their relation to the clinical picture—should be of very real help to the neurologist, radiologist and surgeon in making a preoperative diagnosis. Lastly, some thoughts on the origin of brain tumors have been included.

The special attention given to the clinical aspects of the subject is the result of our close association with the neurosurgical clinics of Dr. W. Tönnis in Würzburg, Berlin, Bochum-Langendreer, and Cologne. This monograph has benefitted greatly from our collaboration and I am much indebted to him.

The data are based upon an analysis of 4000 cases, all of which I myself have examined and classified. As a consequence, emphasis in the text is laid upon personal experience, and citing of authors has been kept to a minimum even when the results of other investigators have been utilized. Nonetheless, references to the most important contributions on each subject and the relatively complete bibliography included in this book will facilitate study of the literature.

With increasing frequency, surgeons and general pathologists have been enabling us to enlarge our experience by sending us material from rare or difficult tumor cases. Certain new insights have thus been made possible from this unusual concentration of material. I maintain the hope that we may be fortunate enough to set up a central tumor registry where these rare cases can be assembled, and in this way fill in the remaining gaps in our knowledge.

The American edition is based on the second German edition, which has been revised and enlarged both to keep abreast of current progress in the field and to record our own increasing experience. In particular, a number of tables concerning biological data on brain tumors have been added. The histological drawings have been replaced by original photomicrographs, all of which were taken with the Leitz-Panphot or Aristophot.

Cologne

July, 1957   K. J. Zülch

TRANSLATORS' INTRODUCTION

The first edition of Dr. Zülch's book on brain tumors appeared in 1951 at a time when both of the translators had, for different reasons, undertaken a study of brain tumor pathology; they found his book so useful that the idea of translating it into English was a natural consequence. Subsequently, the popularity of the first edition (which was sold out by 1952) was sufficient to encourage the preparation of a second German edition, especially in view of interim progress in the field. The translation of the book was postponed until the text of this second edition was available.

The reasons for undertaking this translation were several. Relatively few English-speaking physicians and scientists today are sufficiently familiar with German to make ready use of texts in that language, with the result that much valuable material remains inaccessible. Translation of Dr. Zülch's book provides an opportunity to present a comprehensive exposition of the subject of brain tumors as viewed by the German schools of pathology, neurology, and neuropathology, or at least as viewed by a representative of these fields.

The book has an impressive number of merits of its own. It is comprehensive, up-to-date, and sufficiently detailed to serve as reference for the worker in the field, while at the same time compact and not excessively expensive. On the other hand, most of the other more comprehensive and authoritative monographs on the subject were printed some years ago (e.g., Bailey's chapters on brain tumors in Penfield's Cytology and Cellular Pathology of the Nervous System, or Penfield's contribution to tumor pathology in Nelson's Loose-Leaf Surgery) and are now out of print and very difficult to obtain. Other fundamental contributions to the subject are to be found in various journals, where again they are not readily accessible except in reference libraries. The current texts on neuropathology and clinical neurology can rarely devote enough space to the single subject of brain tumors to provide the details and background so important to the worker in the field.

A word about the manner in which the translation was carried out should be added. Despite the similarity of many of the words, the differences between English and German are often formidable and translation was not an easy task. Our first aim has been clarity. Thus we have felt justified in simplifying some of the original text and omitting some of the modifying words and phrases which enrich meaning at the expense of ease of comprehension. But we have endeavored to preserve the distinctive flavor of the original, retaining Dr. Zülch's critical analyses and comments without resort to the more customary euphemisms of English. The colorful habit in German pathology of describing structures or lesions in terms of common household objects ("size of a tangerine," "consistency of bacon," etc.) has been retained also. German words have been eliminated except in those few instances where they have no meaningful English counterpart (e.g., "Pinselzellgliom"—paint-brush cell glioma) in which case they are sometimes followed by the English translation in parentheses. No German words have been brought over directly into English other than those already in common use (e.g., Anlage). In cases where a descriptive German phrase appeared to correspond to an English phrase using a different set of words, the customary English expression has been used, (e.g., perivascular cuffing instead of perivascular cell-wreath, the literal equivalent of "perivaskulärer Zellkranz"). The use of quotation marks has largely followed the German original; they never indicate a quaint or inexactly translated German word or phrase. When reference was encountered to persons or techniques totally unknown to the majority of English-speaking readers, most examples were simply omitted, but a few persist. Occasionally we have felt the need to supplement the translation with a word of explanation, or to add comments about the subject itself. This has been done in the form of Translators' Footnotes.

Citations in the text are made by name of the author or authors. We added the date where it is necessary to avoid ambiguity or where it has intrinsic interest. The bibliography at the end of the book is identical with that of the German edition. It is complete except for certain old references of primarily historical value and for a few references that have been added in the translation. In the latter case, the actual citation has often been given as a footnote.

Throughout the period of translation we have been able to consult Dr. Zülch on any controversial or poorly understood point; his help has made our task immeasurably easier. Finally, Dr. Zülch has read over the entire English manuscript himself, making improvements when indicated, thus assuring that the translation would be reasonably authoritative and accurate.

Montreal

A. R.
J. O.

CONTENTS

THE HISTORICAL DEVELOPMENT AND PRESENT STATE OF CLASSIFICATION

" . . . The essential criteria for a classification of tumors according to their intrinsic properties can be found only in the study of their chemical nature, their microscopical structure, and the manner and sequence of their development . . . It has always seemed to me that the tumor types most correctly formulated are those that are arranged parallel to normal structures, like the tendinous, fibrous-tissue tumors . . . and the enchondroma, whose structure is parallel to that of cartilage..."
Johannes Müller: *Über den feineren Bau und die Formen der krankhaften Geschwülste*. Berlin, 1838.
" . . . Certainly the neurosurgeon of the present day must take the wide view, if he ever is to attain the goal he should strive for, of foretelling, before the operation, not only the precise situation of a given lesion but its probable character as well..."
Harvey Cushing: *Intracranial Tumors and the Surgeon*. The Cameron Prize Lectures, 1925.

These two quotations seem to characterize so clearly the development of tumor-research over the last 100 years, that I used them to introduce a review article appearing in commemoration of Harvey Cushing's 70th birthday. Johannes Müller indicated the direction the development was to take in the following century. Investigations of the chemical nature of a tumor, with the demonstration of protein-like or gelatine-yielding substances, have developed into micro-chemical demonstrations of the individual components of the tissue and their degeneration products, by the use of various dyes and the tissues' response to impregnation with metallic salts. Chemical and biological investigations of the metabolism of tumors and their respiration followed. The morphological development of tumor tissue has been elucidated to some extent by the application of the tissue culture method. Johannes Müller's idea to compare tumors with normal tissues was further pursued and enlarged upon by taking into consideration the developmental stages of cells. In the hands of Ribbert, Bailey and Cushing, this approach yielded outstanding results in the classification of brain tumors. Thus it happened that Cushing was not only able to formulate his goal in the above mentioned sentence, but also to witness its realization a decade later. This detailed study of individual tumor types had already been forecast and utilized by Johannes Müller. In his own words: "Let us remember the poisonous plants. Useful knowledge about them will not be obtained by considering only those characteristics common to all poisonous plants, because there are as few such characteristics for the latter as there are for neoplastic diseases. Rather, such knowledge can be obtained only by specific information about each individual poisonous plant. I am firmly convinced that the same approach should be applied to the different types of cancer, and, on the basis of certain characteristics that I have observed myself, I have obtained some confirmation of this theory."

In order to understand the present state of brain tumor classification, we had best begin with a historical review of the past century. Such a review—as in most fields of pathological anatomy—must begin with Virchow. Prior to his time there was a lack of basic or systematic knowledge, although, to be sure, there were clear and informative individual descriptions of brain tumors, particularly in the excellent work of Cruveilhier[1]. Indeed, first attempts at classifications were being made—but a precise histological differentiation was still not possible. Classification according to certain external characteristics, such as cyst formation and fatty degeneration, was then customary, but it constantly led to erroneous conclusions.

The lack of any system and the adherence to meaningless external characteristics becomes evident in an attempt at a systematic description of the subject matter as we find it in the encyclopedic descriptions of Bressler. He speaks of "presenting in a concise fashion the disease picture and the etiological and pathological investigations based on the finest contributions" and quotes as authorities for pertinent chapters Abercrombie; Copland; Andral; Calmeil; Schönlein; Louis; Siebold; Walther; Ebermayer; Chelius; and Blasius. However, other authors of that time have not advanced far beyond this point either (for example, Hasse in Virchow's *Handbuch der speziellen Pathologie*, or Leubuscher in *Gehirnkrankheiten*).

Bressler presents a pathological classification including a chapter on "Induration of the Brain" in which we find what were perhaps tumors of cartilagenous consistency, scars, or even just special forms of brain swelling. Certain of his descriptions are meaningless today, but in his "hypertrophy" of the brain, we can easily recognize the classical description of dry brain swelling.

Among the actual space-occupying processes, the "pseudoplasms," Bressler recognizes 45 cases of "brain cancers," including three hypophysial tumors. Most authors of that time still considered brain cancer the result

---

[1] For example (in his book): I/3 Ganglion cell tumors of the sympathetics; II/6 Epidermoids; VIII/1,2,3 Meningiomas, etc.

of an inflammation—a concept to which he himself could not subscribe. Beside brain cancers, he recognized:

1. *Fatty tumors, steatomas, ceromas;* some of these may represent fibrillary astrocytomas, neurinomas, epidermoids, metastases, and tuberous sclerosis.

2. *Fleshy tumors, adenoidea;* possibly these are the meningiomas which have often been described by others as cancer of the calvarium or "sponges" of the meninges.[2]

3. *Bony tumors;* these might have included some hyperostosing meningiomas and osteosarcomas. If they contained "lime and chalk," they were more often found in the pineal (pinealomas?).

4. *Blood tumors, hematomas;* here, by the description of the variegated, spotted surface,[3] we recognize our glioblastoma.

5. *Medullary sarcoma;* this term might have been applied to the ependymoma of the hemispheres and the fourth ventricle.

6. *Melanosis;* we are here probably dealing with metastases of malignant melanomas.

7. *Cystic tumors;* certain cystic astrocytomas, angioblastomas, and also small encapsulated hemorrhages may be hidden here.

8. *Hydatids;* in his accurate description we can recognize cysticercosis, in particular.

The "sponge" of the meninges is well described in a special chapter. It was thought to arise from the inner or outer meninges and be able to break through the bone.

Louis' descriptions in particular served as models for Bressler. The pearly tumors (epidermoids) described by Cruveilhier were also quite well known, and a controversy about their origin had already started.

A new period began with the discovery of the cell by Schleiden and Schwann. The possibility of microscopic study caught the imagination of Johannes Müller who was convinced that the development of the normal cell would repeat itself in pathological processes. Thus he succeeded in making an essential step forward in the approach to tumor study: he was able to compare the tumor tissue with the normal tissue and even with the development of cells in "embryonic formations." We find in Müller's work descriptions of the morphology and composition of individual types of benign and malignant tumors, especially of cancers, and, in particular, descriptions of the form of individual tumor cells and "tailed elements.',

[2] We should like to call attention to the splendid publication by Josef and Carl Wenzel *Über die schwammigen Auswüchse auf der äusseren Hirnhaut*, Mainz, 1811, where they were obviously dealing with metastases, probably from a primary carcinoma of the lung.

[3] Abercrombie provides an excellent description of the variegated appearance of what is now called the glioblastoma multiforme (*see* Globus, 1946).

We have lingered so long over the description of that period because we see anticipated here the development of the coming century. This century has brought about a deeper understanding and improved methods of investigation but it is surprising how few really new ideas have emerged once such men as Johannes Müller had blazed the trail. In Lebert's exhaustive study (1851) the most important contribution was the distinction between the two large groups of "cancer." The real value of this large work is that for the first time the different biological significance of these groups was appreciated, i.e., that life expectancy is longer for one than the other. Contrariwise, the description of "pseudoplasms" by Leubuscher contributes little that is new, but a study of his book may be recommended for the subject of brain swelling and brain edema.

Only with Virchow did the period of systematic classification of tumors begin. In 1835 and 1846 he described the neuroglia and related it to brain tumors; he separated the gliomas from the other "sarcomas" of the nervous system. He recognized hard and soft forms, and cellular, medullary, fibrous, and telangiectatic types which occasionally, through mucoid degeneration, assumed the character of myxogliomas. In general, he found that soft forms were more closely related to myxomas and hard forms to fibromas. He called soft forms with numerous cells and blood vessels gliosarcomas. They were apt to contain spindle cells with long processes, large round cells with single or multiple nuclei (resembling giant cells, with four to five nuclei), and frequently fatty degeneration and hemorrhages as well. It was often difficult to distinguish them from true apoplexy. In addition to fresh hemorrhages, these hemorrhagic gliomas also contained older ones, and in some instances even caseous or fibrinous foci (necrosis?). Moreover, Virchow recognized gliomas of the ependyma in the form of warty structures, sometimes as large as peas (ependymitis granularis?), and larger when located in the fourth ventricle (our ependymomas). He included in these gliomas tumors of the sacral region, which in their histology resembled the cerebellar cortex (therefore probably ependymomas as well). He considered tumors of the acoustic nerve and some of the spinal cord as derivatives of the brain substance originating from perineurium, and therefore neuroglia, too. Finally Virchow offered a new interpretation for the neoplasms of the dura: the presence of psammoma bodies caused him to exclude some of them from the dural sarcomas and to put them in a new group of "psammomas." But by classifying them according to an external characteristic he made an error, in as much as he included other "psammomatous" neoplasms too—e.g., the calcified pinealomas, and "hyperplasias" of the choroid plexus.

This classification by Virchow remained almost unchanged for half a century and found its last major application in Borst's tumor atlas. In this form it has influenced the teaching of German pathology for a long time.

Borst (1902) recognized

Gliomas: Soft and hard gliomas, depending on the number of fibers. The soft gliomas merge without a clear boundary with the gliosarcomas. Special types appear, depending on the number of blood vessels: the "telangiectatic" and "cavernous" glioma—also called "apoplectic"—if hemorrhage is present. Blood vessels can participate in the tumor growth to a high degree. Tumors with a large number of blood vessels are called "angiogliomas." "Gliosarcomas" are mixed tumors which possess neoplastic glial tissue in addition to true mesodermal proliferation. On the other hand, the cellular and fast-growing gliomas belong to "glioma sarcomatodes."

Neuromas: False neuromas, e.g., plexiform neuromas. True neuromas have certainly been proved to occur in the peripheral nervous system but their presence in the CNS is questionable.

There were subsequent attempts to define further the "glioma" entity. The beginning of such endeavours goes back as far as 1874, when Simon described the "spider-cell glioma." Shortly before, Kölliker had discovered the cells with long and short processes, Deiters the fiber-forming astrocytes ("connective tissue cells"), Boll the "brush cells," and Jastrowitz the "spider-cells." Von Lenhossék's investigations of the origin of the ganglion and glial cells of the spinal cord further clarified the subject. We credit him with the concept of "astroma." Golgi (1869), furthermore, described as "gliomas" only those growths that were composed of fiber-producing spider-cells and generally quite benign. Together with Virchow he defined as "sarcomas" tumors that were composed of round undifferentiated (malignant) elements. Here historical comparison shows very nicely how each new discovery in the field of normal anatomy was soon followed by a corresponding one in oncology. In contrast to these views stands the isolated opinion of Klebs, who suspected that the gliomas were "organoid tumors," i.e., a hyperplasia of all parts of the brain (neurogliomas), and explained the different manifestations of gliomas as so many different stages of their development. He nevertheless described certain cases of glioma extremely well, and illustrated them with some excellent pictures.

Another approach was employed by Muthmann and Sauerbeck, who, with the help of serial sections, were able to prove the origin of a glioma of the fourth ventricle from the ependyma. Stroebe (1895) then published an observation that attracted considerable attention and influenced the literature for nearly three decades. He reported on a glioma with cystic spaces formed of cylindrical epithelium which had supposedly been pinched off from the ventricular wall and thus given origin to the tumor. The search for scattered germinal rests became the principal object of many studies (Bonome; Saxer, and others). A more important contribution, however, was made by Storch, who was working on the origin and growth of fibroblastic[4] and brain tumors. He investigated them for signs of an "infectious" stimulus. Noteworthy, also, is the work of Stumpf, who described the penetration of tumor cells into the glial syncytium. Held's views of the reticular (syncytial) arrangement of the glial cell groups have played an important part here. Ranke, too, expressed similar thoughts. It finally became necessary to separate the gliomas from the sarcomas, and to decide whether there really was such a bipotential tumor as the "gliosarcoma." (von Lenhossék; Landau, 1910; Stroebe). This controversy has persisted until today (Spatz, 1938; Hasenjäger, 1938). Most of the authors have expressed their doubts, especially since the sarcomatous nature of certain tumors, that are very similar to glioblastomas, was established (*see* p. 206 ff.).

In the meantime the development of modern neurosurgery had begun. After such original pioneers as McEwen, Ernst von Bergmann, Hahn[5] and von Brammann, came two European surgeons, who may be considered neurosurgeons according to our present definition: Sir Victor Horsley and Fedor Krause. Neurosurgery is indebted to these two for the first descriptions of the most important operative approaches to the brain (chiasm, cerebellopontine angle, and collicular region). Both men, however, lagged far behind in their knowledge of pathological anatomy, which was limited to the information available in the comprehensive clinical monographs of Nothnagel, Duret, Bernhardt, Oppenheim, and Bruns. The excellent chapter by Bruns (1904, 1908) on pathological anatomy accurately reflects the state of knowledge of his time.

The final phase of development is marked by the work of Pick and Bielschowsky, who considered the indifferent neurogliocyte, previously described by Held, as the focal point of cell development. Divergent development led from there to the ganglion, glia, and Schwann cells. The authors maintained that a separation of such multi-potential elements

[4] In discussing "fibroblastic" tumors, Lebert (1851) mentions among other things one of the first successful brain operations—"that performed upon Marcus Aurelius Severinus, a Spanish nobleman of the house of Avalon, who suffered from severe headaches for which many remedies had been applied in vain. He was persuaded to undergo a trepanation which disclosed a protuberance under the bone; after that had been removed the patient was completely cured."

[5] In addition to the "classical" case of McEwen's (1879), which is usually cited as the first report of a brain operation, Oppenheim points especially to the case of Wernicke and Hahn (1882). While McEwen was led to the tumor by external changes in the skull, Wernicke was the first to recommend a surgical attack on a space-occupying lesion (tuberculous) that was localized solely through cerebral symptoms.

from the normal tissue groups could—during the subsequent neoplastic transformation—lead to nerve cells and fibers as well as glial cells and fibers, or even sheath and capsule cells.

The differentiation, however, of tumor cells could stop at any given stage. Theoretically, the development of the gliomas would be possible either from embryonic rests of solely glial potentiality (spongioblasts) or from an indifferent precursor of these cells. Cohnheim's doctrine of the development of tumors from scattered embryonic rests was obviously still very prevalent and here even supported histologically.

This thesis also formed the starting point for the fundamental work of Ribbert who eventually extended it to include other tumors of the body. He proved that the cell rests that form the tumor matrix can become separated during tissue development not only by malformation but also as a result of inflammatory processes.

According to Ribbert (1918), gliomas, like other tumors of the body, developed from tissues that had been arrested at various stages of their anatomical and functional development. The nervous system in particular, has to complete a long period of maturation, and form and position of the cells change frequently during development.

According to his thesis, we can distinguish a diversified series of gliomas: some tumors with mature spider-cells, others with elements that resemble ganglion cells with abundant protoplasm, again others with strands of parallel fibrils, and finally those that consist almost entirely of densely packed nuclei. The latter were customarily (but falsely) called gliosarcomas; they should have been called cellular gliomas. These gross morphological differences could be explained best by correlating the tumor cells with the various developmental stages of the glia. The more cellular a tumor, the earlier it will have to be placed in the development stages of the glia; the more fibrillary it is, the more differentiated the original cell type will be. Ribbert's formulation of the different stages of maturation of the gliomas (spongioneuroblastoma → spongioblastoma → glioblastoma → glioma/neuroblastoma) contained the foundation of present-day classification. With this the stage was set for a basically new classification—one, however, that required the development of completely new methods of research and clinical techniques.

Neurosurgery, in the meantime, had made rapid strides; Cushing had developed it into a teachable discipline and it had branched off as a surgical speciality. The concentration of so many brain-tumor patients in one clinic afforded the pathologist unusual opportunities for research, especially when the clinician himself was interested in pathology, as Bailey was. This kind of research was urgently needed since the available pathological information was insufficient to answer the clinician's principal question—

that of a tumor's biological significance.[6] This, then, supplied the problem for subsequent investigations which used the work of Pick and Bielschowsky; Ribbert (1918); Strauss; and Globus (1918) as a starting point.

These last two authors reported a case of "spongioblastoma" with an unusually rapid course and had mentioned some thoughts about the histogenetic origin of this tumor. A new approach to research now became necessary: a tumor had to be investigated simultaneously from a clinical, surgical, and pathological point of view. This approach had already been anticipated in the works of Cushing on *The Pituitary Body and its Diseases* (1912); the *Tumors of the Nervus Acusticus* (1917), and by Henschen (1910) in his paper *On the Tumors of the Posterior Fossa, especially the Cerebello-Pontine Angle.* The next advance concerned the "gliomas." Bailey and Cushing divided this task between them and ultimately achieved their common goal. Bailey—with the help of the metal impregnation techniques of the Spanish school of Ramon y Cajal and Del Rio Hortega—undertook the demonstration of the **cell** types present in brain tumors. These were compared with the cells of normal tissue and their developmental stages, according to the histogenetic principles established by the German (His) and Spanish schools. It became possible to correlate the different types of glioma with various cell types and their stages of development. The result was that 15 (14) groups[7] of brain tumors were derived from medullary epithelium, with only a few tumors remaining unclassified.

1. Medullo-epitheliomas
2. Medulloblastomas
3. Pineoblastomas
4. Pinealomas
5. Ependymoblastomas
6. Ependymomas
7. Neuroepitheliomas
8. Spongioblastomas   a. multiforme   b. unipolare
9. Astroblastomas
10. Astrocytomas   a. protoplasmic   b. fibrillary
11. Oligodendrogliomas
12. Neuroblastomas
13. Ganglioneuromas
14. Papillomas of the choroid plexus.

[6] " . . . We were at a loss to know how it could be that a patient, from whose cerebellum a large tumor diagnosed "glioma" was removed as long ago as 1906, might prove to be living and well, the father of a family, and a wage-earner 19 years later, whereas another patient from whom a "glioma" happened to be removed in like fashion, supposedly in its totality, might survive for a scant six months before a rapid recurrence took place." Bailey and Cushing, 1926, p. 104.

[7] Spongioblastoma multiforme and unipolare must be considered as two groups.

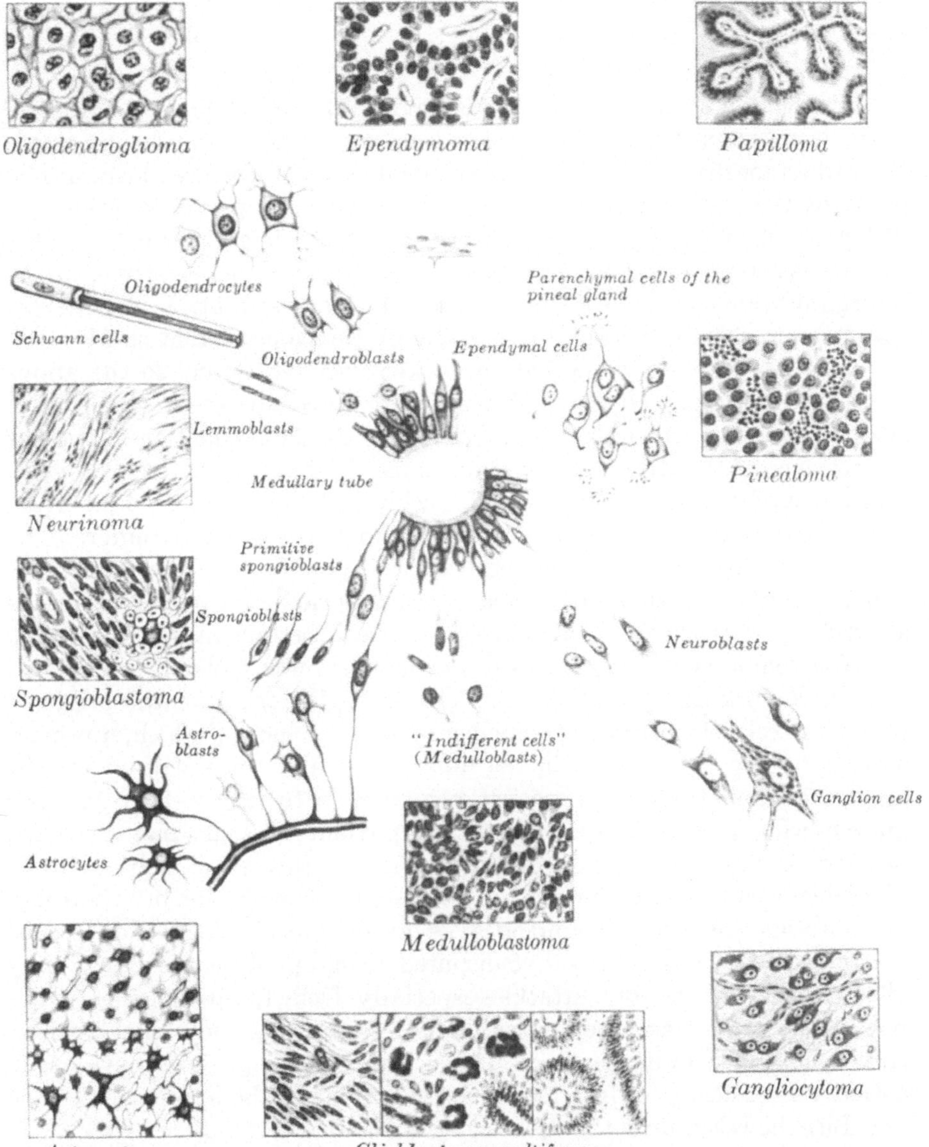

Fig. 1. Development of the cells of the central nervous system from medullary epithelium through various stages of maturation into individual differentiated cell-types. The corresponding tumor types are included. This figure explains the principle of classification of Bailey and Cushing.

This new classification was at first, probably for theoretical reasons, rather inclusive. With increasing experience, however, the desire arose to simplify it, with the result that it was condensed to ten types—as in the German edition of 1930—and finally to eight types, that form the basis of Bailey's contribution to Penfield's *Cytology and Cellular Pathology of the Nervous System* (Fig. 1).

At the same time Cushing was reviewing the clinical histories of patients on whom he had operated at least one year previously; he noted the earliest localizing symptoms, the general signs of increased intracranial pressure, the post-operative course, and the survival period. A review of 254 cases classified by Bailey allowed an approximate estimate of the average survival period for each tumor type and, for the first time, of the biological behavior of these brain tumors. Tumors with little cell differentiation grew quickly, those with more highly developed forms, slowly.

This was the first time that an answer had been found to the above mentioned question. Of equal clinical importance was the recognition of sites of preference of many tumor types, and ᴛhe determination of the age of incidence of the disease. The significance of these results may be summarized as follows: the Bailey and Cushing classification brought order out of the "chaos" of the various forms and types of brain tumors. The classification had biological significance, i.e., the different forms and types could be correlated with a particular survival period. Moreover, the tumors showed a preference for certain age groups and certain sites in the brain.

The comparison with stages of histogenesis was probably considered more as a working hypothesis than an oncologic dogma for the origin of the tumor cells. It provoked a number of attacks, most of which, however, seemed to have originated in the quiet—but also the isolation—of the laboratory, and thus were scarcely comparable to the work of the two authors who, in ceaseless efforts at their patients' bedside, had created a new era in neurosurgery. True, their original theoretical and scientific ideas might, in the long run, not have been entirely adequate, but their new classification was extremely practical as far as clinical work was concerned and became the basis for the undisputed progress of neurosurgery since 1926. In spite of various attacks—especially from the pathologists—this new classification was accepted with only minor changes in all fields where therapy was of primary concern. This is not surprising, since this classification was basically only a logical development of the approach of Pick and Bielschowsky, and the pathologist Ribbert.

THE PRESENT STATE OF CLASSIFICATION

A summary of the controversy about Bailey and Cushing's classification will best explain the existing system in the form we have selected. Because of the vast amount of literature on the subject, only those works are mentioned that have made definite contributions to the classification or delineation of types.

Almost simultaneously with the Americans, the French authors Roussy, Lhermitte and Cornil produced a classification of brain tumors. Since they failed, however, to take impregnation methods into consideration, their classification proved to be deficient. As a basis for subdivision, they, too, utilized the similarity between tumors and mature and embryonic cells. They recognized astrocytomas, cellular and afibrillary gliomas, glioblastomas and spongioblastomas. More important than the classification itself was the *manner* of investigation, which contained an excellent pathological description of the individual groups, including a thorough appreciation of regressive processes or changes.

In 1928 Roussy criticized Bailey's classification, mainly on the grounds that the histogenesis was still insufficiently substantiated, and that a classification from a histogenetic point of view was hypothetical and could not be proved. Moreover, he took exception to the idea that the tumor arises from cells that were arrested at certain stages of their development rather than from cells that underwent anaplastic transformation. Nevertheless, Roussy and Oberling in their 1931 atlas approached Bailey and Cushing's classification very closely—the differences being essentially only in nomenclature.

Classification of gliomas according to Roussy and Oberling

1. Gliomas
   Astrocytomas, oligodendrogliomas, glioblastomas
2. "Ependymo-choroidal" tumors
   Ependymocytomas, ependymoblastomas, ependymogliomas,
   plexus papillomas
3. Ganglioneuromas
4. Neurospongiomas
5. Neuroepitheliomas

The difference in the principle of classification which the authors wished to emphasize was that they spoke only of a *similarity* to embryonic tissue but, unlike Bailey and Cushing, did not necessarily presuppose a *dysembryogenetic* development (aberrant development of fetal cells). In their atlas, which was clearly composed but slightly confusing because of the welter of terms, they distinguished three main groups of tumors derived from nervous tissue: those from the glia, those from the ependyma and choroid plexus, and finally those from the neuronal elements. In addition there were tumors which recalled the primitive neurospongium—neurospongiomas (medulloblastomas). Others duplicated tissues of the earliest developmental stages—neuroepitheliomas.

Actually, all the groups of Bailey and Cushing's system are represented here. Among the ependymo-choroidal tumors, the authors recognized two types—one arising from the ependyma, the other from the choroid plexus. Among gliomas, three subgroups were recognized—astrocytomas, oligodendrogliomas and glioblastomas. The only omissions were the polar spongioblastomas, which (along with Hortega) were considered fusiform oligodendrogliomas, and the astroblastomas, which appeared as a subgroup of astrocytomas.

Penfield (1931, 1932) largely adopted the proposals of Bailey and Cushing. His work on brain tumors contained the same eight tumor groups as Bailey's. In only a slightly altered form, this classification was accepted by the American Neurological Society and the Commission on Nomenclature.

Classification of gliomas according to Penfield

    Astrocytoma
    Glioblastoma multiforme
    Medulloblastoma
    Ependymoma
    Astroblastoma
    Spongioblastoma polare
    Oligodendroglioma and oligodendroblastoma
    Neuroepithelioma
    Pinealoma

Penfield provided a very fruitful critique of the interpretation of certain groups by Bailey and Cushing which we will discuss later in more detail.

In principle Schaffer's classification system was the same as that of Bailey and Cushing, since representatives of the "gliogenetic series" were used as the starting point; it differed only in the grouping of the separate forms and the nomenclature. Schaffer distinguished between the ependymoma, the dendroglioma (macrodendroglioma; whether there is a microdendroglioma, too, has yet to be decided), and lastly the adendroglioma (oligodendroglioma of the usual classification)—each depending on the form and number of processes. He further suggested that the forms derived from immature glia be called hypogenetic, those derived from mature glia, eugenetic, and those from irregular cell types (such as gigantocellular), dysgenetic.

Bergstrand's (1932) suggestions for improvement are understandable from a clinical viewpoint. Olivecrona (1927), whose tumor material Bergstrand had studied, first employed a predominantly biological classification of the cerebral gliomas, distinguishing only "malignant" and "benign" forms according to their clinical syndrome. Bergstrand provided a detailed *morphological* basis for this classification.

Classification of gliomas according to Bergstrand

1. Benign group
     Astrocytoma fibrillare
     Astrocytoma protoplasmaticum
     Astrocytoma gigantocellulare
2. Malignant group
     Glioblastoma multiforme
     Glioblastoma fusiforme
     Glioblastoma protoplasmaticum
3. Ependymoma
4. Oligodendroglioma

He considered a division into two main groups sufficient for the classification of the most common cerebral gliomas: 1) the benign types of astrocytoma (fibrillare, protoplasmaticum, and gigantocellular) and 2) the malignant types of glioblastomas (multiforme, fusiforme, and protoplasmaticum). The third and fourth groups were relatively rare.

He aligned the astroblastoma with the gigantocellular astrocytomas and abandoned the spongioblastoma polare altogether. In a paper published in 1932, Bergstrand pointed out the biological and morphological difference between the cerebellar form of astrocytoma and the cerebral tumor of the same name. Later (1937), however, he blurred the picture by further broadening the description and including some false interpretations. The new names—gliocytoma embryonale and glioneuroblastoma—which he proposed for this tumor (astrocytoma) have not been generally accepted. Moreover, they contradicted his otherwise praiseworthy attempts to simplify the nomenclature.

In 1933 Cox presented his own experience with the Bailey and Cushing classification in a paper which is still worth reading. He employed the nomenclature without changes, but objected to the terminology based on histogenetic cell types, since it was his impression that anaplasia of mature cells played a greater role in tumor growth. Fortunately, he did not yield to the logical consequences of his ideas and refrained from introducing a whole new terminology.

Carmichael, too, on the basis of a study of 75 tumors (62 gliomas) acknowledged in principle the usefulness of Bailey and Cushing's classification, although a simplification stressing two main groups, astroblastic and spongioblastic, seemed desirable to him. (One of the differentiating characteristics was the reaction to impregnation with gold sublimate: the first group was well impregnated, the latter only slightly).

Finally, we have the work of Hortega (1932, 1944, 1945), who presented his experiences with the scientific investigation of intracranial

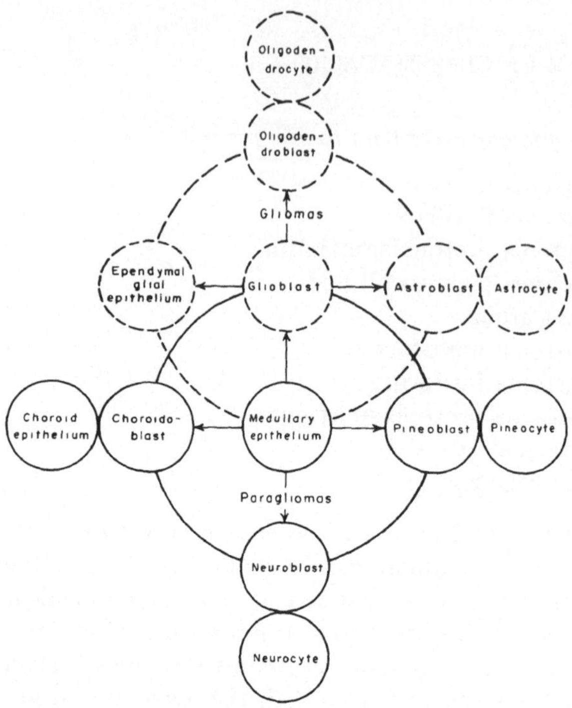

Fig. 2. Hortega's scheme of glial origin which forms the basis for his classification of gliomas.

tumors in two monographs and numerous contributions made during his work in Argentina. From his histogenetic studies he arrived at a developmental system for glia and specific parenchyma which differed from the above only superficially and not in principle (Fig. 2). Of importance was the division of the developmental lines of medullary epithelium into one cell series related to gliomas, and another, related to "paragliomas." This division into gliomas and paragliomas seemed so valuable that we have adopted it ourselves.

Hortega distinguished two main types of immature glioma (glioblastoma): the isomorphic and the heteromorphic, depending on the uniformity of the tumor cells. In the isomorphic group we find some examples of glioblastoma multiforme, ependymoma, and the medulloblastoma; in the heteromorphic group we find most of the examples of glioblastoma multiforme.

One criticism of Hortega's classification must be made, although it in no way detracts from the great service he has rendered by his work on brain tumors. His system fails to include the most essential feature of Bailey and Cushing's classification, whose main advantage was the *parallelism* between the *biological* and *morphological* properties of the different groups.

14

Hortega abandoned this way of classification in favor of a purely histological grouping and for this reason his work unquestionably represent a step backward. He was misled by an analysis of cell types based on metallic impregnation, where it is the form of the individual cells that is most striking. It can also be argued whether or not the cells of the medulloblastoma correspond to the hypothetical neuroblasts of the embryological theory, as he assumed.

Hortega's group of astroblastomas is completely heterogeneous; we encounter some gigantocellular astrocytomas, some polymorphic glioblastomas, monstrocellular sarcomas, and even a few polar spongioblastomas. He also favored a combination of names, like "glioblasto-astroblastoma," or "astroblasto- astrocytoma," i.e., groups which are useless for the clinician. He succumbed to the great danger of constructing his classification purely according to histogenesis and cytology, without having it controlled constantly by those biological aspects which only the *clinic* can furnish. Type of growth, general architecture, and especially biological behavior too often remained in the background. A classification based only on superficial resemblances between cell forms leads to the formation of groups whose members lack any biological uniformity.

In his review of gliomas, F. Henschen (1934) aligned himself—with only minor exceptions—with Hortega's classification, as did Morelli; but in his "Handbuch" article of 1955, Henschen joined the scheme of Bailey and Cushing. H. J. Scherer (1933,1935), who was fundamentally opposed to all current classifications, also found it still the most acceptable. At the beginning of his comprehensive study of intracranial tumors, Scherer took up the problem of existing classifications and thought, from the example of a small special group of tumors (glioblastoma multiforme ganglioides of Foerster and Gagel), that they would all lead to absurdity. He was unwilling to admit that any valid classification was possible. He deplored the fact that classifications as arrived at by "enthusiasts of histogenesis" had made of the glioma question a pure "problem of cell diagnosis" which had "degenerated more and more into a mere cytological game."

The first objection to Scherer's work is that, in most instances, he did not adopt the names of the "American" classification. Consequently, it is frequently hard to see to which tumor type a given observation refers. The second objection concerns Scherer's approach which depends *exclusively* upon *morphological* characteristics without any reference to clinical experience. The following "conclusions" (Scherer, 1940; De Buscher and Scherer) would otherwise have been impossible: there are no circumscribed astrocytomas; these tumors, because of their diffuse spread, can scarcely be differentiated from brain swelling and brain edema; most of them undergo de-differentiation spontaneously (without operation); 20% of glioblastomas are sufficiently demarcated to assure a successful operation, so that pessimism on the part of neurosurgeons is not warranted; and finally, ependymomas are the only operable gliomas which do not recur. This is not true, however, of the ependymomas of the cerebral hemispheres; on the other hand, in every neurosurgical clinic the cerebellar astrocytomas (spongioblastomas) consistently produce the longest postoperative survivals[8].

One final objection may be made as to the manner in which Scherer criticized the work of Bailey and Cushing. His style, the acerbity of his polemic against the classification (which his own suggestions for improvement failed to support), and the presumption of his assertions have often detracted from the respect which his work deserves. Nonetheless, it must be said in conclusion, that the wealth of his observations on the morphology of brain tumors has not yet been fully assimilated or evaluated, and that, in particular, his demand for a "total" investigation of the whole tumor in serial sections deserves serious attention. This method, following the traditions of Nissl and Spielmeyer, had been used in Gagel's department of the Foerster Institute and is also our method of choice.

It was possible to apply Bailey and Cushing's system of classification to tumors of the spinal cord without essential change. Kernohan (1932) reported a study of 52 primary spinal tumors, among which he found all the intracranial types, after Bailey and Foerster (1936, Jubilee volume of Davidenkow) had already described seven primary spinal cord tumors. We are indebted to Foerster and Gagel (1934) also for a condensed description of spinal tumors. An attempt to apply the same principles of classification to the tumors of the eye seems not only ontogenetically justified, but has actually shown itself to be possible in practice (Grinker; Verhoeff, 1932).

In the meantime, tissue culture methods gave new support to the Bailey and Cushing classification of gliomas. Investigations by Kredel (1928); Canti, Bland and Russell; Cox and Cranage; Buckley and Eisenhardt; Benedek and Juba (1943); Costero and Pomerat; and Lumsden were able to show, in fact, that individual morphological and biological properties (for instance, movement and form) persist in tissue culture of tumor cells. This was shown particularly well by a demonstration of growth in motion pictures. While very real differences existed, for example, between astrocytomas and oligodendrogliomas, such differences were not as striking between astrocytomas and glioblastomas as might have been

---

[8] Nor can we disregard the statistical data of Bailey and Cushing and of their co-workers Cairns, van Wagenen, and Eisenhardt; or of Olivecrona and Tönnis; or Davidoff.

expected on the basis of the fixed material. The importance of such studies becomes clear when we remember that Russell and Bland (1934) felt justified doubting that the polar spongioblastomas were a separate group; studies of tissue cultures had shown that the cells growing out were really "piloid" astrocytes (in the sense of Penfield), which looked bipolar or spindle-shaped only because of their usual position of lying one beside the other.

Cox and Cranage even succeeded in culturing tumor cells from meningiomas, neurinomas, and angioblastomas, as well as from gliomas that had been successfully cultured before. The forms of the cultured cells were generally similar to the pictures seen in the usual histological preparations.

Among recent articles on classification those by Maffei; Chiovenda; and Jequier-Doge, as well as several by Globus, Kuhlenbeck and co-workers are worth mentioning. To discuss them in detail, however, would be repetitious; strict adherence to the histogenetic interpretations of tumors just does not seem possible. This interpretation was intended only as a basis for organization, but the authors never meant—as Bailey later strongly emphasized—that the tumor cells *really* consisted of embryonic spongioblasts, astroblasts, etc.[9] This histogenetic interpretation has proved to be so defective as a doctrine (most recently through the new classification of astroblastomas and spongioblastomas) that there is no justification for its further expansion or the introduction of new terms. Similarly, to deduce a histogenetic system for normal development by basing it on the findings in tumors seems to be putting the cart before the horse. Kernohan was liable to this error when he used certain morphological resemblances in oligodendrogliomas and ependymomas to explain the normal stages of glial development.

Recently Kernohan (1949) and his group proposed a new simplified classification based upon a revised histogenetic interpretation. This proposal grew out of the commendable desire to make the classification of brain tumors comprehensible and acceptable also to the pathologists. Kernohan looks upon the different tumor types as having arisen not from particular tissues and their developmental stages, but by anaplasia of cellular development. The latter had already been assumed by Roussy, Lhermitte and Cornil; and Cox (1933), and has been adopted by us for classification of the glioblastomas. Kernohan also believes that there is a continual series of gradations going from fibrillary and protoplasmic astrocytomas through astroblastomas to glioblastomas, and that a com-

---

[9] This controversy is reminiscent of the time in the history of dogma when the question of "similar" versus "identical" came up. For the *theory* of tumor origin it may be of some significance whether tumor cells were really cells of some developmental stages or were merely "similar" (i.e., comparable) to them.

parable series of stages may be demonstrated for ependymomas and other
tumor types, although he has not worked the latter out in detail for every
group.

His system looks as follows:

New names	Old names (with new names in parenthesis)
Astrocytoma grades 1-4	Astrocytoma (astrocytoma grade 1) Astroblastoma (astrocytoma grade 2) Spongioblastoma polare (left out) Glioblastoma multiforme (astrocytoma grades 3 and 4)
Ependymoma grades 1-4	Ependymoma (ependymoma grade 1) Ependymoblastoma (ependymoma grades 2-4) Neuroepithelioma (left out) Medulloepithelioma (ependymoma grade 4)

Oligodendroglioma
    grades 1-4
	Oligodendroglioma (oligodendroglioma
	    grade 1)
	Oligodendroblastoma (oligodendroglioma
	    grades 2-4

Neuroastrocytoma	Neurocytoma Ganglioneuroma (neuroastrocytoma Gangliocytoma grade 1) Ganglioglioma Neuroblastoma Spongioneuroblastoma (neuroastrocytoma Glioneuroblastoma grades 2-4)
Medulloblastoma	Medulloblastoma

A detailed discussion of Kernohan's proposed classification appears in
the section on definition of individual tumor types. Suffice it here to make
a few general remarks. By and large, his classification follows cytological
criteria, and an over-all evaluation of the tumor (as an "organoid" unit)
is hinted at only by an occasional reference to the blood vessels. Regressive
cell changes are not even considered as possible causes for a particular cell
or tissue pattern, though I myself have repeatedly tried to call attention to
the changes which occur in the "normal" tissue of various tumors through
regressive processes.

We need only mention that the cerebellar astrocytoma (spongioblastoma), so decidedly benign, may acquire a very polymorphic structure
through purely regressive changes (Zülch, 1940, 1956).

A histological investigation and interpretation of a small area of tissue and a prognosis as to the apparent grade of malignancy are very difficult if the matter of regressive processes is not taken into account. In addition, the same tumor can show different histological pictures in different regions, without this influencing its over-all biological significance. This was shown in the oligodendroglioma (Zülch, 1941, 1955, 1956), where the small-cell normal structure and the spindle-cell or large-cell variant can be found right next to each other in the same tumor. Here it is purely a matter of chance which of these three tissues comes from the operating room to be studied and diagnosed.

The same applies to monster-cell sarcomas (Zülch, 1953, 1956) and other tumors. The new classification of "neuroastrocytomas" is particularly confusing; benign tumors of ganglion cells with a very long history and many years of post-operative survival (*see* p. 183ff.) are here placed in the same group as the very malignant cases, described as gangliogliomas, which we have shown to be monster-cell sarcomas.

There is a parallel in pathology worth mentioning—namely, the problem of kidney tumors. Apitz (1943) has described these tissue inter-relationships in a series of fundamental contributions and has called attention, with many illustrations, to the extraordinarily variable cell and tissue types contained in a single tumor as well as in its various metastases. Each of these types would require a completely different biological evaluation. Apitz was able, on the basis of these observations, to demonstrate the development of renal carcinomas from benign growths. Here, too, the attempt at "grading," which goes back to Broders, must *a priori* be considered questionable as it was in the case of brain tumors.

This theoretical concept of Kernohan's, based, to be sure, on very extensive histological and biological experience with brain tumors, will yet have to stand the test of time; in the meantime it has found many supporters.

A similar classification with three grades has just been published by Ringertz (1950), based on Olivecrona's material. In general, this classification agrees with Kernohan's. Ringertz' conception, however, of the origin of glioblastomas from malignant degeneration of ependymomas and oligodendrogliomas will certainly require additional confirmation.

CHAPTER II

BASIS OF OUR CLASSIFICATION

The following is a survey of the simplified classification of space-occupying lesions of the brain that was used in our institute. It permits the classification of practically all existing space-occupying processes, with the exception of a few "unclassifiable" tumors.

Four families may be distinguished:

A. Neuroepithelial (neuroectodermal) tumors
B. Mesodermal tumors
C. Ectodermal tumors
D. Congenital and embryonic tumors

A. NEUROEPITHELIAL TUMORS

The following ten types which are found in all modern classifications, though sometimes under different names, are adequate for a classification of the central and peripheral derivatives of neuroepithelium. The types presented here enjoy the widest use and are most generally accepted, particularly in the Anglo-Saxon literature. Omission of some types found in Bailey and Cushing's classification will be justified later.

The ten types

1. Medulloblastoma	6. Ependymoma
2. Spongioblastoma	7. Plexus papilloma
3. Oligodendroglioma	8. Pinealoma
4. Astrocytoma	9. Neurinoma
5. Glioblastoma	10. Gangliocytoma

An attempt to assemble these types into four main groups, according to their kinships and tissue differentiation, results in the following grouping:

I. Medulloblastomas
II. Gliomas
III. Paragliomas
IV. Gangliocytomas

According to degree of maturity:

Undifferentiated

I. Medulloblastomas

Retinoblastoma—pineoblastoma—medulloblastoma cerebelli—sympathoblastoma

Differentiated

II. Gliomas	III. Paragliomas	IV. Gangliocytomas
Spongioblastoma	Ependymoma	Gangliocytoma cerebri
Oligodendroglioma	Plexus papilloma	Gangliocytoma cerebelli
Astrocytoma	Pinealoma	(Gangliocytoma of the
	Neurinoma	sympathetic trunk)

Anaplastic

Glioblastoma	Anaplastic ependymomas and pinealomas?	Anaplastic gangliocytoma?

The reasons for this arrangement are as follows:

I. Medulloblastomas

1. *Medulloblastomas:* This main group includes a number of undifferentiated growths with a series of common characteristics; for instance, the well-known *medulloblastoma of the cerebellum.* In the past, an undifferentiated developmental stage of neuroepithelium (medulloblast, "indifferent cell") was considered to be the cell that corresponded to that of the medulloblastoma. Medulloblasts supposedly were able to develop into either ganglion or glial cells, i.e., have bipotential properties. This was reflected also in the French term "neurospongioma" and Gagel's term "neurogliocytoma." Such an interpretation, however, of the tumor's histological structure, which supposedly contained mature glial and neuronal cells together with undifferentiated ones, is scarcely justified. On the contrary, I have had to assume that the ganglion and glial cells recognizable in the tumor are local cerebellar cells included in the neoplasm. But the comparison with undifferentiated cells of the neurocyte series generally may be correct. In his new classification, Kernohan, too, retains medulloblastomas as a special group, but adds tumors which he had previously classified as medulloepitheliomas (*see* above).

In addition to these undifferentiated tumors of the cerebellum in children there are similar tumors of the *pineal* region, the *retina* and the *sympathetics.* Of these, the pineoblastomas behave like the cerebellar tumors with respect to tissue type, growth, and metastasis, and Bailey therefore placed them close to each other. The retinoblastomas and sympathoblastomas are biologically of the same type as the cerebellar tumors and Bailey thus termed them "analogous" tumors. Histologically, all four can be so similar—especially with respect to formation of pseudorosettes—that even the experienced pathologist cannot distinguish one from the other, although the presence of "true rosettes" allows the definite identification of the retinoblastoma. (This, however, applies only to *some* of the retinal tumors.) The two *peripheral* representatives differ from their *central* counterparts in the degree with which they metastasize to tissue of different embryologic origin (retinoblastoma to bone; sympathoblastoma to lymph nodes, bone, and liver). The biological significance of all four types is about the same.

After more detailed study, the neoplasms previously described as medulloblastomas of the cerebrum proved to be tumors of other subgroups, mostly oligodendrogliomas (Cushing, 1932). The concept of the medulloblastoma as a sarcoma (Nishii) has in the meantime been abandoned. The demonstration of argentophil fibrous connective tissue in this tumor can be explained by the latter's infiltration of the leptomeninges of the numerous cerebellar folia.

II. Gliomas[1]

This main group previously included practically all neuroepithelial tumors occuring in the brain. Today, however, the term neuroglia—the corresponding normal tissue—is restricted to two types of astrocyte and the oligodendroglia. The neuroglia may be contrasted with the paraglia—the special parenchyma of ependyma, choroid plexus, pineal body, and the neurilemma of the Schwann cells. This contrast is reflected in our classification. Hortega (1932) was the first to introduce the paragliomas (Fig. 2), a concept which we have developed further. No reference is made here to microglia. Its significance in the origin of tumors will be discussed below.

2. *Spongioblastomas (polar):* There are still difficulties in the interpretation of this tumor. The corresponding normal cell, according to orthodox teaching, is taken to be the spongioblast, a bipolar cell in the developmental series whose morphological and staining properties could not be agreed upon (Zülch, 1939). Moreover, such a comparison with a relatively undifferentiated cell (Russell and Bland, 1934) would not correspond to the biological benignity of these neoplasms. In addition, there occur—besides elements similar to spongioblasts—many "more highly developed" cells with multiple processes, some of them resembling astrocytes. Hortega (1932, 1945) considered these cells to be oligodendroglia and described the tumors as "fusiform" oligodendrocytomas.

[1] As a clinical term the name "glioma" will remain temporarily applicable to all neuroepithelial tumors, until further subclassification is achieved by histological study.

Kernohan (1949) decided against listing the spongioblastomas as a separate group and included them under astrocytomas. As far as I can tell, the infundibuloma of Globus (1942) also belongs to the spongioblastoma group.

In my opinion, any determination of the origin of spongioblastomas must begin with their site which, rather like the ependymomas, is always close to the ventricles. A specific property of the spongioblastomas is, furthermore, the formation of Rosenthal fibers. These are peculiar degenerative forms of fibrous cell-processes, which relate this tumor to a whole series of pathological changes occurring in the subependymal glia after inflammation, degenerative states, and even syringomyelia. There is thus considerable justification for relating spongioblastomas to a proliferation of the mature subependymal glia. Morphologically this glia occupies a position between the ependymal cell and the astrocyte and corresponds, as described by Opalski (1934), to the tumor cells of the spongioblastoma.

Also, the inflammatory-degenerative changes of ependymitis granularis and plastica closely resemble some of the spongioblastomas, as we have been able to demonstrate again and again in our own preparations.

Today we include among the spongioblastomas the so-called cerebellar astrocytomas, whose special position among and difference from the cerebral astrocytomas was established more than a decade ago. The cerebellar astrocytomas form the bulk of the so-called piloid astrocytomas, and have often been diagnosed spongioblastomas of the cerebellum. However, no morphological or biological difference exists between these tumors, some of which have been designated astrocytomas, some spongioblastomas. It would be ridiculous to split up a homogeneous group simply because at some times bipolar spongioblast-like forms predominate among the different cells and astrocyte-like forms at others. Consequently I consider all so-called cerebellar astrocytomas spongioblastomas. Though the term spongioblastoma still does not reflect the comparison with the subependymal glia, I have temporarily refrained from changing the name until the new interpretation has been thoroughly accepted.[2]

3. *Oligodendrogliomas:* It is important to point out the three different types of tissue which occur in oligodendroglioma: a) those with the classical honey-comb architecture and the characteristic round cells; b) spindle-cell types, reminiscent of the spongioblastoma; and c) large-cell types with a certain resemblance to the giant-cell astrocytoma. In spite of this I cannot agree with the practice of Cooper; de Buscher and Scherer; and Hortega

---

[2] Names, such as "ependymoglioma" or "subependymoma," may be worth considering. The former, however, has already been used by Roussy and Oberling for specific ependymal tumors.

(1945), who speak of mixed forms, i.e., oligoastrocytomas.[3] Kernohan thinks, furthermore, that he can distinguish four types of oligodendrogliomas according to malignancy. The question of whether the oligodendrogliomas occur in the cerebellum seems to have been answered in the affirmative in the report by Juhász from Gagel's laboratory. However, these are certainly very rare cases. The majority of cases described as oligodendrogliomas of the cerebellum are probably really spongioblastomas undergoing mucoid degeneration, with architectural patterns that, because of regressive changes, are deceptively similar to those of oligodendrogliomas (*see* p. 138).

4. *Astrocytomas:* The astrocytoma group used to consist of three subgroupings: the protoplasmic, fibrillary, and gigantocellular types, to which I have added a fourth, the astroblastoma. The latter is difficult to distinguish macroscopically and has the same biological significance. The *malignant* astrocytoma forms the fifth subgrouping. It includes cases which still have the characteristics of astrocytomas but also are beginning to show a malignant degeneration in several regions that imperceptibly shades into glioblastomas. The so-called astrocytomas of the cerebellum are now listed under the spongioblastomas.

I hope a better subdivision will eventually be possible, taking into consideration the amount of fibers and the cell size. For instance, a distinction could be made between small- and large-cell fibrillary, small- and large-cell afibrillary, and malignant astrocytomas.

The limits of the astroblastoma group in Bailey and Cushing's classification were at first inadequate. If one adhered strictly to the cytogenetic approach (i.e., looked for "astroblastic" cells) one could often find them in tumors having the malignancy of glioblastomas. If, on the contrary, one used as the distinguishing characteristic Bailey's description of the perivascular arrangement of astroblast-like cells, one soon included tumors similar to astrocytomas (Teltscharow and Zülch, 1948). Consequently, I have classified astroblastomas with astrocytomas, as did Bergstrand (1932; 1933). Kernohan (1949), however, has followed the former, more cytogenetic interpretation. His astroblastomas therefore appear in the second grade of astrocytomas, and point to a development in the direction of the glioblastoma.

In an especially informative case, I have described the transition of an astrocytoma, circumscribed and fiber-forming, into an adjacent tumor of the glioblastoma type (*loc. cit.*, 1948). In 10% of our material I have found tumors that showed evidence of malignancy, similar to that of the glioblastoma ("the malignant astrocytoma"), in addition to their astrocytic

---

[3] On the contrary, after silver staining both the spindle-cell and the large-cell parts can be definitely recognized histologically as tissue of the oligodendroglioma.

characteristics. Scherer (1940), too, has called attention to cases of this sort which he clearly distinguishes from the primary glioblastomas by referring to them as "secondary glioblastomas." Our "malignant astrocytomas" correspond roughly to Kernohan's grade 3 astrocytomas.

In order to eliminate the classification of the glioblastoma as a separate group, three related groups could be set up: astrocytoma, malignant astrocytoma, and glioblastoma—much as Kernohan suggested. But I consider it basically undesirable to give up the established classification in favour of this new attempt, since from this sequence it would be easy to conclude that *all* glioblastomas develop anaplastically from astrocytomas, which is certainly not the case. Scherer, therefore, justifiably makes a strong genetic distinction between the two tumors, the "primary" and the "secondary" glioblastoma.

5. *Glioblastomas:* Here are gathered a series of tumors that are dissimilar in their cell type, but similar macroscopically and biologically, and in their growth. We can, if we wish, distinguish three kinds of tumors according to the predominant cell type: the globuliform (consisting of small round cells), the fusiform (spindle-cell form), and the multiform. This subdivision has no biological significance. According to present-day investigations, the concept of gliosarcoma can be rejected, especially since we were able to separate a not inconsiderable series of true sarcomas (sarcoma monstrocellulare), that previously had been considered glioblastoma ganglioides or gangliocytomas (*see* p. 206 ff.)

Kernohan's (1949) conception of glioblastomas as grade 4 astrocytomas has already been mentioned. Busch and Christensen (1947) have divided the glioblastomas into three subtypes in a paper which provides interesting information about this group and goes into the question of preferential location of these tumors. Their principle of subdivision is not consistent (angionecrotic, multicellular, and magnocellular glioblastoma), and the magnocellular group behaves much more favorably biologically than the two others. It corresponds principally to the large-cell astrocytoma or to the malignant form of what is ordinarily considered the large-cell astrocytoma.

In my experience, the new classification of glioblastomas by Davis, Martin, Goldstein, and Askenazy into angioproliferative and angiothrombotic glioblastomas is not based on fundamental characteristics; indeed, this classification can not be adhered to in the examination of large sections, since the thromboses naturally lead to necroses, and angioproliferations arise right on the border of the cysts and necrotic areas (Zülch, 1939).

III. Paragliomas

This name was apparently introduced by Hortega (1932). However, I have removed the gangliocytomas from his paraglioma group and added instead the neurinomas, which are related to the "peripheral glia" (Schwann cells), (Fig. 1).

6. *Ependymomas:* No further subdivision of ependymomas, either biological or morphological, is necessary; their differentiation from the neuroepitheliomas will be presented further on.

Like many authors before me, I gave up the subdivision into ependymoblastomas, and also have not accepted Kernohan's subdivision of ependymomas into three groups (1937). I have, however, pointed out that the ependymomas of the cerebral hemispheres in children are biologically much more unfavorable than other ependymomas. The latter differ only in their rate of growth, as measured by the number of mitoses (Zülch, 1940), and can not be distinguished morphologically.

Furthermore, I have noticed that the ependymomas around the foramen of Monro and the third ventricle show the usual architecture (nucleus-free spaces around the blood vessels) to a lesser extent than the others, and that ependymal tubules can be observed in large numbers only in the ependymomas of the aqueduct and the spinal cord. However, I have been unable to discover a biological difference between these last two subtypes.

Kernohan (1949) proposed a morphological subdivision into four grades, while at the same time abandoning his previous definition (1937) which included the plexus papillomas. His present grade 1 shows a structure similar to the one we have seen in the ependymomas around the foramen of Monro; in this respect it is somewhat atypical of ependymomas. His grades 2 and 3 correspond to the classical description of ependymomas. In his illustrations and descriptions we can not find any difference between them—unless it be the mitoses in grade 3, which might make them correspond to our ependymomas of the cerebral hemispheres. His grade 4 seems to be extremely rare; I have seen it on occasion in recurrences and described it as a stage of dedifferentiation (Zülch, 1940). He also includes with grade 4 the medulloepitheliomas, which I have refused to consider a separate group from the outset.[4]

It should also be mentioned that I would classify the ependymal spongioblastomas of Globus and Kuhlenbeck (1944), which probably correspond to the ependymoblastomas of Kernohan, differently. Some of these tumors are glioblastomas (e.g., case No. 3, 1942); some ependymomas of the cerebral hemispheres (e.g., case No. 3, 1944), or of the foramen of Monro (case No. 6, 1944), and another a plexus papilloma of the lateral ventricle (case No. 7, 1944—"papillary ependymoma"). It seems to me that an attempt to lump biologically different tumors together into a

---

[4] ZÜLCH, K. J. u. KLEINSASSER, O.: Ortsgebundene Abweichungen in der Histologie und im biologischen Verhalten der Ependymome. Zbl. Allgem. Path. 1957, in press.

single group has no practical purpose and is also unconvincing from a morphological point of view.

The cells of Scheinker's subependymoma (Scheinker, 1948) according to his description are supposedly indistinguishable from those of the normal subependymal glia. But judging by the pictures in his book (Figs. 120, 121), it seems that they are partly ependymomas with regressive changes, as described in 1937 by Giampalmo, and partly infiltratively growing tumors. Here again biologically different tumors have been gathered into a single group—something that we consider undesirable.

7. *Plexus papillomas:* I have kept these histologically well-characterized tumors in a group by themselves since even their localization differs from the ependymomas. A further subdivision is unnecessary. Malignant plexus papillomas that behave like true carcinomas of the brain occur rarely. If they do, they are usually metastases from cancers elsewhere. However, a diffuse spread of an otherwise benign plexus papilloma can occur by way of the cerebrospinal fluid (implantation metastases). The term "plexus carcinoma," often used by pathologists, seems therefore inappropriate for this group of plexus papillomas.

8. *Pinealomas:* After transferring the pineoblastomas to the medulloblastoma group, there still remain two histological subtypes of pinealomas, which are only slightly different biologically—the isomorphic and anisomorphic pinealomas. I have seen a 72-year-old man with a pineal tumor whose pleomorphism required that it be considered an *anaplastic* type of pinealoma (Zülch, 1956).

9. *Neurinomas:* The neurinomas can be treated briefly, although considerable variations in nomenclature and interpretation still exist (perineurial fibroblastoma, neurofibroma, etc.). I am not convinced that the neurinomas are derived from connective tissue as has been claimed by Mallory and Penfield. Peculiar silver-staining fibers can be demonstrated, but these appear to be specific for neurinomas. In my experience these fibers are not the same as ordinary reticulin fibers. I also consider tumors of peripheral nerves to be neurinomas where the abundantly present epi- and endoneurial connective tissue proliferates as stroma. The peripheral nerve tumor of von Recklinghausen's disease, although distinguished by its content of connective tissue, usually is fundamentally of the same nature.

IV. Gangliocytomas

10. *The gangliocytomas* of the cerebral hemispheres and brainstem are fundamentally different from the tumors of the same name in the cerebellum and peripheral nervous system. The first group, despite a large number of case reports, is still difficult to characterize. Biologically the individual cases show little uniformity, especially since they are apt to lie in inacces-

sible sites deep in the brain. However, the group in the mediobasal temporal lobe, described by Tönnis and Zülch (1939), differs from the others and is also readily amenable to surgical treatment. In naming gangliocytomas in neurosurgery, we do not have to indicate the content of glia, axis-cylinders, and myelinated fibers by particular names (e.g., "ganglioglio-neuroma amyelinicum").The typical gangliocytomas of the cerebellum comprise a rare but definite subtype. Gangliocytomas of the sympathetics are well-known to general surgeons as predominantly benign tumors, most commonly encountered in the thorax. The malignant sympathoblastomas of the adrenals and of the sympathetics are now grouped with medulloblastomas.

As Scherer (1934) pointed out correctly, in making the diagnosis of gangliocytoma, particular care must be taken not to misinterpret preexisting ganglion cells, a mistake that is particularly apt to occur in the region of the nuclei around the third ventricle. The demonstration of ganglion cells actually infiltrating the leptomeninges will prevent such a mistake. I have separated from the gangliocytomas certain tumors which were first described in 1914 by Schmincke and later by Wätjen; Paul; Scherer; Alpers; Foot and Cohen; and Foerster and Gagel, and which the latter referred to as spongioblastoma ganglioides. I now believe, as Foot and Cohen did previously in another connection and for different reasons, that these tumors are really sarcomas, biologically very similar to glioblastomas; and I think I have demonstrated this satisfactorily (Zülch, 1953, 1956). The term "ganglioglioma" therefore, found in the literature, provides an erroneous notion about these tumors.

Considerable confusion still prevails about the definition, subdivision, and biological evaluation of gangliocytomas. Kernohan proposes to group all the gangliocytomas together under the term "neuroastrocytoma," again with a subdivision into four grades of malignancy. Not only are there no definite criteria for this subdivision, but there are also instances of overlapping. For instance, the first, most benign group includes not only the ganglion cell tumors of the cerebral hemispheres (the group described by us in the temporal lobes) but also the above-mentioned, highly malignant tumors (actually sarcomas although in the literature they are called gangliogliomas). The classification of Globus and Kuhlenbeck (1946) contains a continuous series, ranging from spongioneuroblastomas through "transitional gliomas" to "glioneuromas." In their spongioneuroblastoma group we find periventricular tumors of tuberous sclerosis beside glioblastoma multiforme (case No. 13) and "gangliogliomas" (i.e., the monstrocellular sarcomas of our classification), whereas the glioneuromas could not always be recognized from the illustrations or descriptions.

(From this group, for instance, I would classify case No. 4 from their 1942 paper as a spongioblastoma.)

Despite these authors' efforts, I must emphasize again that tumors which seem closely enough related to be put into one group be morphologically and biologically uniform.

Neuroepitheliomas; medulloepitheliomas: We have omitted these names from our classification. They were included by Bailey and Cushing mainly for theoretical reasons. Certain structures in rare tumors, for instance of the retina, were interpreted as medullary epithelium, and the "true rosettes" of the retinoblastomas considered neuroepithelial rests. However, only part of these retinoblastomas form true rosettes (and those only in the eye and never in the metastases). It is impossible to find a biological difference between those that do and those that do not. If, therefore, we were to separate them because of this one characteristic, we would break up a biologically uniform group of tumors. In any case, a "neuroepithelioma" would be a most malignant tumor.

The neuroepitheliomas which have been described mostly by pathologists (most recently Seifarth) are benign tumors of the ependymoma group.

The justification for considering them neuroepitheliomas was to be found in the infrequent presence of ependymal tubules. Thus the "true rosettes" have been falsely identified with ependymal tubules (*see* Table 2). However, ependymomas with or without ependymal tubules are biologically indistinguishable from each other. Subdividing them according to this characteristic would again mean breaking up a uniform group. To make the confusion complete, the ependymomas of the hemispheres in the young, tumors whose behavior is the most nearly malignant, never show ependymal tubules.

Nor can we form a clear picture of neuroepitheliomas from other cases briefly presented in the literature, as for instance those of the experienced brain tumor pathologist Penfield (1932). In any case, these tumors of peripheral nerves are malignant neoplasms. Numerically they are insignificant. Further information may be found in our own detailed publication (Zülch, 1939).

Microgliomas: On the basis of pertinent cases described so far (Benedek and Juba, 1941; Russell[5]), this classification does not seem to be sufficiently justified and such tumors should, therefore, remain unclassified for the time being. I have never been able to relate a tumor to the microglia with any assurance. Moreover, Russell's demonstration did not convince me of their microgliomatous nature.

[5] RUSSELL, D. S., A. H. E. MARSHALL and F. B. SMITH: Microgliomatosis: Form of reticulosis affecting the brain. Brain **71**, 1–15, 1948.

B. MESODERMAL TUMORS

The meningiomas: The meningiomas are the most important representatives of the mesodermal tumors. Macroscopically uniform, they can be subdivided histologically into three, ten or 22 subtypes. Biologically, as Cushing himself admitted (Cushing and Eisenhardt), this subdivision has no significance. We are content, therefore, to recognize three subtypes, for which the traditional names still seem suitable—endotheliomatous, fibromatous and angiomatous. However, even these three groups scarcely differ in biological significance. It is important, though, to distinguish between these subtypes and the rare, unencapsulated, meningioma-like tumors of the dura, which infiltrate the adjacent tissues. Such tumors, if the capsule is absent and the histological picture appropriate, should be termed fibrosarcomas.

The angioblastomas: The angioblastomas of Lindau are well-defined. The name "angioma of the cerebellum" should be avoided because of the danger of its being misunderstood. Bailey had already rejected the idea of considering certain tumors of this group as "angiogliomas" (Roussy and Oberling, 1930) whereas the "angioglioma" of Bergstrand (Bergstrand, Olivecrona, and Tönnis) was only a vascular so-called cerebellar astrocytoma. The "angioglioma" of Scheinker (1938) was an oligodendroglioma, and the "angiogliomas" of Koella are not convincing as a homogeneous group.

Fibromas and sarcomas: Fibromas rarely occur in the brain. Within the sarcoma group, which figured prominently in the older literature and included meningiomas, glioblastomas, oligodendrogliomas and medulloblastomas, the process of clarification has made considerable progress. We have now attempted a new division into five subtypes. The first and second are types of diffuse sarcomatosis. In one case the tumor spreads via the cerebrospinal fluid pathways, from where it extends into the brain —along the vessels—only slowly: *diffuse meningeal sarcoma* or *sarcomatosis of the meninges;* in the second it spreads around the adventitial space of the intracerebral vessels and rarely reaches or invades the cerebrospinal fluid space—the so-called *adventitial sarcoma* or *sarcomatosis of the vessels.*

The next two types are circumscribed sarcomas. Only a few cases of circumscribed sarcomas of the cerebellar arachnoid have been described (Lhermitte and Duclos; Foerster and Gagel, 1933, and others), and I have had no experience with them myself. In the last group we are dealing with tumors which were first described by Schminke in 1914 as "ganglioglioneuromas," and were subsequently named "spongioblastoma multiforme ganglioides" by Foerster and Gagel (1931). The sarcomatous nature of these neoplasms was first suggested by Foot and Cohen; I mentioned it in 1940 and demonstrated it in 1947 and 1953 on the basis of 42 cases.

(The malignant fibrosarcomas of the dura have already been mentioned with the meningiomas.)

Chondromas; lipomas; osteomas; chordomas: These growths are sufficiently defined in pathology and need, therefore, no detailed description. Only in the case of chordomas is it clinically important to distinguish between benign and malignant forms according to their growth. Histologically, they are difficult to differentiate.

C. ECTODERMAL TUMORS

Craniopharyngiomas; pituitary adenomas: No detailed discussion is required of the classification and subdivision of the ectoderm derivatives or the different embryonic layers. The division between the chromophobe and the chromophil pituitary adenomas is not always a simple matter. There are mixed forms—transitional adenomas—that might belong more to one or the other, and malignant forms that are characterized by rapid growth (many mitoses). The basophilic adenoma is not a neurosurgical problem. The craniopharyngiomas, a biologically benign group, have already been described. The cell pleomorphism which arises through regressive processes —the effect of cholesterin—does not justify the interpretation "squamous-cell cancer." I have included here the cylindromatous epithelioma of the base, of which we ourselves have observed six cases around the Gasserian ganglion and two on the crista galli.

D. CONGENITAL AND EMBRYONIC TUMORS

Epidermoids and dermoids are sufficiently defined in pathology; and in the case of teratomas, to split off "teratoids" is without biological significance.

E. VASCULAR MALFORMATIONS AND TUMORS
OF THE BLOOD VESSELS

Angiomas and aneurysms: For our basic classification we have taken over Virchow's old system which has been revised by Bergstrand, Olivecrona and Tönnis. For blood vessel tumors I have uniformly used the term "angioma" (with corresponding qualifications) in order to reserve the name "aneurysm," as is done in pathology, for the *secondary* enlargements of arteries. An arteriovenous *aneurysm* is, therefore, in the true sense of the word, a *secondary* communication between arteries and veins, both of which have undergone enlargement. The corresponding congenital malformation, on the other hand, will be termed the arteriovenous *angioma*. In order to use uniform terminology, we prefer to use the term capillary (ectatic) angioma of general pathology instead of the name telangiectasis. From the pathological point of view, Sturge-Weber's disease is a calcified capillary and venous angioma of the leptomeninges.

The venous angioma, moreover, must be clearly separated from the venous varix. Among the secondary malformations of the blood vessels there remain the arterial aneurysms, the varices of the veins and sinuses, and the secondary arteriovenous aneurysms; among the latter the main representative is the so-called cavernous sinus-carotid aneurysm. The existence of the purely arterial angioma has still not been conclusively proved.*

F. OTHER SPACE-OCCUPYING LESIONS

Under the "unclassified tumors" we have assembled those growths whose neoplastic nature can be demonstrated, but which, through lack of material, cannot be classified accurately. Moreover, we find here tumors that have not yet been classified at all, and which appear to be somehow related to the ependymomas and spongioblastomas. We have characterized such a similarity by an additional term, such as unclassified "ependymoma-like," "spongioblastoma-like," etc., (Zülch, 1950).

In our classification we have included ependymitis and arachnoiditis, as these lead to marked hydrocephalus and in that sense become space-occupying lesions, i.e., the cases of ependymitis of the aqueduct, large arachnoidal cysts, and cystic arachnoiditis of the cisterns. This attitude seems justified, since other inflammatory space-occupying processes like gummas, tuberculomas and those caused by parasites are also listed in neurosurgical statistics, even though, strictly speaking, they are not neoplasms of the brain.

The selection of names for classification[6]

A prerequisite for any understanding between clinician and pathologist is the existence of a universally valid and comprehensible language, with

---

* Translators' note: We have altered the names used in K. J. Zülch's classification slightly in accordance with the prevailing American and English terms, in particular to avoid long, cumbersome Latin terms. These latter names, along with other synonyms, are included in the special section in parentheses after the term chosen for ordinary usage.

It is also apparent that the author's classification, even though it makes a useful and convenient distinction between *angiomas* and *aneurysms*, is still controversial. Thus, certain aneurysms, such as the fusiform aneurysms of old age, are clearly acquired or secondary, and would therefore deserve the name *aneurysm*. However, berry or sacular aneurysms are commonly thought to be of congenital origin, even though much or their enlargement takes place post-natally. In a strict sense, then, the term "aneurysm" —denoting an acquired condition—is inappropriate; however, to call such a lesion an angioma—to denote a lesion of congenital origin—is even less satisfactory.

[6] In order to eliminate controversy over nomenclature, serious consideration should be given to the replacement of names by letters or numbers, as suggested by Nissl for the ganglion cell changes that were named after him. Endless repetition of the same inadequate names, simply because of their priority, would thus be avoided.

terms that do not change yearly.[7] Up to now the giving of names in tumor pathology has served as an exercise field for those with a passion for changes.

Names once introduced should be retained until everybody feels an improvement is needed (e.g., the so-called cerebellar astrocytoma); tumor groups classified according to morphology should also have clinical significance, i.e., only biologically similar tumors should be grouped together. A classification based on purely histological considerations without such (biological) value has no place in clinical medicine.

Tumor pathology, more than any other branch of pathology, is an applied science. Its estrangement from the clinic, often so pronounced today, leads to an isolation of general pathology, with the undesirable result that the clinician again becomes his own pathologist. This is happening more and more in the specialities of ophthalmology, otology and dermatology, while in neurology it has been the practice from the very beginning. The resulting difficulties can be surmounted only by teamwork in which the pathologist once again shares the interests of the clinician.

Summary of our classification of brain tumors
and other space-occupying lesions

A. Neuroepithelial tumors
   I. Medulloblastomas
      1. Medulloblastomas
         a) Retinoblastoma
         b) Pineoblastoma
         c) Cerebellar medulloblastoma
         d) Sympathoblastoma
   II. Gliomas
      2. Spongioblastomas (including the so-called cerebellar astrocytoma)
      3. Oligodendrogliomas
      4. Astrocytomas (fibrillary, protoplasmic, and gigantocellular astrocytomas; astroblastomas and malignant astrocytomas)
      5. Glioblastomas (globuliform, fusiform, and multiform)
   III. Paragliomas
      6. Ependymomas
      7. Plexus papillomas
      8. Pinealomas
      9. Neurinomas

[7] "Time, however, will doubtless bring order, agreement and simplification out of existing confusion. What is important for the surgeon is to know the kind of glioma he has brought to view, whatsoever its "alias." A medulloblastoma by any other name is just as unfavorable." Cushing, H., *Intracranial Tumors*, p. 16, Thomas, Springfield, Ill., 1932.

IV. Gangliocytomas
    10. Gangliocytomas
        a) of the cerebrum, medulla, and spinal cord
        b) of the cerebellum
        c) of the sympathetics

B. Mesodermal tumors
    11. Meningiomas (endotheliomatous, fibromatous, angioma-
        tous)
    12. Angioblastomas
    13. Fibromas
    14. Sarcomas
        a) Sarcomatosis of the meninges (diffuse)
        b) Sarcomatosis of the vessels (diffuse)
        c) Sarcoma of the cerebellar arachnoid (circumscribed)
        d) Sarcoma of the vessels (circumscribed)
           —equivalent to the monstrocellular sarcoma
        e) Fibrosarcoma
        f) Primary diffuse melanomatosis—reticular sarcomas
    15. Chondromas
    16. Lipomas
    17. Osteomas
    18. Chordomas

C. Ectodermal tumors
    19. Craniopharyngiomas
    20. Pituitary adenomas
        a) eosinophil ⎫
                  ⎬ chromophil
        b) basophil ⎭
        c) chromophobe
    21. "Cylindromatous" epitheliomas

D. Congenital and embryonic tumors
    22. Epidermoids
    23. Dermoids
    24. Teratomas

E. Vascular malformations and blood vessel tumors
    25. Angiomas and aneurysms
        a) Cavernous angioma
        b) Capillary angioma (telangiectasis)
        c) Venous angioma
        d) Arteriovenous angioma (congenital)

e) Sturge-Weber's disease (angioma capillare et venosum calcificans)

f) Aneurysms, varices, and arteriovenous aneurysms (acquired)

F. Other space-occupying processes

26. Unclassified tumors
27. Metastases
28. Parasites
    a) Cysticercosis
    b) Ecchinococcosis
    c) Other parasites
29. Granulomas
    a) Tuberculomas
    b) Gummas
    c) Mycoses
30. Arachnoiditis and ependymitis
    a) Cystic adhesive arachnoiditis
    b) Ependymitis

CHAPTER III

THE ORIGIN OF
BRAIN TUMORS

Review of current concepts

In the preceding historical review I have presented the most important concepts concerning the origin of brain tumors. Now I shall repeat only the key features of what the knowledge of brain tumors can contribute to general oncology. Cohnheim's theory as regards the origin of tumors is still very applicable to brain tumors. He stated "that the real cause of the subsequent development of tumors should be sought in a fault, an anomaly of the embryonic anlage . . . and that tumors often develop at sites where certain complications have occurred at some stage of embryonic development . . . ." Ostertag's (1936, 1941, 1952) investigative aim was to prove that the gliomas arise in ontogenetically disturbed portions of the brain. But despite Marburg's (1921) findings and Ostertag's analogies, this theory has not been proved. (A very important contribution, however, was Ostertag's observation on the characteristic sites of neuroepithelial tumors.) Proof of such a theory would require a convincing demonstration to the effect that a transformation actually does take place and a new "race of cells" develops in a split-off group of cells which had persisted heretofore without forming neoplastic tissue. To show this would require a case of a tumor that was just beginning, and to find such a favorable situation would depend entirely on chance. The demonstration of "split-off embryonic rests" has repeatedly been attempted (Stroebe, 1895, Pfleger; Yaskin and others). Pathologists and surgeons (Hamperl, 1937, and more recently, K. H. Bauer, 1949, and others) have increasingly moved away from this theory of Cohnheim's, which was elaborated by Ribbert and has survived to some extent in Fischer-Wasels' (1927) "misregeneration theory."

On the other hand, the proposal advanced especially by Virchow, that tumor growth is induced by chronic internal and external irritation, has obtained considerable confirmation in experimental investigation. I list here only those irritants which are now proved "carcinogens": parasites poisons, viruses, physical irritants—especially radiation of various sorts—

exogenous and endogenous chemical substances (hormones, products of intermediary metabolism). In addition to these external factors in tumor origin there are also internal factors of a predisposing sort which are necessary for the induction of a tumor, as we have learned particularly from experimental tumor transplantations. For a long time it seemed as if genetic factors, at least for animal tumors, were playing a decisive role. However, studies of the significance of the "milk factor" in the rearing of progeny changed much of this. Nevertheless, certain genetic influences in animals still cannot be denied (Gottschewski, 1953). In man, this has been demonstrated in particular in the familial hamartoblastomatoses and the retinal neuroblastomas.

According to some authors' concepts about tumor growth, numerous internal and external carcinogenic factors are *simultaneously* involved in the induction of the tumor, with certain preneoplastic states appearing as precursors of carcinoma formation (K. H. Bauer).

A detailed description of the attitude of pathologists was given by Apitz in his five papers on kidney tumors. On the one hand he affirms the origin of certain kidney tumors from a dysontogenetic matrix (as in tuberous sclerosis), but on the other he rejects anything so simple as a separation of embryonic rests as in Cohnheim's theory. He believes that it is rather a matter of a locally inherited or acquired precancerous disposition of tissues, i.e., neoplastically-destined cells which must go through a certain number of generations before they emerge as true neoplastic growths. A speeding up of this process can be brought about by external stimuli, or possibly, through an exhaustion of hormonal growth-inhibiting mechanisms.

Büchner too is an adherent of the "misregeneration theory" of Fischer-Wasels for certain tumors (1950, p. 270). He explains the appearance of carcinomas partly by loss of the ability to differentiate, an involutional occurrence based probably on a chemical alteration of the cells. A "carcinoma signifies a catastrophe of form, and the essential nature of form is its capacity for differentiation and thus restriction of growth . . . ." Willis (1953, p. 199), to quote only one of the better-known tumor pathologists, adheres to a similar view of modern biology (Nicholson, 1933) which sees in tumor formation essentially an alteration of the normal relationship between growth and inhibition. In summary, tumor formation is the end-product of a cell's response to the stimulus of its environment. But when it comes to particulars of these processes, Willis too admits the ignorance of science.

Because of the poor opportunities for observation, we have not yet been able to recognize local "precancers" in the brain, nor have we had the good fortune to prove the existence of "dysontogenetic" embryonic rests (*see* p. 36) at least in statistically significant numbers.

To be sure, K. H. Bauer considers the hereditary systematic neoplasms to be due to inheritance of preneoplasms, but otherwise attaches only slight importance to the genetic factor. In fact he is right in pointing out "that a selection based on the cases' particular interest (cases from so-called cancer families) always yields a distorted picture." But he himself takes the view, in contrast to many other authors (e.g., Schönbauer, 1952, 1953), that "hereditary predisposition plays no role in cancer." He proposes —as a rule of thumb—that "carcinoma is practically always acquired." According to Bauer, therefore, cancer is always primarily a local disease, and no matter how far back its cause may be traced, it is still almost invariably acquired from cancer-producing injuries of one type or another.

It seems to me questionable whether the findings in twins and in familial brain tumors can be so lightly dismissed, as is done so often in the literature. The theories concerning syncarcinogenesis (the composite action of carcinogenetic factors) developed for other carcinomas cannot be applied to brain tumors. We recognize no occupational tumors of the brain. We know nothing of any local tissue stresses which could conceivably be exerted via the cerebrospinal fluid circulation. We know of no definite local precancers, with the exception of the systematic hamartoblastomatoses (see p. 42). We know nothing of radiation damage to the brain, except for cases of X-ray overdosage which, up to now, has never produced tumors.

Only further study will show us the importance of a case which I observed together with Klar (Heidelberg), in the evaluation of the carcinogenetic effects of X-rays. Tönnis totally removed an ependymoma of the cerebral hemisphere in a 15-year-old girl. In the following year the site of operation was systematically radiated. Six years later a nodular tumor, which on biopsy proved to be a fibrosarcoma, arose in the region of the bone flap. At autopsy it was shown that this tumor was continuous with the dura of the operative site. There was nothing left of the primary tumor.

On the other hand, the model system of Fischer-Wasels (the simultaneous action of a general and a local factor) can be applied particularly well to brain tumors.

The importance of a *general* factor in the origin of brain tumors is supported by the predilection of all tumors for certain age groups (see p. 58). Tumors of youth (puberty), and the upper age brackets (involution) are almost mutually exclusive. The age peak of certain malignant tumors (medulloblastomas, glioblastomas) falls at the times of hormonal adjustment and shows a predilection for males as well.

The occurrence of hereditary systematic tumors indicates the importance of the general factor in the origin of tumors of the central and peripheral nervous system. There definitely are hereditary tumors of the hemispheres (or its derivatives, the eyes) and in the cerebellum; these are not only familial but can be followed through many generations.

The *local* factor in the origin of brain tumors is impressive to a degree which is unparalleled in other organs, where the same tumor does not keep appearing at the same site with almost photographic faithfulness (*see* p. 62 ff.). Moreover, tumors arise especially often in those brain regions that lie along the raphé where the neural tube closed.

Suffice it to say that general theories about carcinogenesis are presently of little use in explaining the origin of brain tumors. All that can be said is that the presence of many factors is probably necessary for a brain tumor to develop: a *local* factor involving an abnormal anlage, revealed by the predilection of brain tumors for specific sites; and a *general* factor involving an abnormal humoral or endocrine constitution. On the other hand, the co-action of other factors, particularly *external* ones, upon the brain cannot be assessed at this time. These ideas are found more and more in general pathology, where Dietrich (1955) deserves special mention ("... for the initiation of the altered growth no new external circumstance is necessary other than an alteration in homeostasis, particularly of the endocrine system . . .").

Lastly, I shall summarize a few observations made in the field of brain tumors which can contribute to our knowledge of general oncology.

Experiments with carcinogenic substances

The experimental production of neoplasms with carcinogenic substances has been successful in the brain. Using such substances, a number of authors (Pigalew; Roussy, Oberling and Raileanu; Oberling and Guérin; Zondek; Ilfeld, Weil and co-workers; Mulligan, Neubuerger *et al.*) have succeeded in producing a variety of tumors in the mouse (where spontaneous gliomas are almost unknown)[1] and other animals. Tumors most closely resembling human brain tumors have been produced by Zimmermann and Arnold (1940), Seligman and Shear; they have been classified histologically by Alexander.

Seligman and Shear used small pellets of 20-methyl cholanthrene which they introduced through burr holes in the skull of mice. Brain tumors developed after 227 to 511 days. According to Alexander, the following tumors were found: glioblastoma, oligodendroglioma, ependymoma, neuroepithelioma, pinealoma, spongioblastoma, fibrosarcoma, etc. However, our own study (naturally of limited value) of their pictures and descriptions suggests that most of them were glioblastomatous growths. Nevertheless,

---

[1] According to Maud Slye, only three brain tumors were found in sections of 11,188 mouse brains; one endothelioma, one papillary ependymoma and one pituitary adenoma.

one case (No. 3 C) resembled an oligodendroglioma, another (No. 11 B) an astrocytoma, and there were also definite fibrosarcomas.

Peers too was able to produce 32 tumors in 87 mice; specifically, 15 gliomas and 17 mesodermal tumors. Some could be transplanted and were still growing after five and 11 generations. Zimmermann (1943, 1955) has reported similar results in transplanting tumors.

There was an interesting relationship between the type of tumor which arose and the site at which the carcinogenic agent was applied. When the agent was put on the ventricular wall, ependymomas developed; in the white matter, glioblastomas or, more rarely, astrocytomas arose. Oligodendrogliomas usually grew in the occipital lobe; polar spongioblastomas in the corpus callosum, medulloblastomas in the cerebellum. In this way the distribution of experimental tumors resembled that of spontaneous tumors in man (Zimmermann and Arnold, 1941, 1943; Arnold and Zimmermann).

The transplantability of brain tumors. Brain has shown itself to be a good host for heterologous tissue, especially tumors. Only the anterior chamber of the eye is an equally suitable host site. Upon homologous transplantation, mature and embryonic tissue, as well as malignant tumors, grow, whereas benign tumors and precancerous tissue does not take. Upon heterologous transplantation, however only embryonic tissue and malignant tumors survive. The experiments were carried out on rabbits, guinea pigs, rats, and mice. Further particulars may be found in the contributions of Greene (1951 and 1953). The guinea pig and the mouse are particularly suitable for transplantation experiments.

It has been possible, moreover, to culture neuroepithelial tumors on chick embryos and to transplant them for eight generations. However, the tumor lost its characteristic architecture in the process and regained it only upon being transplanted back into mice (Cohn and Zimmermann, 1955).

The carcinogenic action of thorotrast. Until the end of World War II, thorotrast was considered to be the medium of choice in cerebral angiography. Doubts were expressed about its use quite early, since it supposedly damaged blood vessels. Roussy; Oberling, and Guérin (1936) were able to show that thorotrast had a carcinogenic effect upon mesoderm. In fact, a few cases of liver and kidney sarcoma have already been reported. However, these involved the use of the massive doses that had been employed earlier for the demonstration of liver and spleen (MacMahon *et al.*, 1947; Matthes). Doses of less than 10 cc. are apparently without carcinogenic hazard (Kuntzmann *et al.*).

The significance of hereditary factors in tumor formation

TUMORS IN TWINS

Even the most recent branch of genetics, the study of twins, has been employed in the investigation of brain tumors. The statistics in the older literature on brain tumors are unfortunately of only limited value to us, because the diagnoses are obsolete. Nevertheless, Thums mentions 45 verified cases of intracranial tumors, among them a pair of identical twins, both of whom were operated on for brain tumor at about the same time, and an instance of triplets of the same sex, two of whom developed pituitary tumors.

Geyer and Pedersen reviewed six pairs of identical twins with concordant disease. Of those the pair with medulloblastomas of Leavitt (1928) is the best known. Also mentioned is another pair of twin girls, originally reported by Joughin, each of whom developed a glioma of the base of the brain. Geyer and Pedersen themselves added a new pair of non-identical twins where brother and sister at nearly the same age (43 and 44) developed cerebral gliomas, probably glioblastomas. In addition, the authors collected three identical but discordant pairs from Tönnis' clinic. One member of the first pair of twins developed a sphenoid wing meningioma at age 40; one of the second pair had a ganglion cell tumor at the age of 12[2], and one of the third pair developed a pituitary tumor (diagnosed only by X-ray) at the age of 24, while their twins apparently had no tumor at that time. However, the brother of the patient with the sphenoid wing meningioma subsequently became concordant and died of a glioblastoma in 1951 (*see* Hoppe, 1952). We attach less value, consequently, to subsequent reports of non-identical discordant pairs of twins. In addition, Geyer and Pedersen reported the first case of identical twins with von Recklinghausen's disease (28 years old at the time, but affected from puberty). All presently known cases have been clearly summarized in a table by G. Koch (1954). He was able to find in the literature 12 pairs of twins affected with brain tumors. Among them were nine identical pairs, of which the concordant occurrence of brain tumors was observed in five. Out of 20 unselected pairs of twins from his clinical material (one partner with a brain tumor) concordancy was never found (i.e., the other partner never had a brain tumor).

Our colleague Lüders (Berlin)[3] was kind enough to send us the histological sections of a pair of identical female twins both of whom died of medulloblastomas of the midline cerebellum at the age of not quite three months. One of the partners also had a pigeon-egg sized metastasis in a clavicular lymph node with spread to the pulmonary apex, as well as other small lymph node metastases. The other partner had remained free of metastases.

FAMILIAL AND HEREDITARY BRAIN TUMORS

The best-known "hereditary" brain tumors were described by Bender and Panse, and Hallervorden (1936) for the siblings G. Of the three

---

[2] Erroneously classified by us at first as an astrocytoma.

[3] *See* GRIEPENTROG, F., and H. PAULY: Intra- und extrakranielle, frühmanifeste Medulloblastome bei erbgleichen Zwillingen. Zbl. f. Neurochir. **17**, 129, 1957.

brothers, Hermann G., appears to have suffered from a polar spongio-blastoma or a tumor very close to diffuse spongioblastomatosis. Reinhold G. obviously had a diffuse oligodendroglioma. The other brother had changes of a sort related to tuberous sclerosis. Hallervorden subsequently reported on another pair of siblings where the brother died of a giant-cell glioblastoma; and all that is known of the sister is that she died of a brain tumor at the age of 42. Böhmig reported briefly on a similar case.

In our collection of cases, the brothers B. are particularly noteworthy; both of them died of glioblastomas of the parieto-occipital region. Of these, Willi B. died at the age of 54 with a right parietal glioblastoma, while George B. died of a parietal glioblastoma at the age of 61. G. Koch has furnished tables on the familial brain tumors known until 1953. He himself was able to find six instances of familial brain tumors.

Pass investigated the families of 30 patients with brain tumors, totaling 220 members, and found tumors in 11.1%. Three families belonged to the group of von Recklinghausen's disease. Of the 30 patients, 40% had second tumors, most of which were benign and produced clinical signs in only five cases. In one family a glioma in one sibling and a malignant esophageal tumor in the mother were observed simultaneously. In another case of a patient with a glioblastoma, the father had a carcinoma of the larynx, the mother carcinoma of the stomach, and a sister had a myoma of the uterus.

In the literature, the family of Gardner and Frazier is considered a particularly impressive example of a familial disease. This is a study of five generations with 217 members in whom bilateral deafness was inherited as a Mendelian dominant. In the entire sibship, 38 individuals were af-fected; 15 of these became blind and four of them—on closer investigation—showed optic atrophy secondary to papilledema. Two members were autopsied and had bilateral acoustic neurofibromas. Of the deaf members, the authors were able to study seven; of those, five were unresponsive to the Barany test. It is interesting that the average age of survival of the affected members of each generation decreased rapidly. The second gen-eration died at an average of 72 years, the third at 63 years, the fourth at 42 years and the fifth finally at 28 years. There were never any signs of von Recklinghausen's disease.

There are many examples of pedigrees with hereditary retinoblastomas (Benedict; Badtke).

The familial systematic hamartoblastomatoses*

We recognize three systematic tumor groups, in part at least definitely familial and/or hereditary: neurofibromatosis (von Recklinghausen's disease), tuberous sclerosis (Bourneville's disease), and the angiomatoses

of the central nervous system (von Hippel-Lindau's disease). For the sake
of completeness the calcifying capillary and venous angiomas of the face
and brain should be added (encephalotrigeminal angiomatosis or Sturge-
Weber's disease), although the hereditary nature of this latter condition is
uncertain. Van der Hoeve called them phacomatoses and suggested a
corresponding change of name for the morphological manifestations (instead of adenoma sebaceum, phacoma cutis facie, etc.). We prefer the well-
known pathologico-anatomical terms of hamartoma and hamartoblastoma
(for the latter cases with autonomous growths) and apply the term hamartoblastomatosis to the widespread systematic occurrence of developmental
abnormalities combined with partly autonomous neoplastic growth.

1. Neurofibromatosis

Von Recklinghausen's disease is a systematic hamartoblastomatosis of
various connective and supporting tissues of the body; it shows a female
preponderance. In the full-blown syndrome we find neurofibromas of
myelinated and unmyelinated nerves, plexiform neurofibromas of the skin,
racemose angiomas, pigmented nevi and a variety of intracranial tumors,
particularly multiple meningiomas, neurinomas of the cranial nerves,
spongioblastomas of the midline, ependymomas, and numerous heterotopic
rests of the parenchyma. Families whose members had single or multiple
tumors and other signs of von Recklinghausen's disease have often been
described in the literature.

Especially interesting is Schaltenbrand's report (1933) on the family
D. from Hamburg. It has been possible to observe this family over three
generations (the grandmother had "Jacksonian epilepsy;" a daughter and
granddaughter died from von Recklinghausen's disease with multiple
meningiomas, acoustic neurinomas, intramedullary spongioblastomas,
peripheral neurofibromas, etc.). In 1948 I had the opportunity to see
Walter D. in the University Neurological Clinic (Prof. Pette). In addition
to a neurofibroma of the peroneal nerve which he was known to have had
for a long time, he had a cerebello-pontine angle syndrome with enlargement of the internal acoustic meatus and a tangerine-sized calcified olfac-
tory-groove meningioma. Since he had no symptoms of increased intracranial pressure, he declined operation.

In von Recklinghausen's disease, the tumors of the dura are meningiomas of the three subtypes; the tumors of the cranial nerves are true
neurinomas, and the central gliomas—which usually occur in the midline

* Translators' note: The term "systematic" used here pertains to the tendency
of these disorders to manifest themselves regularly in certain characteristic organs or
tissues rather than to appear throughout the body at random. It is used in preference
to the term "systemic," which suggests involvement of the entire organism.

—are spongioblastomas, and lie most frequently around the optic nerve and chiasm (Schaltenbrand, 1933; Tegerter and Smith; Busch and Christensen, 1937). Ependymomas occur particularly in the spinal cord.

Furthermore, there is a series of so-called "central changes" that have been described extensively by Bielschowsky; Henneberg; Gamper; and their co-workers. These include varying degrees of rachischisis, syringomyelia, heteropias of nerve cells, displacement of the cortical layers, plaques fibromyeliniques, excessive atypical glia, and small angiomatous malformations, as well as connective tissue inclusions (Foerster and Gagel, 1932). These changes show a loose kinship with tuberous sclerosis and familial hypertrophic neuritis. The diffuse changes are particularly important in the interpretation of the diffuse gliomas (*see* p. 74) whose origin can be understood on the basis of Bielschowsky's description of the migration of cells from the neural crest and the disturbances that occur during this process.

The circumscribed spongioblastomas of von Recklinghausen's disease have generally been described in the past as "central neurinomas" (*see* p. 134).

It may be stated in summary that in neurofibromatosis there occur disturbances of *cytogenesis* and *cytokinesis*, which lead in part to stationary and in part to neoplastic malformations.

The diffuse infiltration of misdirected and malformed cells is indicated by the finding of Rosenthal's fibers scattered diffusely in the white matter (Hallervorden, 1952). These fibers ordinarily occur as degenerative forms of the subependymal glia (*see* p. 23).

The question of why, in this combination of neoplasia and disturbed cytokinesis, only a part should receive the stimulus for autonomous growth, and why this stimulus does not lead to tumor growth immediately but only years later (Gamper), must still remain an open one. (Study of a number of cases from our own collection has failed to shed any new light on this problem.)

2. *Tuberous sclerosis*

Here we find a series of central and peripheral changes characterized mainly by the triad of adenoma sebaceum, tumors of heart and kidneys, and the central changes in the brain. The brain changes consist of the well-known gross nodules of the cortex (tubera), macro- or microgyria, maldevelopment of the histological structure, heterotopias, glial nests, monster cells developing into either glial or ganglion cells or cells of ambivalent character, as well as ependymal nodules. In certain instances the ependymal tumors reach the size of space-occupying lesions. Indeed, lacking the otherwise characteristic clinical syndrome (Stender and Zülch), they can appear merely as a ventricular tumor at the foramen of Monro, with a general increase in intracranial pressure resulting from the hydrocephalus of the lateral ventricles.

Other sites are unusual; as an example we may cite our own case of a nine-year-old boy (No. 3704). In addition to multiple tubera and numerous small or minute ventricular nodules of no neurosurgical significance, he had a hen's-egg-sized cylindrical tumor on the *lateral* wall of the ventricle in the parieto-occipital region, where it did not produce a significant obstructive hydrocephalus.

3. Systematic angiomatosis of the central nervous system and eye (von Hippel-Lindau's disease)

This disease is described more thoroughly in the section on mesodermal tumors where it is introduced as a special form of angioblastoma. Among the hereditary cases of Lindau's disease, the Møller family is particularly well-known. This family can be traced through four generations; in the last three generations six male and four female members were affected. Of these, five patients had a cerebellar angioblastoma, four had combined retinal and cerebellar disease, while in one the retina alone was involved. The site of the angioma in the affected member of the first generation could not be accurately established.

4. Maloney has added *Sturge-Weber's disease* as a fourth type of familial systematic hamartoblastoma to the three mentioned above. (*See* Brouwer, Van der Hoeve, Maloney). For a detailed description of this condition see the section on Vascular Tumors.

Circumscribed developmental malformations of the brain and spinal cord

The literature of the last 50 years contains numerous attempts to prove that tumors originate from embryonic rests isolated by a developmental disturbance. In a glioma from a 64-year-old woman, Stroebe described cystic spaces which were partly lined with "ciliated columnar epithelium," and which he considered to be detached fragments of the neural tube or ventricular epithelium. The glioma supposedly had developed from these fragments, and this concept of tumor origin was to dominate the literature for a long time. But Stroebe's findings were not in the least convincing. Neither his illustrations nor his descriptions eliminated the possibility of a *secondary* development of these histological structures by regressive changes. Stroebe himself spoke of numerous "softenings" in the vicinity. Between those holes, the walls of which were partly softened, were single cystic spaces which stood out because they were lined with regular, simple "high cuboidal or columnar epithelium."

Our own findings in oligodendrogliomas (case No. 269 and No. 1182, Zülch, 1941) show how easy it is to make this sort of error if ependyma and choroid plexus are included in the tumor (*see* p. 54).

From Bonome and from Henneberg's (1921) particularly illustrative case of an 18-year-old man (apparently with an ependymoma of the cerebral hemispheres) that path leads to Ostertag (1941), who was mainly responsible for developing and supporting this concept of dysontogenic origin. He was primarily interested in finding the origin of the disturbance in more or less malformed embryos, and, where possible, in searching out the tumor anlage. I consider his proof still inconclusive and believe that his observations on tumors of the floor of the anterior horn of the lateral ventricle (1936, Fig. 105), consisting of "neuroepithelial structures" (1936, Fig. 122) or a "mixture of connective tissue with neurospongioblasts" (1936, Fig. 53), could also be explained in a different way.

While I do not yet consider the origin of tumors from developmental malformations an established theory, I must admit that there is a convincing element in the fact that, statistically, tumors are often located at sites which are embryologically vulnerable, as, for instance, the dorsal raphé.

I agree, therefore, with the importance of a local factor, the formation of a focus or "germ," in the origin of brain tumors, even though proof for this is not yet at hand. Such local abnormalities of brain tissue need not be of a morphologically recognizable nature, though some are (*see* Zülch and Schmid, 1955). How easy it is to produce disturbances in differentiation of the central nervous system experimentally (e.g., by anoxia) has been shown by the school of Spemann and Büchner (Büchner, 1952; Rübsamen, 1948 and 1951; Mushett, 1953).

Comprehensive studies, extending the findings of Hassin; Yaskin; and Pfleger, might eventually furnish the true percentage incidence of malformations of the brain. We will then have at our disposal sufficient critical support to solve the question of tumor origin from morphological malformations.

A further possibility to learn more about the origin of brain tumors lies in the study of the relationship between accidents and brain tumors. This involves the problem of the traumatic origin of tumors which might be conceived of as being due to the splitting-off (during trauma) of a tissue fragment that subsequently undergoes faulty regeneration and becomes the "germ" of a future tumor.

Accidents and brain tumors

At present we are faced with the numerous brain injuries of two world wars and those resulting from highly developed industrialization and dense traffic. It is, therefore, particularly important to clarify the possibility of a causal relationship between brain trauma and the development of tumors. This relationship was emphasized in the title of Marburg's book: *Accidents and Brain Tumors*. Springer, Vienna, 1934.

The possibility of the traumatic origin of brain tumors has been considered ever since the time of classical neurology and pathology (Adler; Buck; Bramwell; Gerhard; Gowers; von Monakow; Müller; Paulson; Second; Starr). The figures quoted vary between two and nine per cent of cases. Parker and Kernohan wrote one of the best critical reviews of the significance of head injury in the development of brain tumors. In a large series of tumor cases they found 13.4% with a head injury but after critical evaluation found that in only 4.8% could a connection between the trauma and the tumor be seriously considered. For comparison, however, they produced a group of 431 patients of corresponding age with other diseases, of whom 10.4% had a history of head trauma. Finally, in a corresponding group of healthy individuals of the same age and occupation, 71 (i.e., 35.5%) had a similar history of head trauma.

If we try to settle the question of the possible connection between trauma and brain tumor according to our present conception of brain tumor origin, our thoughts first turn to the effect of a *general* carcinogenic factor on tissue which has been altered *locally* to form a "germ" (Fischer-Wasels). (*See* p. 38). Thus we must assume the presence of both a local and a general factor. But trauma, according to our present knowledge, can never lead to a *general* change in the sense of a general predisposition to cancer. Trauma is, however, capable of producing under certain circumstances, a *local* alteration of tissue which provides the basis for the "germ." Just as we are uncertain about the significance of developmental malformations in the origin of brain tumors, we must assume with Fischer-Wasels—when it comes to the question of the traumatic origin of brain tumors—that a suitable tissue alteration can occur only in the course of chronic regenerative processes ("misregeneration").

The effects of scar formation after infected brain wounds, particularly around foreign bodies (metal fragments, bone splinters, gauze sponges), might thus be well worth considering.

It is difficult for us today to understand the concepts of the origin of tissue damage as proposed by Herrmann, and Beneke. Of these authors, the first has credited the origin of a cerebral glioma to the effect of a sciatic nerve lesion. The prolonged peripheral stimulus was supposed to have led to the death of ganglion cells in the brain and to glial proliferation. Beneke's idea, on the other hand, is best expressed in the following quote: "In some cases one must consider externally acting injuries (mechanical, thermal, electrical) or *sudden psychic trauma* (italics mine) as indirect causes of the injuries which then may be considered a cause of tumors of the brain, spinal cord and meninges."

Marburg (1934) has carefully collected all such cases that had been reported in the literature. He has accepted the traumatic origin of brain tumors with little reservation ("There is no doubt about the existence of a connection between trauma and the development of brain tumors . . .").

At the beginning of World War II the problem aroused renewed interest. In publications by Ostertag and Buschmann (eight gliomas out of 14,400 brain injuries), Scheid (from the school of Fischer-Wasels) and Dietrich, the cases reported during the war years were critically reviewed, and in only 12 cases (Dietrich) was a connection considered likely. This series included, among others, two cases each of Neubürger and Beckmann and one case each of Hasselbach, Fischer-Wasels, and de Martel. Of these only the tumors described by Neubürger; Fischer-Wasels; and de Martel and Guillaume were regeneration-neoplasms (growths which developed out of regenerative hyperplasias). To these should be added the pre-World War I cases of Rössle (1911), and Reinhardt.

A critical review of the cases reported in the literature and of those mentioned above eliminates certain cases from the outset: for instance, Neubürger's case, dealing with a congenital disorder of the tuberous sclerosis type, that of Hasselbach, and others. Beckmann's observations are entirely unconvincing; neither can Marburg's first case stand up to serious criticism:

This was a case of a ten-year-old boy who fell on the back of his head while skating but did not lose consciousness or vomit. Fourteen days later he developed neurological symptoms, and four weeks after the accident he was thoroughly investigated. The circumference of his head was 57 cm. at that time. At autopsy, a little more than four weeks after the fall, a tumor was found—a medulloblastoma of the cerebellum. It was 4.5 x 5 cm. and quite hemorrhagic. Histologically it was a typical medulloblastoma showing characteristic subpial spread. Only in the folia next to the tumor was there an infiltration of the meninges (limited to the pia); this Marburg considered to be a persistent external granular layer. He believed that this "embryonic germ" had been caused to "proliferate" by trauma.

It should be noted here that according to our knowledge of the growth of medulloblastomas, it seems impossible that a tumor could grow from nothing to 4.5 x 5 cm. within four weeks. The time requirements are therefore not met. As regards the embryonic rest, it can be stated that Marburg's illustrations do not contradict the idea of a persisting external granular layer, but neither do they exclude the subpial spread of the tumor—a typical characteristic of the medulloblastoma. He himself mentions that this layer persisted only in the immediate vicinity of the tumor, and that the tumor infiltration of the meninges merged "gradually" into the "external granular layer."

The most important case, in my opinion, and the only one that is really convincing is that of Reinhardt:

A 57-year-old man had had a four-year clinical history of a brain tumor. At autopsy, the brain was adherent to the cribriform plate. There was an extra-cerebral, tangerine-sized tumor which extended from the frontal pole to the chiasm.

In the middle of the tumor lay a metal wire 1 cm. long and ⅓ cm. wide, which—as it turned out later—had been driven in during a boiler explosion 20 years previously. Histologically, it was a "sarcomatous" meningeal tumor, which, according to Reinhardt, developed from a granuloma.

A case of H. R. Müller ought to be mentioned here. I was able to examine the material from this case and am grateful to have had this opportunity:

A 46-year-old man had 22 years ago suffered a superficial skull injury from a grenade explosion which had rendered him unconscious for two days. Half a year before his death, he began to have more severe symptoms which exceeded his usual complaints. Autopsy revealed a meningioma in the Sylvian fissure the size of a small apple. Also visible at autopsy was a "well-healed depressed fracture of the left temporal bone", not demonstrable roentgenologically during life.

It would be possible to consider this a key case, if it could be proved with assurance that the "depressed fracture" did not simply represent the hyperostotic bone changes known to be associated with this kind of tumor (*see* p. 192). In the literature these changes have many times been misinterpreted as fractures of the inner table (e.g., the case of Leszynsky).

The traumatic origin of meningiomas, therefore, will have to be accepted as established only in those few cases that can be proved; M. Müller[4], too, has reported similar cases.

The origin of other connective tissue tumors from chronic regenerative processes should also be kept in mind. Here again I should like to cite a case of H. R. Müller (who was kind enough to send me case history, photographs, and histological sections):

This was the case of a 57-year-old man who had had several trepanations following a brain injury of the right parietal region and who at that time presented the picture of hemiplegia and Jacksonian epilepsy. Twenty-two years later the hemiplegia returned. At autopsy (death from status epilepticus) there was found a meningo-cerebral cicatrix together with a missile track from the temporal region to the falx, along which lay grenade

[4] Zschr. Krebsforsch. **52**, 113–123, 1941.

splinters. There was a tumor situated occipitally with "two cherry-sized nodules directly in the missile track." Histologically, the structure was variable and large necrotic areas were present. It was a typical monstrocellular sarcoma (*see* p. 206). The two well-delineated nodules, which were supposed to have lain in the missile path, were composed of densely cellular portions of tumor far removed from the main tumor mass. However, one could see no remnants of the missile path in them. If this local relationship could really have been proved, this case, too, would be worthy of serious consideration, since such missile tracks, as experience shows, have a considerable admixture of connective tissue in the scar. This peculiar kind of tumor, which is discussed in detail in the special part, might thus have developed from a connective tissue scar.

The case of Schellenberg should also be mentioned, even though the tumor showed only very slight autonomous growth.

The question of the origin of *neuroectodermal* tumors from traumatic foci is more difficult to answer. As yet there are no cases in the literature that are not questionable. Marburg's first case, as shown above, is not without serious objections. Not even the case of Hallervorden (1948), though well substantiated, is beyond criticism. This was an oligodendroglioma intimately related to an area of traumatic destruction which contained bony splinters as well. The plant fiber which was described in the marginal zone of the tumor could have been introduced into the brain substance during the autopsy, as the author subsequently stated. Further information about the "open brain wound" was also unavailable, the case history was not known, and the brain was sent without the general autopsy findings. Hallervorden felt, however, that with the exception of this point the evidence still held. Staemmler's case also is unconvincing. In the meantime there have appeared the cases of N. Wolf (1951) and of Noetzel (1953) (a glioblastoma of the posterior corpus callosum which was in contact with the margin of an old bullet track). Although both these cases would be difficult to dismiss from a legal viewpoint, I would still like to regard them as coincidental. The same applies to the very interesting case recently published by Heyck in which a glioblastoma of the anterior corpus callosum developed in the immediate vicinity of two cysts which were the result of a bilateral leukotomy performed five years previously.

In order to accept the traumatic etiology of a neuroepithelial tumor, the following should be demanded of the "local" findings: the effects of trauma are not simply to be assumed from the direction of the force applied, but have to be demonstrable in the tissue. At this point we should draw upon our knowledge of the histology of particular tumor types. Even though remains of old hemorrhages, brown-pigmented cysts, and macrophages with hemosiderin are found, we must remember that such findings are quite common, even *without* trauma, in spongioblastomas of the cerebellum and the third ventricle, in angioblastomas, in oligodendrogliomas, and in glioblastomas, etc.[5]

It is particularly difficult to interpret certain types of brain scars which can occasionally be observed as a result of hyperplasia of leptomeningeal tissue carried into the depths of the wound. It arises, of course, during the formation of the scar, but withers away very rapidly, leaving psammoma bodies (Zülch, in Tönnis and Griponissiotis, 1939). It must also be noted that proliferation of astrocytes often occurs in scars; this cannot be distinguished from an astrocytic tumor by examining merely a small piece. This should be borne in mind when evaluating numerous "cicatricial gliomas." Also, a foreign body granuloma is not yet an autonomously-growing tumor (Marburg, 1935; *see* Peters, 1952).

Even greater caution about assuming the traumatic origin of neuro-epithelial growths should be exercised than was indicated in the case of mesodermal tumors.

Legal evaluation of cases with "post-traumatic" tumors

Ewing; Jordan; Masson (quoted by Radermecker); von Monakow; Reinhardt; Scheid; Second; Thiem and others have assembled a list of pertinent points, which, when clarified, should facilitate the decision about the "traumatic" origin of a tumor. They have also been critically discussed by Marburg. Taking into consideration this previous work as well as our own knowledge of the biology of brain tumors, the following prerequisites should be demanded.

1. The patient should have been well before the accident. This requirement should be insisted on even though the decision may be difficult, because brain tumors often grow for years without symptoms and can even elude ventriculographic demonstration during this time (Pennybacker and Meadows).

2. The head trauma must have been adequate, i.e., sufficient to produce a destruction of parts of the brain or its coverings leading to chronic regenerative processes. Even a minor trauma can lead to considerable pathological changes (a snowball in the case of Koopmann, and one of our own, 1950). Furthermore, loss of consciousness and other signs of *commotio cerebri* are not obligatory, as severe brain damage can occur without these.

---

[5] Knowledge of the general morphology of tumors should also be taken into account in evaluating the literature; very accurate diagnoses can be made from the frequently excellent descriptions supplied. For instance, Merzbacher's and Uyeda's cases of a "gliosarcoma," and Bielschowsky's (1914) case of an "atypical example of tuberous sclerosis" are really oligodendrogliomas; Marburg's case with the "post-traumatic development of a glioma" in the vicinity of a revolver bullet is an ependymoma of the cerebral hemisphere, etc.

Consequently a thorough investigation of each individual case is necessary (Zülch, 1950).

3. The site of tumor formation must correspond to that receiving the trauma. It is not enough merely to state that the tumor lies at the site of external skull injury or at a region of supposed contre-coup injury. The proof of injury to the meninges, bone, or brain substance must be based upon morphological findings.

4. The time interval between the trauma and the development of the tumor should be adequate. At present we know enough about the rate of brain tumor growth to answer that question. Criticism based on this point leads to rejection of Marburg's case, referred to above. Fischer-Wasels (1932) proposes a very long latency, 4–20 years, for the growth of tumors. In individual cases where a meningioma, cerebellar spongioblastoma or even a large medulloblastoma occurs a few weeks after an accident, trauma may be dismissed as a cause. On the other hand, glioblastomas or medulloblastomas might theoretically develop as a result of trauma even many years after the accident.

5. The tumor has to be proved histologically at autopsy or by biopsy. Here we must caution particularly against misinterpreting the simple glial or connective tissue portions of the scar. The meningocerebral cicatrix affords a good demonstration of this problem. Very frequently small regions of the glial scar cannot be definitely distinguished from astrocytomas.

6. The external force should be defined as sufficient to be considered true trauma. The definition might be as follows: an accident is "a single externally-produced mechanical bodily injury which produces alterations in the structure and function of the body and was not intended by the victim." The trauma must be proved without question. Interval symptoms seem to me to be without significance, since we cannot expect the onset of the tumor immediately after the trauma (*see* point 4, Fischer-Wasels).

According to this strict definition, a traumatic etiology can be accepted for only a few brain tumors. Rather, an *aggravation* of the clinical picture might be found, or an *actual participation* of the trauma in eliciting the clinical manifestations prematurely. This is illustrated by the following professional opinion from our institute (Sprockhoff):

A previously healthy 41-year-old truck driver received a blow to the back of his head during work. This produced headaches, but no loss of consciousness. On the following day the man was admitted to a hospital because of a series of epileptic seizures. He became an invalid, as the attacks recurred regularly. After eight years his condition became worse, and one year later he was referred for operation by the neurological department.

At operation "peculiar changes in the form of many large cysts lying frontal to a parasagittal meningioma the size of a small apple" were found. No such changes were seen behind the tumor, but the brain here was atrophic. The cysts were opened, and the tumor extirpated along with "cicatricial strands of the surrounding tissue and the damaged portions of the brain." The patient was cured. It was assumed that through the effects of the blow to the back of the head a compression of the brain took place when it was thrown against the tumor. The proof lay in the immediate appearance of the clinical symptoms and in the operative findings. The accident was thought to have had a definite influence upon the clinical course of the disease.

Peters (1952), incidentally, concurs with my conservative opinion about the possibility of the development of tumors from brain trauma (*see* details in Zülch, 1953), and has summarized prevailing opinions in a review of this subject.

Brain tumors in animals

These are so rare that we have few opportunities to draw analogies between human and animal brain tumors. Brain tumors, for instance, are much rarer in monkeys and mice than in humans; the mouse is considered to be free from spontaneous gliomas. In general, three-quarters of the tumors are primary and one quarter is metastatic, the latter appearing particularly frequently in the horse. Tumors of the following histological structures (or at least similar structure) have been described: glioblastoma, astrocytoma, pinealoma, gangliocytoma, as well as choroid papilloma, pituitary adenoma, meningioma, lipoma, melanoma, and growths like epidermoids (Jungherr and Wolf; Neubuerger and Davis), the last especially in the horse. Moreover, retinal gliomas are not rare. In cattle, neurinomas and a type of neurofibromatosis have been described (H. J. Scherer, 1944; Jungherr and Wolf; Frauchiger; and others). Animal tumor nomenclature does not yet correspond to that of human pathology. Through the courtesy of Prof. Frauchiger, Bern, I had the opportunity to study 22 cases of brain tumors in animals (horses, cows, dogs, cats and chickens). When I started to compare them with human tumors and classify them accordingly, I realized the difficulties of this task[6]. The same applied to the tumors produced artificially with carcinogenic substances which I

[6] We have made diagnoses of medulloblastomas, astrocytomas, glioblastomatous or sarcomatous tumors, periadventitial and meningeal sarcomatoses, meningiomas, and a chromophobe adenoma. Details have been published in E. FRAUCHIGER's monograph (*See* FRAUCHIGER, E., und. R. FRANKHAUSER: Vergleichende Neuropathologie des Menschen und der Tiere. Springer, Berlin, 1957). In another case, a fibrosarcoma in an elephant was sent to me through the courtesy of Prof. Veit, Cologne.

have mentioned earlier (p. 39) and which we have been able to reproduce in our institute in the meantime (B. Schiefer).

The spontaneous development of tumors of the central nervous system

What can observations on brain tumors contribute to general oncology? The derivation of craniopharyngiomas from the craniopharyngeal duct is an established fact even today, just as is the derivation of epidermoids, dermoids, and teratomas from certain errors of closure of the skull and brain; we refer to this latter group, therefore, as "malformation-tumors" (congenital and embryonic tumors). Similarly, the origin of meningiomas from the meningeal granulations (M. B. Schmidt; Ferner), or other leptomeningeal rests, may be considered proved. However, Stroebe's observations (of ependyma-lined spaces in a glioma) which he related to the tumor's origin have so far been misinterpreted. I nearly made such a misinterpretation myself:

I submitted a paper on the origin of an oligodendroglioma from displaced embryonic ventricular lining to the 1939 German Pathological Congress, which was not held, however, because of the outbreak of the war. An accurate study by serial sections of the brain from this case showed later (Zülch, 1941) that this seemingly crucial observation had to be explained differently. Actually we were dealing with the epithelium of the choroid plexus of the lateral ventricle which had been engulfed by the large thalamic tumor. Since this tumor, occurring in a three-and-a-half-year-old boy, was already fist-sized, this premature judgment was probably an excusable misinterpretation; it had fitted current theories all too well.

A review of our large collection of unoperated brains revealed beyond doubt that the majority of brain tumors arise in sites of predilection (*see* p. 62 ff.) and are not distributed uniformly over all portions of the brain (thus implying the action of a *local factor* in the tissues). Moreover, their relative frequency at certain sites is a regular occurrence (*see* p. 69 ff.). At some sites one can correlate certain frequently-occurring tissue rests with the growth of a tumor at that place. The ependymomas of the foramen of Monro (Zülch and Schmid, 1955) grow at a site where ependymal rests very frequently lie normally. However there still have been no systematic serial-section studies of the occurrence of displaced embryonic rests. A statistical evaluation of our tumor material has given us certain indications that *"general" factors* are also involved in the production of tumors. All brain tumors—with the exception of primary sarcomas—have a pronounced tendency to manifest themselves at a certain age (*see* p. 58 ff.). Also the regular sex predilection of certain tumors suggests that there are endocrine factors which have an effect upon the production of the tumors. The two large groups of malignant gliomas show this particularly clearly: the medulloblastomas occur up to and including puberty, while the equally highly malignant glioblastomas occur predominantly when various involutional changes are beginning. Both tumors are more common in males (*see* p. 77 ff.). On the other hand, the benign tumors of the brain coverings —meningiomas and neurinomas—are more common in females. We can deduce from that, along with Fischer-Wasels, that a local factor of tissue predisposition and a general constitutional factor may be involved in the origin of brain tumors, the latter having probably something to do with age and sex as they occur in the life cycle (*see* p. 39).

On the other hand, we do not know any exogenous factors which might play a role in the origin of brain tumors. The development of brain tumors from the local tissue changes produced by trauma is practically non-existent. Moreover, no tumors have been seen following inflammatory processes. At the present time we cannot admit the possibility of a specific chemical influence (carcinogen) upon the brain and spinal cord in humans, even though it is effective experimentally in animals. In cases of occupational cancers produced by chemical substances, brain tumors were never seen. We know nothing about the possible effects of radiation of various wave-lengths upon the brain and spinal cord, with the exception of deliberately administered X-ray irradiation, which might, in single cases, have contributed to the production of tumors (*see* p. 39).

We still do not know then how brain tumors really originate *spontaneously*. We can consider a universal explanation of tumor origin as established only when it can also account for the behavior of that particularly well-protected organ, the "central nervous system," and can explain the "spontaneous" formation of tumors there, too. As regards brain tumors, I think the soundest theory of tumor origin is that which takes into account a) *a general factor*—the interplay of hormonal controls with the possibility of a derangement in this equilibrium, and b) *a local factor*—a local morphological or metabolic tissue derangement which developed in an individual during embryogenesis. This local factor, acting during embryological development at least of the nervous system is responsible for certain predilections as to site, etc. An hereditary factor plays a role only in the exceptional case (hamartoblastomatosis, retinoblastomas).

CHAPTER IV

GENERAL STATISTICAL AND BIOLOGICAL DATA ON BRAIN TUMORS

Incidence

Reliable data on the incidence of brain tumors has so far been lacking. The percentage of general hospital admissions of patients with brain tumors seems to vary between 0.2% and 2.6% (McLean, 1936). In 1928 the mortality from cancer and other malignant tumors of the brain in the U:S. was 0.06%.

Specifically, we find 4.6% of patients with brain tumors out of 12,000 admissions to the Wenzel-Hanke Hospital (O. Foerster, 1934); and Bailey (1933) quotes the corresponding figure for three London hospitals as 1.8% of 15,500 admissions, while the statistics of the Royal Infirmary at [Leeds show 167 brain tumors (1.34%) out of 13,000 cases; however, the brain was examined in only 27% of autopsies. Finally, Peers (1936) at Boston City Hospital had 10,592 autopsies in 38 years; tumors were the cause of death in 16.8% of cases. Of these, 188 were tumors of the central nervous system, with 43.1% gliomas, corresponding approximately to the relative frequency in Cushing's (1932) material. However, the brain was removed in only one half of all the autopsies.

According to McLean (1936) there were 367 patients with brain tumors out of 300,000 admissions to a large American hospital. Because of the increase in specialization, it is difficult to provide more recent data.

According to Klebs in Prague (1877), pathological statistics showed 64 brain tumor cases (1.76%) out of 3,622 autopsies; Gruber in Göttingen reported 79 intracranial tumors (1.3%) in 6,000 autopsies. Schmincke had 2.07% brain tumors out of 7,642 cases in Tübingen (Rapp), and 1.4% primary brain tumors out of 31,698 autopsies (1854–1931) in Heidelberg. Rudershausen described Schmincke's material in detail and found 444 primary tumors of the brain and 102 metastases in 546 cases. Among 232 cases of glioma, there were 139 males and 93 females. Granulomas were not included.

Gärtner (1955) continued the series from Heidelberg for 21 years. During this time, 710 space-occupying intracranial lesions were recorded, of which 654 could be properly evaluated. The results have been compared

TABLE 1. REVIEW OF THE CLASSIFICATION OF 4,000 (AND 6000*) BRAIN TUMORS, COMPARED WITH CUSHINGS (1932) AND OLIVECRONA'S (1955) SERIES

| | Our series of 4000 | | Our series of 6000 | | Cushing's | Olivecrona's |
	cases	% of total	cases	% of total	%	% (5250 cases)
Medulloblastomas	161	4.0	230	3.8	4.3	
Spongioblastomas (incl. the so-called cerebellar astrocytoma)	292	7.1	419	7.0	6.1	46.5†
Oligodendrogliomas	312	7.8	490	8.2	1.3	
Astrocytomas	283	7.1	381	6.4	9.8	
Glioblastomas	530	13.3	738	12.3	10.3	
Ependymomas	184	4.6	259	4.3	1.3	
Plexus papillomas	20	0.5	30	0.5	0 6	0.3
Pinealomas	16	0.4	25	0.4	0.7	
Neurinomas	297	7.5	451	7.6	8.7	8.0
Gangliocytomas	15	0.4	27	0.4	0.2	
Meningiomas	723	18.1	1079	18.0	13.4	19.2
Angioblastomas	60	1.5	78	1.3	1.2	2.4
Fibromas	5	0.1	7	0.1		
Sarcomas	74	1.9	162	2.7	0.7	
Chondromas	11	0.3	20	0.3	0.1	
Lipomas	1		4	0.1		
Osteomas	16	0.4	29	0.5	0.7	
Chordomas	9	0.2	14	0.2	0.1	
Craniopharyngiomas	107	2.7	150	2.5	4.6	1.7
Pituitary adenomas	282	7.1	478	8.0	17.8	8.5
Cylindromatous epitheliomas	8	0.2	12	0.2		
Epidermoids	61 }66	1.5	94	1.7	0.7	0.7
Dermoids	5	0.1	10	0.2		
Teratomas	12	0.3	14	0.2	0.2	0.3
Angiomas and aneurysms	83	2.1	151	2.5	1.0	7.0
Unclassified tumors	151	3.8	221	3.7	9.6	
Metastases‡	163	4.1	242	4.0	3.2	3.4
Parasites	6	0.2	9	0.1	0.1	
Granulomas	32	0.8	45	0.7	2.2	1.0
Arachnoiditis and ependymitis	53	1.3	92	1.5	1.1	
Miscellaneous: (myelomas, Schüller-Christian's disease, etc.)	28	0.8	39	0.6		1.0
Total	4000	100.0	6000	100.0	100.0	100.0

* The series of 6000 brain tumors includes the series of 4000. *See* Zbl. Neurochir. **17**, 1957.

† Neuroectodermal tumors excepting plexus papillomas and neurinomas.

‡ Translators' note: Dr. Percival Bailey points out that the percentage of metastatic tumors is too low because the material utilized in preparing the table came mainly from neurosurgical services.

with our collection of 4,000 cases and differ only in unimportant details
Our figures, therefore, can be considered as fairly typical. Moreover, the
results in 248 intracranial tumors presented by Link and Schleussing (1950)
vary but little from these figures.

Germany, with a population of 70 million, had about 800,000 deaths
per year, 140,000 of which were due to malignant tumors. Recent figures
(1950) gave a cancer mortality rate of 26:10,000, compared to a general
mortality rate of 106:10,000. Since the central nervous system's share of
tumors is about 2% (Naffziger and Boldrey, 1948), we can calculate the
death rate from brain and spinal cord tumors at about 1:20,000 or 1:25,000
population per year, with the then existing age distribution.

We are better informed about the *relative* frequency of brain tumors,
particularly of the different kinds; it is quite constant in all large series.
Differences exist in details, according to the interest of the particular surgeon or investigator, the composition of the clinical material, or the
peculiarities of classification.

Collections of cases from psychiatric clinics are high in frontal lobe
tumors, with meningiomas of the olfactory groove, the sagittal sinus, and
falx prevailing; collections from chronic mental hospitals, on the other
hand, abound in brain tumors which produce early seizures but do not
lead to increased intracranial pressure until later (oligodendrogliomas).
Malignant glioblastomas predominate in pathological institutes but rarely
remain in neurosurgical clinics. In some clinics, tumors of special locations
or age groups accumulate if the surgeon is particularly interested in them,
or develops particular operative skills (Cushing: pituitary adenomas).

Of our collection, about 75% came from the neurosurgical clinics of
Tönnis, and 25% from other sources: Hafenkrankenhaus, Hamburg (Prof.
Brütt), Department of Psychiatry of the University Hospital in Munich
(Prof. Spatz), Pathological Institute of the Charité, Berlin (Prof. Rössle
and Hamperl), and the mental hospital in Berlin-Buch; and from private
referrals.

It may be assumed that the data of our series—as shown in the table
—come closest to the average incidence frequency in the general population, since the selection was less restricted and the sources were "mixed."

Age incidence

Determination of the age incidence of the individual tumor types was
one of the most important achievements in the biology of brain tumors.
Such relationships had already been indicated in Starr's (1894) first large
statistical analysis. In childhood and adolescence (up to the age of 20)
tuberculomas were four times as frequent as in the higher age groups. The

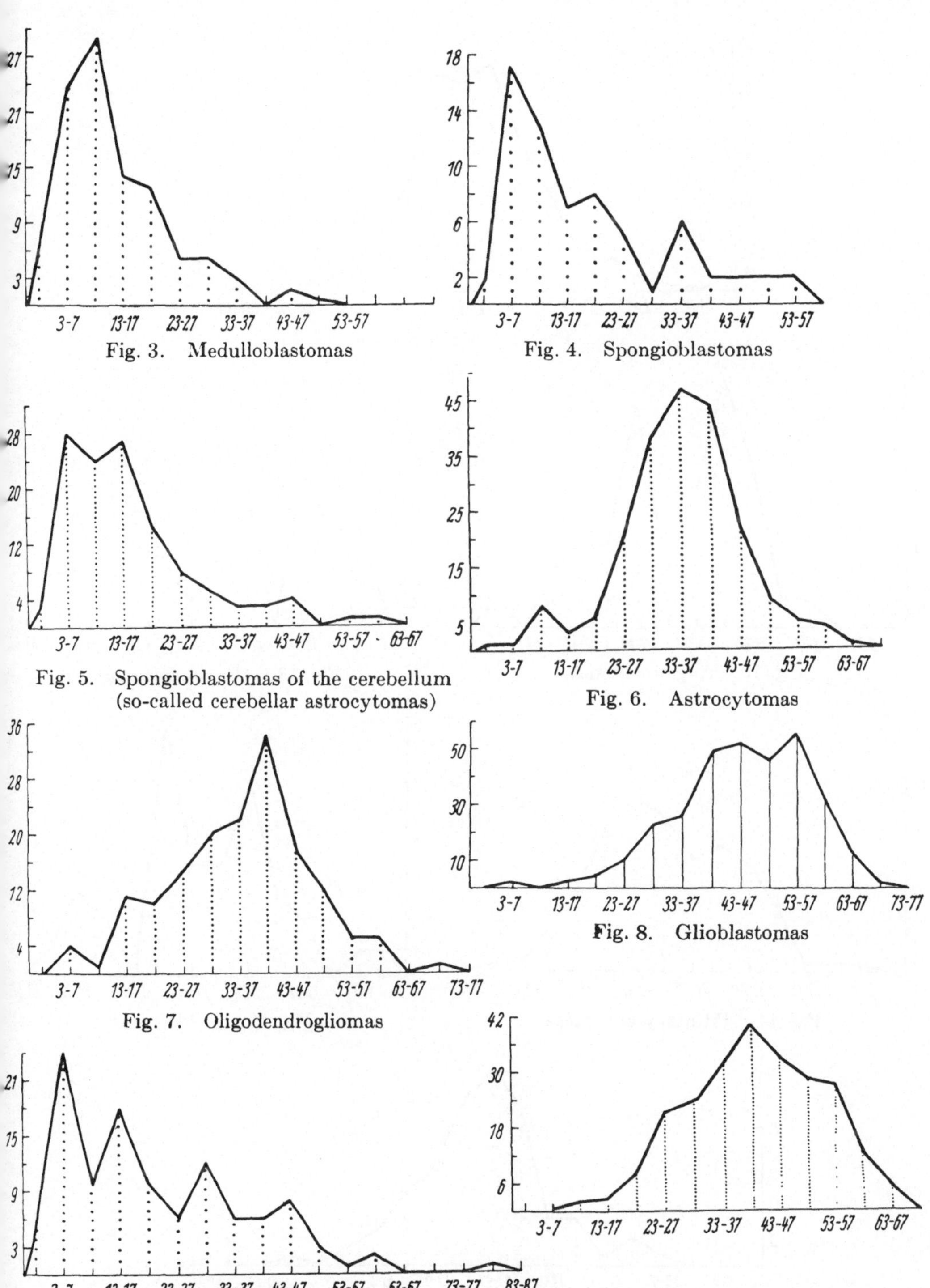

Fig. 3. Medulloblastomas

Fig. 4. Spongioblastomas

Fig. 5. Spongioblastomas of the cerebellum (so-called cerebellar astrocytomas)

Fig. 6. Astrocytomas

Fig. 7. Oligodendrogliomas

Fig. 8. Glioblastomas

Fig. 9. Ependymomas

Fig. 10. Neurinomas

Incidence of individual tumor types according to age groups

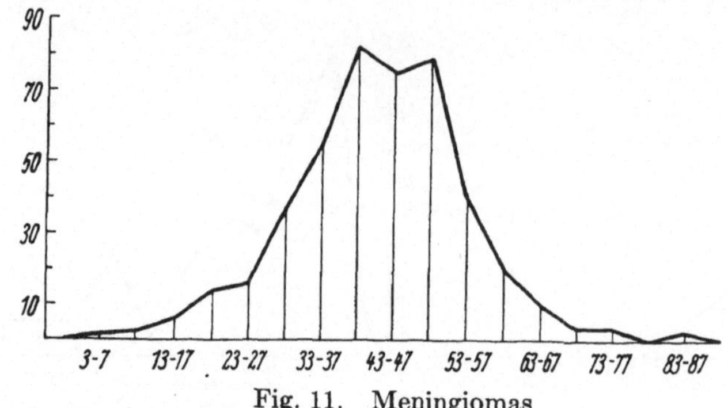

Fig. 11.   Meningiomas

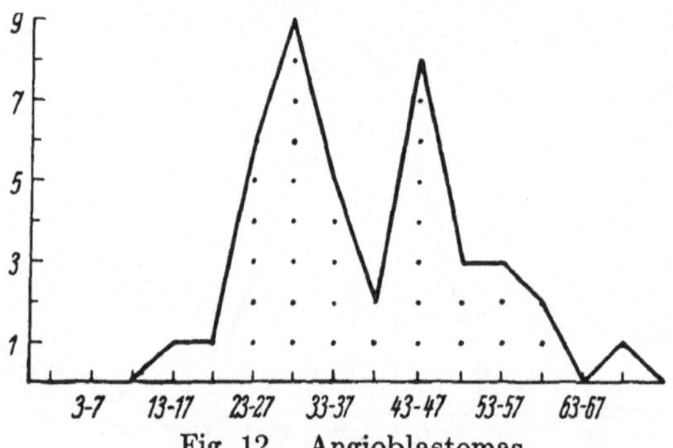

Fig. 12.   Angioblastomas

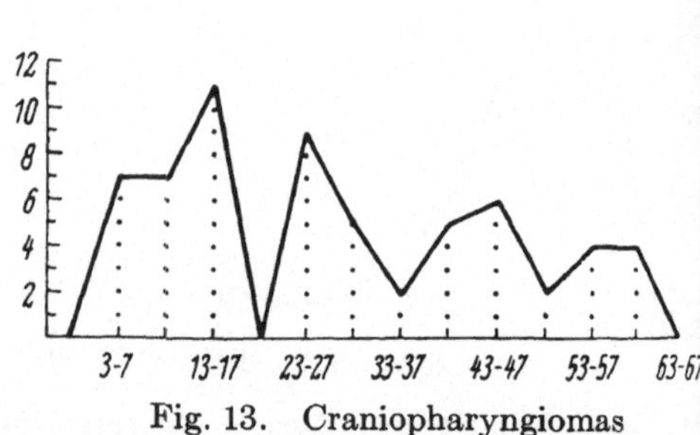

Fig. 13.   Craniopharyngiomas

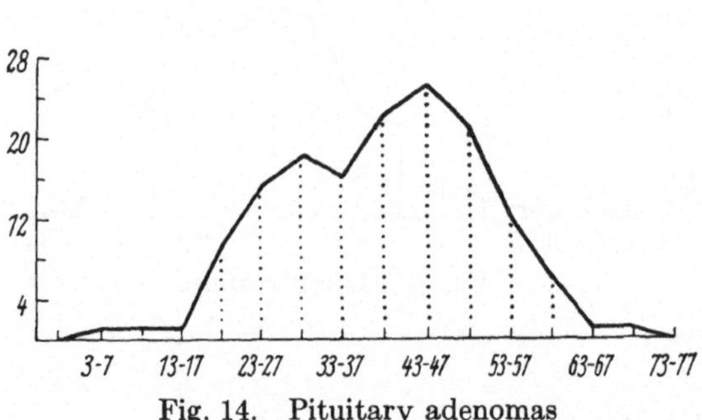

Fig. 14.   Pituitary adenomas

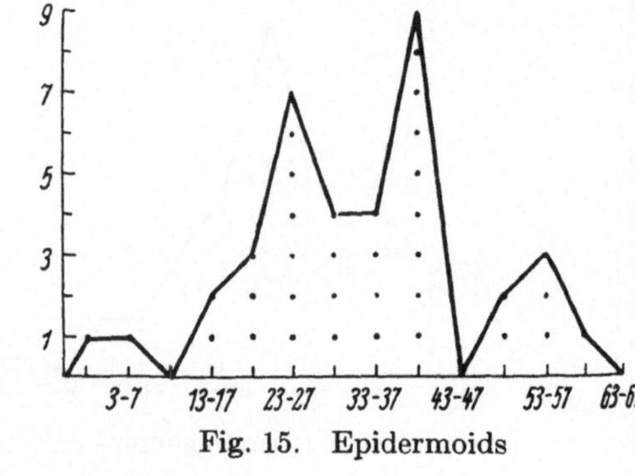

Fig. 15.   Epidermoids

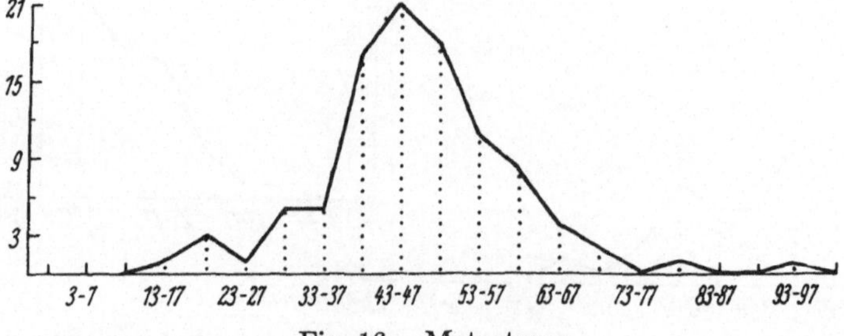

Fig. 16.   Metastases

Incidence of individual tumor types according to age groups

precise definition of tumor groups, i.e., entities with similar location, age
incidence, and tissue type we owe to Cushing (1930, 1931) in his description of cerebellar tumors (medulloblastomas and the so-called astrocytomas). If the age of incidence is plotted against the frequency of all tumor
groups, the resulting curves show characteristic age peaks (Figs. 3–16).
Since the actual time of tumor onset cannot be determined, we use the
age at the time of admission to the hospital, or—where there has been no
hospital treatment—the time of death. The discrepancy between that time
and the actual beginning of the tumor growth can obviously be quite
considerable in the case of astrocytomas, oligodendrogliomas, some gangliocytomas, as well as meningiomas, craniopharyngiomas, epidermoids, etc.

With all the age curves plotted together on a single ordinate, we notice
a crossing of many of the curves at around age 20, i.e., the ascending and
descending limbs of a number of curves here cut across one another. This
again indicates the biological significance of this age period which represents the end of childhood and adolescence.[1]

We also see that certain tumor types show a predilection for the third
and fourth decades, and that the fifth and sixth decades, too, are preferred
by certain kinds of tumors. These interrelations have recently been described in detail. We define as childhood and adolescence the ages between
1–20 years, middle age from 21 to 45, the age of involution from 46–65,
and old age from 65 on (Zülch, 1949; Borck and Zülch; Zülch and Borck,
1952).

If we evaluate a large series of patients from the point of view of age
incidence, we come to the following conclusions: in childhood and adolescence, the most common tumors in the cerebral hemispheres are ependymomas, with the other gliomas and ganglion cell tumors appearing less
frequently. Monstrocellular sarcomas are also encountered. On the other
hand, we see only a few of the meningiomas, which form the single largest
group in the higher age groups. In the chiasmal region craniopharyngiomas
and spongioblastomas are frequent, while pituitary adenomas are nearly
absent. The complete absence of neurinomas is very impressive, while in
the cerebellum itself the bulk of all tumors occurring in the younger age
groups is made up of medulloblastomas and spongioblastomas (so-called
astrocytomas).

The angioblastomas of the fourth ventricle are not very evident as
yet. In the region of the quadrigeminal plate, teratomas and pinealomas
occur in this age group; nearly all spongioblastomas (so-called astro-

---

[1] The age curves of individual tumor types however are not "pure," as they include
groups with mixed age incidences. For example, the oligodendroglioma, which occurs
mostly in the third and fourth decades, also includes a definitely adolescent type, the
oligodendroglioma of the thalamus, which blurs the age peak to some extent.

cytomas) around the aqueduct occur under the age of 20. Other tumors of childhood and adolescence are the oligodendrogliomas of the thalamus, and astrocytomas and spongioblastomas of the pons.

The middle decades of life (third and fourth decades) are characterized by the frequent occurrence of gliomas of the cerebral hemispheres (astrocytomas and oligodendrogliomas), meningiomas of various sites, pituitary adenomas, the neurinomas of the cerebello-pontine angle, and the angioblastomas of the cerebellum. The two cerebellar tumors of the younger age groups are met with only rarely.

The latter decades of life (fifth and sixth decades) show a more frequent occurrence of malignant glioblastomas and of metastatic tumors, while oligodendrogliomas and astrocytomas, as well as meningiomas, angioblastomas and neurinomas are also encountered.

In the sixth and seventh decades, glioblastomas, meningiomas, and neurinomas comprise 82%, and together with the metastatic tumors, clearly predominate. According to Moersch, Craig and Kernohan, 20% of all brain tumors occur in the sixth decade and 8% beyond the age of 60 (*see* also Kloss). We have little information about comparable data in the aged, who seldom come to autopsy (W. Fischer, 1947). Also in the very youngest age groups the distribution of brain tumors does not follow the usual type (Russell and Ellis).

The relative frequency of the various tumor types within each age group and their sex distribution can be read from the three graphs in Figures 20–22 (Zülch and Borck, 1952). The above-mentioned predilection of tumors for childhood, middle age, involution and old age is very evident.

The preferential site of brain tumors

Brain tumors may occur singly and circumscribed, multiple, diffuse or limited to a system. The systematic neoplasms have been dealt with above (p. 42 ff.). Most brain tumors, however, are single growths.

It is a matter of long experience, (and easily understandable from what we know of embryology) that pituitary adenomas, pinealomas, and craniopharyngiomas occur at one site only and that the neurinomas (of the cerebello-pontine angle) prefer the eighth nerve. Meningiomas and cerebellar tumors, too, show a similar regularity in their occurrence (Cushing 1931, 1938). To Ostertag (1932, 1936) and P. Schwartz (1932, 1936) goes credit for having demonstrated similar relationships for the other types of glioma. Unfortunately, though, both authors paid little attention in their classification to the characteristic that is most decisive for the neurosurgeon: the tissue type of the tumor. Occasionally tumors of the same location but of a different type were grouped together—an understandable

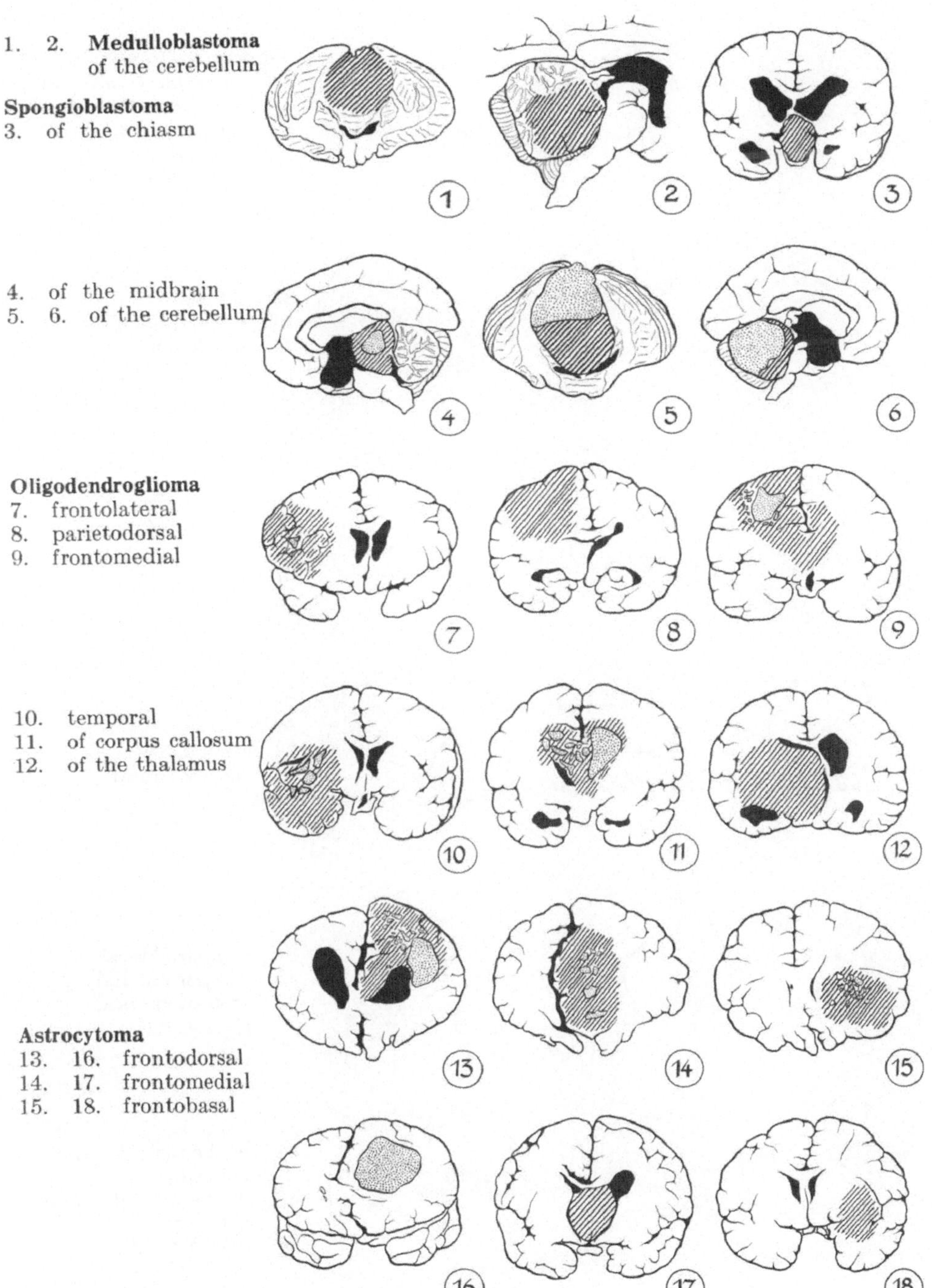

Fig. 17. Preferential sites of brain tumors

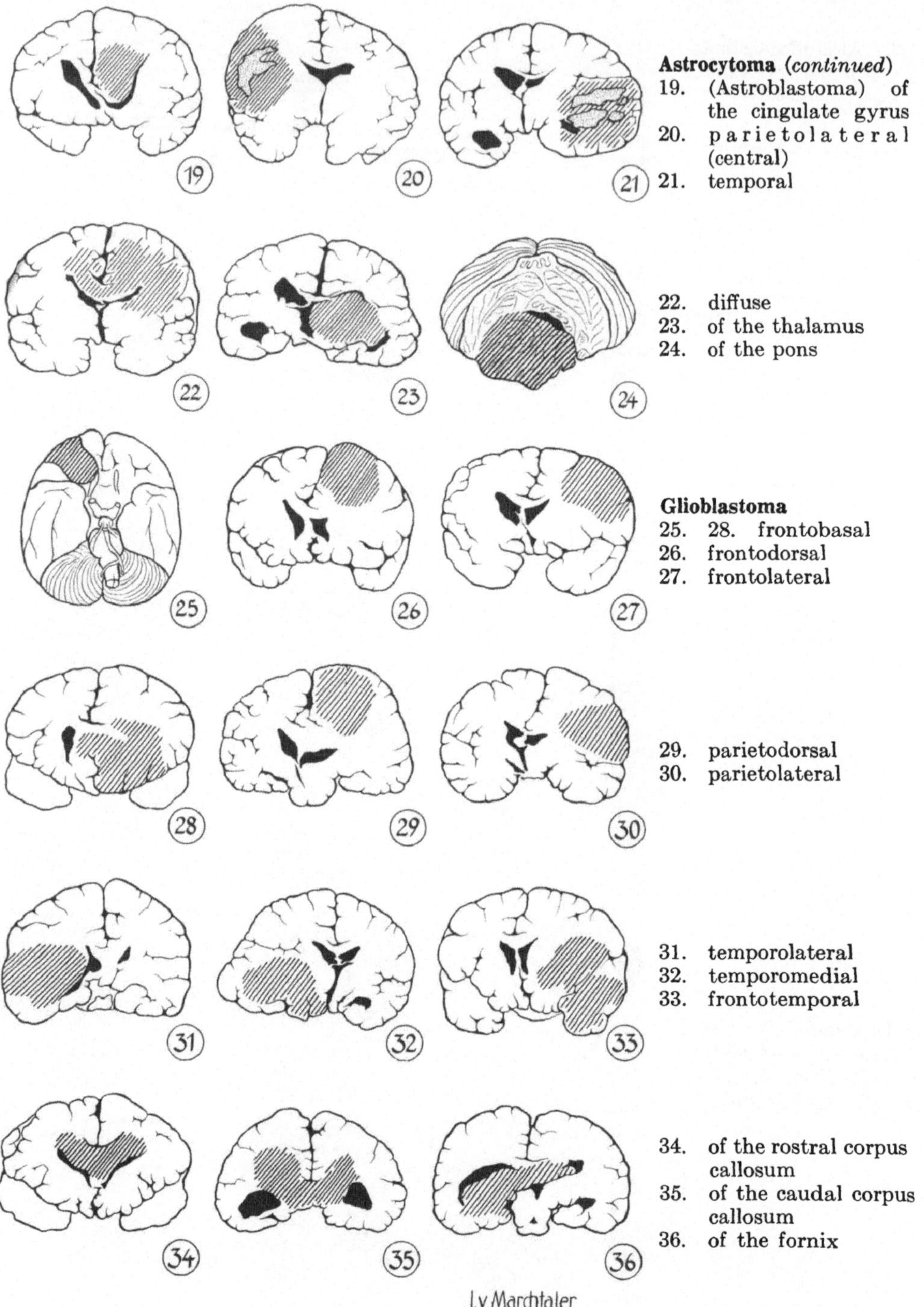

Fig. 17.   Preferential sites of brain tumors (*continued*)

Glioblastoma (*continued*)
37. of the rostral radiation of the corpus callosum
38. of the caudal radiation of the corpus callosum
39. of the thalamus

40. of the midbrain

Ependymoma
41. of the cerebral hemisphere
42. of the lateral ventricle (foramen of Monro)

43. of the third ventricle (region of the quadrigeminal plate)
44. of the fourth ventricle
45. of the spinal cord

46. **Ependymal cyst** of foramen of Monro

47. **Pinealoma**

48. **Neurinoma** of the cerebello - pontine angle.

Meningioma
49. of the falx, bilateral
50. of the falx, unilateral
51. of the anterior third of the sagittal sinus, bilateral

52. of the middle third of the sagittal sinus
53. of the posterior third of the sagittal sinus
54. of the convexity

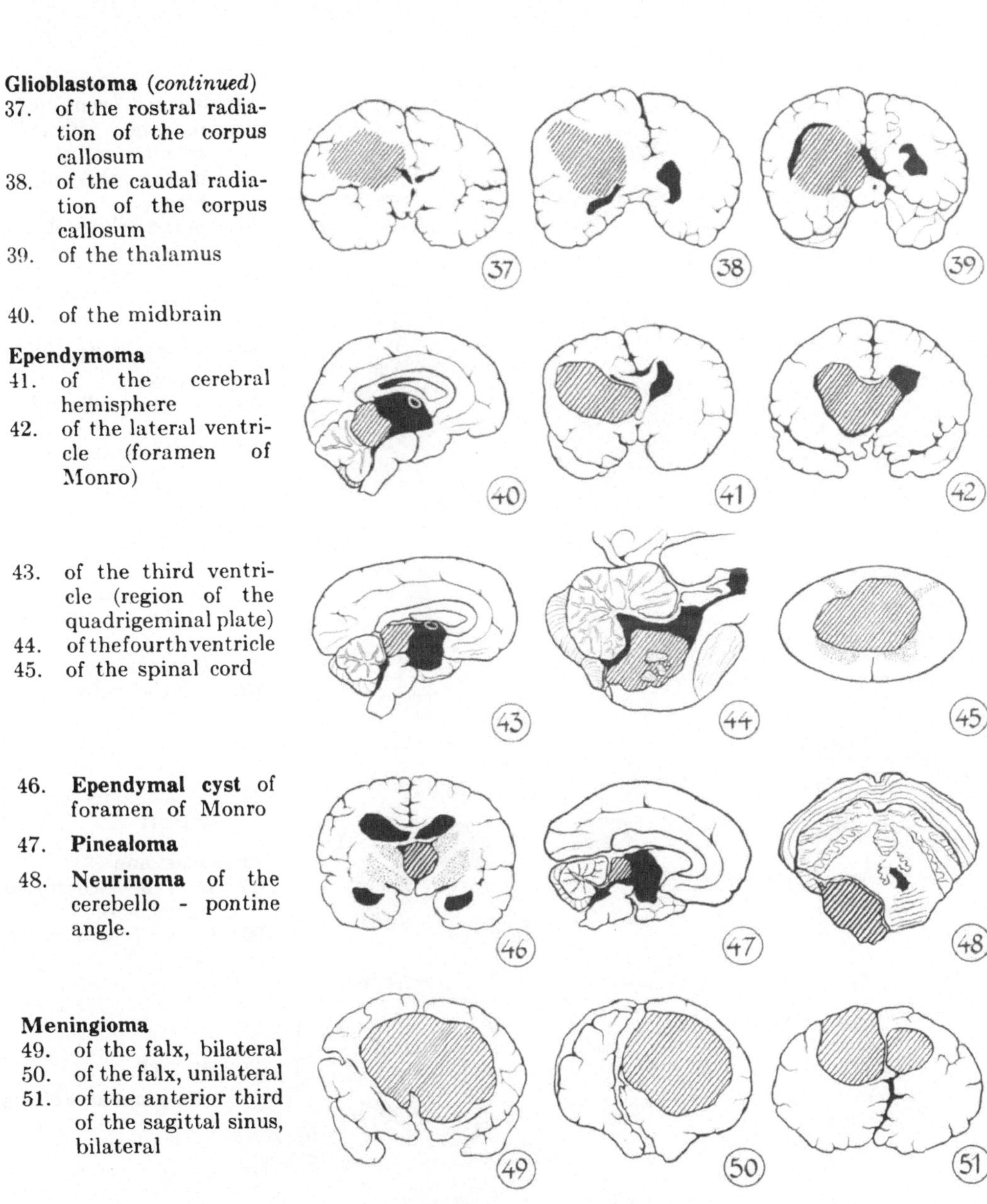

Fig. 17. Preferential sites of brain tumors (*continued*)

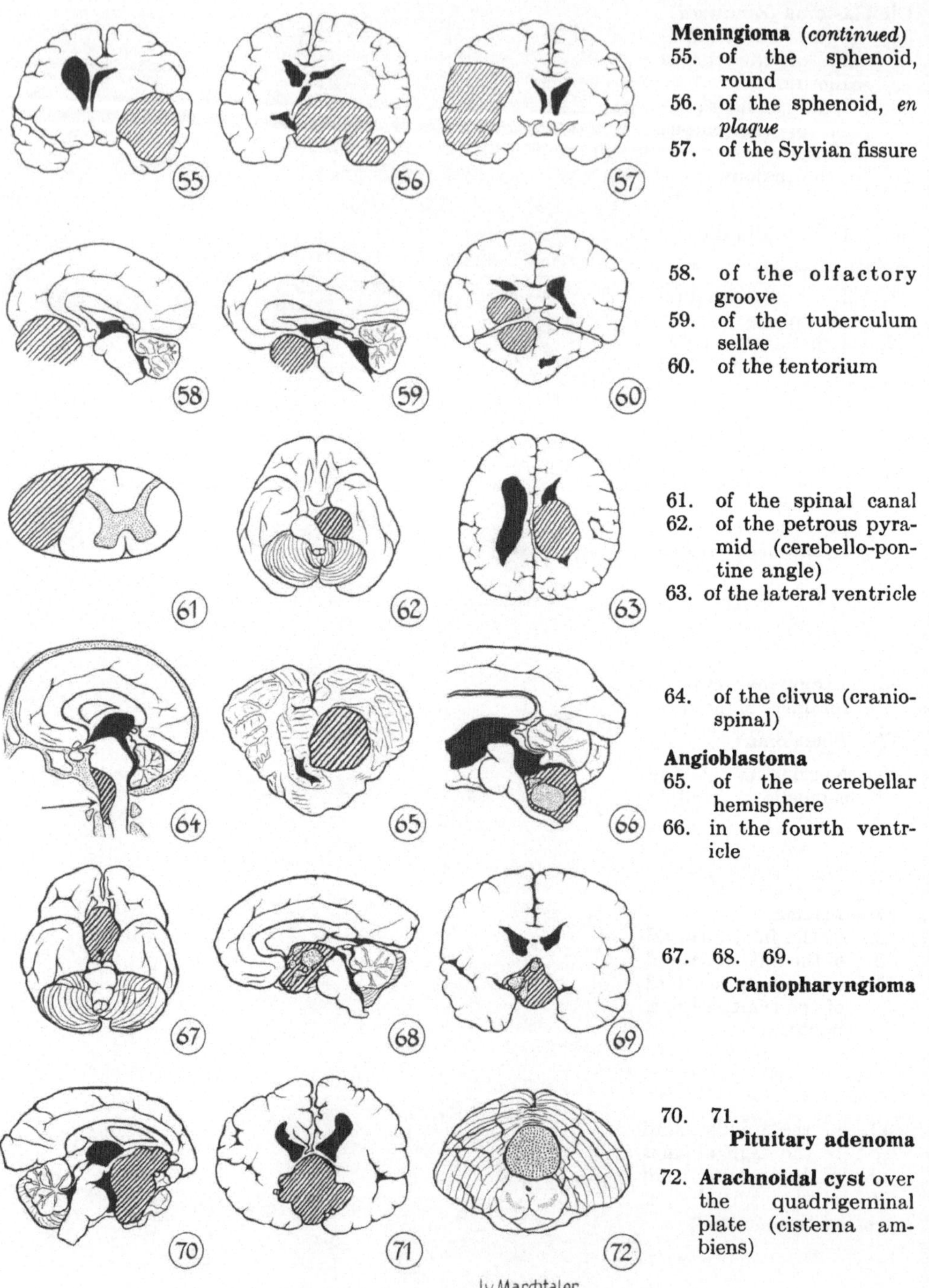

Fig. 17.   Preferential sites of brain tumors (*continued*)

1. Meningioma of the anterior third of the sagittal sinus—frontodorsal meningioma.
2. Frontodorsal astrocytoma
3. Frontodorsal glioblastoma

4. Parasagittal oligodendroglioma (frontomedial oligodendroglioma)
5. Meningioma of the convexity (frontolateral meningioma)
6. Frontolateral astrocytoma

7. Frontolateral glioblastoma
8. Frontolateral oligodendroglioma
9. Olfactory groove meningioma (frontobasal meningioma)

10. Frontobasal glioblastoma
11. Meningioma of the falx (frontomedial meningioma)
12. Frontomedial astrocytoma

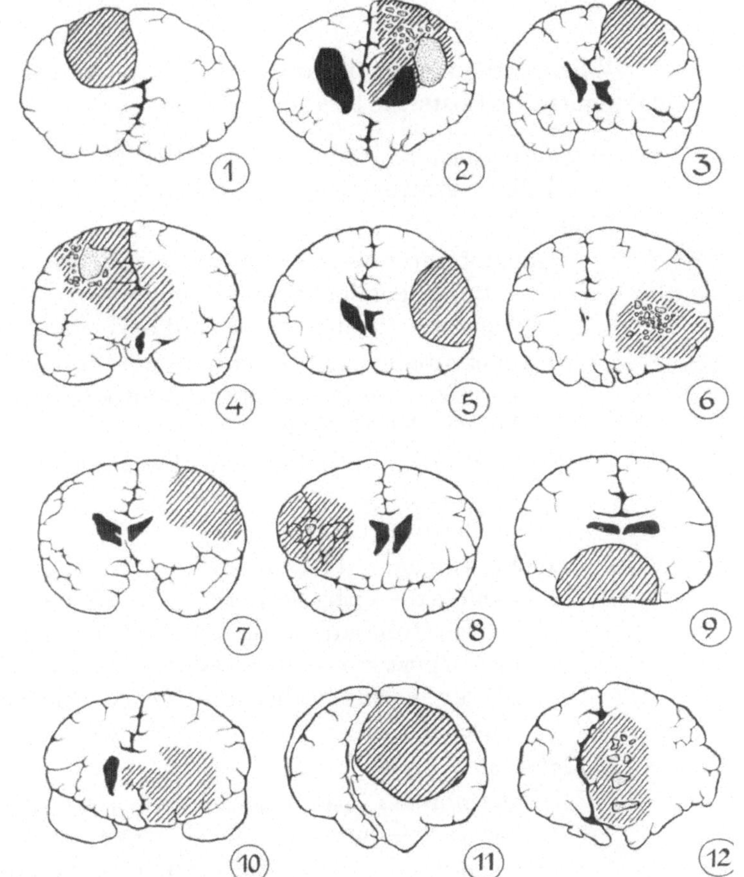

Fig. 18.   The principal brain tumors of the frontal lobes.

oversight since the idea of dysontogenetic origin was uppermost in the author's minds.

I have reversed the former procedure by starting with the tumor types and then establishing their site of predilection. On the basis of considerable experience, I can confirm the concept of preferential sites for brain tumors in the overwhelming majority of instances and—like Ostertag—have recently found it especially pronounced in glioblastomas.

The preceding diagrams (Figs. 17–18) present the results in schematic form; a detailed description of the sites is to be found in the chapters dealing with these specific tumors.[2]

[2] The topographical terms were chosen in agreement with the roentgenological ones of Lysholm.

Whereas the figures illustrate only the commonly occurring types, the subsequent text lists the location of the other (less common) types as well[3]:

Medulloblastomas: Retina—quadrigeminal plate/pineal body—cerebellar vermis—sympathetic trunk

Gliomas:

Spongioblastomas: Cerebral hemispheres—hypothalamus/chiasm —quadrigeminal plate—aqueduct—cerebellar vermis—floor of fourth ventricle—spinal cord and cauda equina

Oligodendrogliomas: Frontolateral—frontomedial/parasagittal— corpus callosum—temporal/temporo-occipital—parietal—thalamus—[cerebellum]

Astrocytomas: Frontodorsal—frontomedial—frontolateral—parietolateral (parietomedial)—diffuse—temporal—thalamus— midbrain—pons

Glioblastomas: Frontodorsal—frontolateral—frontobasal—parietodorsal — parietolateral — [occipitodorsal — occipitolateral —occipitobasal] — temporolateral — temporomedial — anterior/posterior corpus callosum—anterior/posterior radiation of the corpus callosum—fornix—[thalamus—quadrigeminal plate—pons]

Paragliomas:

Ependymomas: Cerebral hemispheres—lateral ventricle—third ventricle—fourth ventricle—spinal cord and cauda equina— ependymal cyst of the foramen of Monro

Plexus papillomas: Lateral ventricles—third ventricle—cerebello-pontine angle—fourth ventricle

Pinealomas: Quadrigeminal plate

Neurinomas: Acoustic—[trigeminal]—spinal nerve roots (usually dorsal)

Gangliocytomas: Hemispheral, temporobasal—infundibulum—brain-stem—medulla—cerebellum—sympathetics—[spinal cord]

Meningiomas: Sagittal sinus ("parasagittal meningiomas")—sphenoid ridge and the Sylvian fossa—olfactory groove (meningiomas of the cribriform plate)—tuberculum sellae (suprasellar or of the anterior chiasm)—tentorium (or peritorcular meningiomas, supra- or infratentorial)—middle fossa and Meckel's cave—falx—cerebello-pontine angle—ventricles—clivus (and cranio-spinal meningiomas)—spinal canal

---

[3] The sequence in which the tumors are listed does not indicate their relative incidence; the less commonly occurring types are in brackets.

Angioblastomas: Cerebellar hemispheres—at the exit of the fourth ventricle ("calamus scriptorius")—spinal cord

Sarcomas: With diffuse meningeal spread—large circumscribed sarcomas without any preferential site

Chondromas: Falx—lateral ventricle—middle fossa

Lipomas: Corpus callosum—infundibulum—quadrigeminal plate—choroid plexus—spinal cord

Osteomas: Only a few cases reported, with sites in paranasal sinuses and frontal bone

Chordomas: Clivus—odontoid—sacrococcygeal region—[nasopharyngeal region with intracranial extension]

Craniopharyngiomas: Intrasellar—surprasellar

Pituitary adenomas: Intrasellar, with extension into the third ventricle

Epidermoids: Cerebello-pontine angle (parapontine)—chiasmal region (parapituitary)—region of the quadrigeminal plate (posterior corpus callosum)—Sylvian fissure—lateral ventricle—third and fourth ventricles—longitudinal fissure (anterior corpus callosum)—diploe

Dermoids: Parapituitary—parapontine—orbito-frontal sulci

Teratoids and teratomas: Pineal region—parapituitary—lateral ventricle—spinal

THE RELATIVE FREQUENCY OF TUMOR TYPES IN DIFFERENT LOCATIONS

If we reverse the basis for matching and proceed from each of the various tumor sites, we obtain the following list of tumors typical for a given location. Tumors located in the frontal lobes are illustrated in Fig. 18, for the base of the skull in Fig. 19.

Unfortunately, it was impossible to provide data on all the above-mentioned subtypes (frontodorsal, frontobasal, frontolateral astrocytoma, etc.), but figures happen to be available for a series of 127 frontal lobe tumors[4], subdivided as above.

Frontodorsal

Meningiomas (of the anterior third of the sagittal sinus)	11
Astrocytomas	9
Glioblastomas	6

Frontolateral

Meningiomas (of the 3rd frontal convolution)	2
Astrocytomas	13
Glioblastomas	4
Oligodendrogliomas	21

[4] *See* the doctorate theses of Engels, Esslen and Wolff, Hamburg, 1950–1951.

Frontobasal
    Meningiomas (olfactory groove)   3
    Glioblastomas   4
Frontomedial
    Meningiomas (of the falx)   1
    Astrocytomas   2
    Oligodendrogliomas   21

Total cases:		
	Meningiomas	17
	Oligodendrogliomas	42
	Astrocytomas	24
	Glioblastomas	14

The preceding text has dealt with the commonly-occurring tumor types, irrespective of their degree of frequency. In order to give some idea of the relative frequency with which specific types occur at each of the various locations, the corresponding data are listed in Table 2; they are based on an analysis of our collection of 3,000 cases[5].

Frontal lobes (Fig. 18)
    Frontodorsal: Astrocytomas—glioblastomas—meningiomas (parasagittal, uni- or bilateral)
    Frontolateral: Oligodendrogliomas—glioblastomas—meningiomas (of the convexity)—astrocytomas (with spread to the insula)
    Frontomedial: Oligodendrogliomas (parasagittal with extension into the corpus callosum)—astrocytomas (with spread to the septum)—meningiomas (of the falx, uni- or bilateral)
    Frontobasal: Glioblastomas—meningiomas (of the olfactory groove)
    Diffuse: Astrocytomas

Temporal lobes
    Temporolateral: Oligodendrogliomas—glioblastomas—meningiomas (Sylvian fissure)—astrocytomas
    Temporobasal: Gangliocytomas—meningiomas—chordomas
    Temporomedial: Glioblastomas—oligodendrogliomas

Parietal lobes
    Parietolateral: Astrocytomas—oligodendrogliomas—glioblastomas—ependymomas and spongioblastomas (in adolescence)—meningiomas (of the convexity)
    Parietodorsal: Glioblastomas—astrocytomas—meningiomas (parasagittal)
    Parietomedial: Astrocytomas

[5] *See* Krause and Zülch, Zbl. Neurochir. **11**, 222–230, 1951.

Occipital lobes
> Glioblastomas spreading from the corpus callosum or its radiation —meningiomas (posterior third of the sagittal sinus—tentorium/torcular)—[astrocytomas and oligodendrogliomas spreading from the temporal or parietal region]

Chiasmal region
> Spongioblastomas and craniopharyngiomas (adolescence)—pituitary adenomas—meningiomas—epidermoids—adhesive arachnoiditis—chordomas—aneurysms of the anterior communicating and carotid arteries (parasellar)—parasellar teratomas

TABLE 2. THE RELATIVE FREQUENCY (IN PER CENT) OF TUMOR TYPES FOUND AT THE VARIOUS LOCATIONS

	Frontal (629 cases)	Temporal (414 cases)	Parietal (345 cases)	Occipital (130 cases)	Region of the chiasm (352 cases)	Third ventricle (28 cases)	Lateral ventricle (41 cases)	Upper brainstem (87 cases)	Quadrigeminal plate (49 cases)	Aqueduct (24 cases)	Cerebellum and fourth ventricle (482 cases)	Pontocerebellar angle (282 cases)	Lower brainstem (27 cases)	Spinal cord (96 cases)
Medulloblastoma									10.1		24.8	0.4		1.2
Spongioblastoma	0.6	1.2	0.3	3.7	6.5	39.6	7.3	2.3	6.1	29.4	28.8		7.4	9.2
Oligodendroglioma	15.7	12.4	8.7	5.1		3.6		12.6	2.1		0.2		3.7	
Astrocytoma	17.4	11.8	12.2	6.6		10.8		10.4	6.1	4.2	0.2		22.2	3.2
Glioblastoma multiforme	19.4	28.8	21.8	25.6				52.9	2.1				22.2	2.2
Ependymoma	2.4	2.6	7.5	6.6		18.0	16.9		12.1		11.1	0.4	14.8	7.2
Plexus Papilloma		0.2				3.6	14.5				2.0			
Pinealoma									26.1					
Neurinoma		0.2										79.2		15.2
Gangliocytoma	0.3	1.0	0.9	1.5			4.9		2.1					2.2
Meningioma	30.6	26.2	31.3	27.0	9.9		9.7	1.1			5.3	6.7	3.7	22.2
Angioblastoma		0.3									11.6	0.4		4.2
Fibroma	0.5				0.4							0.4		
Sarcoma	1.3	1.4	1.7	1.5	0.4		2.5	2.3	2.1		0.6			6.2
Chondroma	0.2	0.5										0.7		
Lipoma														2.2
Osteoma	0.6	0.5	0.3	0.7										
Chordoma					1.2							0.4	3.7	
Craniopharyngioma					21.9									
Pituitary adenoma					52.2									
Epidermoid	0.2	1.9		1.5	0.7		9.7	2.3	4.1		0.6	4.6	7.4	2.2
Dermoid		0.2									0.6			
Teratoma		0.5			·				14.1		0.4			
Angioma & aneurysm	0.9	1.4	2.9	8.8	1.2			2.3			0.6	0.4	3.7	
Unclassif. tumors	3.2	4.8	6.4	2.9	4.0	10.8	14.5	4.6	6.1		2.7	2.5	7.4	11.2
Metastases	5.4	2.9	5.2	6.6	0.4			5.7			2.5	1.4	3.7	4.2
Parasites											0.2			
Granuloma	0.5	0.2	0.3	0.7				7.3	3.5		1.9			2.2
Adhesive arachnoiditis	0.3	0.5	0.3		0.7				6.1		5.3	0.7		1.2
Ependymitis										46.2				
Misc.	0.3	0.2		0.7	0.4		12.1			21.0	1.7			
Colloidal cyst						14.4								
Neurofibroma														1.2
Cyst														1.2
"Glioma"														1.2

Third ventricle
> Ependymal cysts (foramen of Monro)—ependymomas—spongio-blastomas (of the hypothalamus)—plexus papillomas—[epidermoids]—meningiomas of the velum interpositum

Lateral ventricles[6]
> Ependymomas—meningiomas—plexus papillomas—epidermoids—[chondromas—teratomas—lipomas—the ventricular tumors of tuberous sclerosis]

Corpus callosum and septum pellucidum
> Anterior: Glioblastomas—oligodendrogliomas—astrocytomas (diffuse—[lipomas]
> Posterior: Glioblastomas—oligodendrogliomas—[lipomas]
> Tumors of the septum pellucidum

Spongioblastomas (which have generally grown in from the surroundings) — astrocytomas — oligodendrogliomas — glioblastomas —cysts of the septum pellucidum

Rostral brain stem and basal ganglia
> Glioblastomas—oligodendrogliomas (adolescence)—astrocytomas (often bilateral, growing across the massa intermedia)

Region of the quadrigeminal plate
> Pinealomas — medulloblastomas/pineoblastomas — spongio-blastomas—[glioblastomas]—ependymomas (aqueduct and posterior third ventricle)—ependymal cysts—arachnoidal cysts—teratomas—meningiomas—[capillary angioma]

Aqueduct
> Spongioblastomas (adolescence)—ependymitis—malformations—[ependymomas]

Cerebellar vermis
> Medulloblastomas—spongioblastomas (so-called astrocytomas)—[epidermoids — dermoids — teratomas] — meningiomas (torcular)

Cerebellar hemispheres
> Medulloblastomas—spongioblastomas (so-called astrocytomas)—angioblastomas—meningiomas (tentorial)

---

[6] We divide them as follows: Primary, true tumors of the lateral ventricle are those which develop from the ventricular lining (the ependyma and subependymal glia), from the epithelium of the choroid plexus along with arachnoidal supporting tissue, or from misplaced tissue—epithelium, adipose tissue, or embryonic rests. They leave the ventricular wall intact except for their place of attachment.

Secondary tumors are infiltrating tumors of the brain substance which bulge into the ventricular lumen.

Fourth ventricle
> Ependymomas — plexus papillomas — spongioblastomas — angio-blastomas (calamus scriptorius)—adhesive arachnoiditis

Cerebello-pontine angle
> Neurinomas—meningiomas—epidermoids—[plexus papillomas—ependymomas—ependymal cysts—adhesive arachnoiditis]

Caudal brain stem (pons and medulla)
> Astrocytomas — spongioblastomas — glioblastomas — ganglio-cytomas—chordomas—meningiomas (clivus/craniospinal)

Spinal tumors
> Intradural: Ependymomas—spongioblastomas—astrocytomas—oligodendrogliomas — meningiomas — neurinomas — angio-blastomas—epidermoids—lipomas—[teratomas]
>
> Extradural: Sarcomas—cavernous angiomas of the vertebral bodies and epidural space, especially in the thoracic region—metastases—[tumors of thyroid origin—dumbbell neurinomas]—gangliocytomas of the sympathetics

Tumors of the optic foramen
> Spongioblastomas—meningiomas

Tumors of the retina
> Medulloblastomas (retinoblastomas)—melanoblastomas

Tumors of peripheral nerves
> Neurinomas and neurofibromatosis (von Recklinghausen's disease)—plexiform neuromas—sarcomas—(neuroepitheliomas?)

Tumors of the sympathetic trunk
> Medulloblastomas (sympathoblastomas)—gangliocytomas—para-gangliomas

Leptomeninges
> Sarcomas, diffuse and circumscribed—melanomatosis—carcinoma-tosis (secondary)

Diffusely growing tumors
> Spongioblastosis — oligodendroblastosis — sarcomatosis of the vessels

Tumors without preferential location
> Metastases—primary circumscribed sarcomas of the brain—granulomas

Calvarium
> Osteomas—osteosarcomas—cavernous hemangiomas—Paget's disease—Schüller-Christian's disease—eosinophilic granulomas—tuberculosis and syphilis—epidermoids.

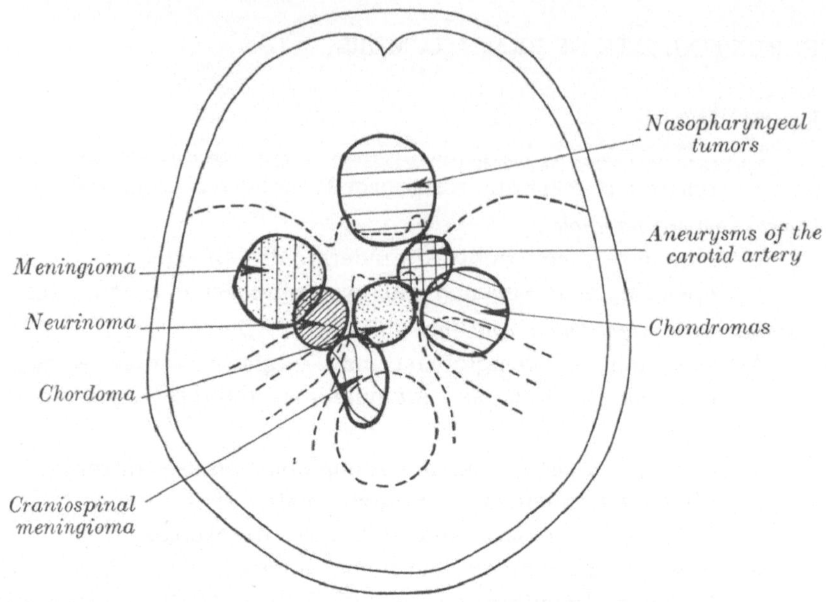

Fig. 19. Schematic representation of the site of rare tumors of the base of the skull. (The typical meningiomas and other common tumors of the base of the skull are represented in Figs. 63, 76, 77, 79, 81).

Base of the skull (Fig. 19)

> Medial group: Chordomas—nasopharyngeal tumors (fibromas of the nasopharynx, "cylindromas," squamous cell carcinomas, lymphosarcomas, reticulum cell sarcomas)
>
> Paramedial group: Chondromas/osteochondromas of the petrous tip—neurinomas of the Gasserian ganglion—aneurysms of the carotid (infra- and suprasellar)—meningiomas of Meckel's cave—craniospinal meningiomas and meningiomas of the clivus—parasellar teratomas—"cylindromas"

DIFFUSE AND MULTIPLE BRAIN TUMORS

The name "diffuse glioma" has been applied to various different pathological processes. In a broad sense, it includes gliomas, growing diffusely throughout one or both hemispheres like oligodendrogliomas (Landau, 1910) and astrocytomas (Scherer, 1940). In a narrower sense, it is presently understood to include diffuse neoplastic proliferation, such as has been described under the terms gliosis, glioblastosis, lemmoblastosis, and central diffuse Schwannosis. However, the whole group needs further study and clarification.

To improve both the understanding and classification of these conditions, I would like to propose the following grouping:

1. Diffuse gliomas, i.e., diffusely growing astrocytomas, oligodendrogliomas, etc.

2. Diffuse glioblastosis (spongioblastosis)—an independent entity.

3. Multicentric gliomas, i.e., tumors of a single type with multiple, independent growth centers.

4. Multiple brain tumors, i.e., multiple tumors of either similar or different type (multiple meningiomas, combinations of different brain tumors) without any histological connection.

Diffuse glioblastosis: In attempting to describe diffuse glioblastosis (spongioblastosis) certain rare cases—such as Foerster and Gagel's (1934), and von Sántha's—stand out. These cases (having occurred in adolescents with more or less definite signs of neurofibromatosis) showed a diffuse enlargement of the white matter and brain stem as a result of tissue infiltration by elongated cells which conformed to the local fiber architecture. The true nature of these cells cannot be clearly established. They do not form fibers, nor do they give any clear indication of their origin. They are probably maldeveloped, spongioblast-like cells which Gagel assumed to be Schwann cells because of certain characteristics of form and growth. In our own case (No. 3449) an 11-year-old boy showed a typical diffuse tumor spread with increased concentration of tumor cells in and around some fiber bundles. The characteristics of the cells were similar to those of Foerster and Gagel's case. (Schwartz and Klauer; Scheinker, 1936, 1943; v. Sántha; Evans and Scheinker; Kautzky, 1939; Einarson and Neel).

Such diffuse neoplasms might be explained as arising from cells "cut off" from normal development at some earlier period of embryonic determination. Other diffuse gliomas of the rostral brain stem, particularly of both thalami in older people, form a transition between diffuse glioblastosis and the diffusely growing astrocytomas and glioblastomas. The peculiar, apparently subependymal tumor spread in the case of Kino remains unexplained.

Multicentric gliomas: Certain gliomas can grow in the form of multiple nodules, connected by thin cellular bridges (Zülch, 1941). But there are instances where these cellular bridges are lacking (Köhlmeier, 1943).[7] In our own material we have seen four cases of glioblastoma occurring simultaneously in the second and third frontal convolutions and the occipital lobe (*see* Bertha, 1942, who placed his case at our disposal). In these cases the manner of growth has not been elucidated.

Case No. 496 may serve as an example: a 40-year-old man had one glioblastoma, the size of a tangerine, in the left second frontal convolution

---

[7] The distinction between multicentric and multiple tumors is not too sharp. Usually one speaks of "multicentric" gliomas even if there is no cellular interconnection, but calls several meningiomas in one case "multiple."

and another, the size of a chestnut, in the left occipital region lateral to the posterior horn. Cellular connections between the two were absent (*see* also Bertha, 1942).

We have no explanation for the growth of another peculiar, unclassified spongioblastoma-like tumor which was found growing in one temporal pole and in the superior cerebellar vermis without any cellular interconnections (case No. 874, a 37-year-old woman).

Some authors appear to have observed these cases quite frequently. Courville (1936) states that 10% of glioblastomas and 6% of astrocytomas are multiple. But many tumors that seem "multiple" can be explained by the growth of the tumor along winding fiber bundles. For instance, the glioblastoma of Hasenjäger (1938), which lay close to the lateral ventricle, could best be designated a glioblastoma of the fornix. Also, the possibility of metastases along some pathway as yet unknown to us—via the sub-arachnoid cerebrospinal fluid, for instance—has to be considered (*see* above).

Multiple brain tumors: We see the occurrence of multiple tumors of different types most frequently in the systematic hamartoblastomatoses (von Hippel-Lindau's disease, von Recklinghausen's disease). In the latter condition meningiomas, neurinomas, and spongioblastomas form a well-known triad, sometimes associated with ependymomas and angiomatous malformations as well (Foerster and Gagel, 1934). But other combinations also have been described: gliomas and connective tissue tumors (Myerson); meningiomas and astrocytomas (Hosoi, 1930, 1931); meningiomas and glioblastomas (Feiring and Davidoff); pituitary adenomas and oligodendrogliomas; meningiomas and oligodendrogliomas, etc. I have observed the combination of meningiomas with a monstrocellular sarcoma (case E 1662) and with a pituitary adenoma (case No. 6545).

In addition to cases of multiple meningiomas and neurinomas in von Recklinghausen's disease, I have seen the combination of malignant tumors of the brain (monstrocellular sarcoma) and ovary (carcinoma) in a 64-year-old woman. In this case the cerebral tumor, the size of a finger-tip, was found only by accident (Case E 539). The coincidence of benign and malignant tumors in a single individual is an old observation in pathology and has usually been explained by Cohnheim's theory. More recently, Guleke (1946) has pointed to the amazingly frequent occurence of multiple malignant tumors in the same patient. K. H. Bauer (1949), however, does not believe that there is an increase in the number of cases with multiple tumors.

TUMORS OF THE SPINAL CORD

It is thought that the tumor types that occur intracranially are also found in the spinal canal, but there are some that occur more frequently than others. Spongioblastomas, ependymomas, and angioblastomas among the intramedullary tumors, and meningiomas and neurinomas among the intradural extramedullary tumors, seem to dominate the picture. Furthermore, there are the tumors of the vertebral column.

The largest series (979 cases) is provided by Kernohan and Sayre (1952). Here 29.9% were neurinomas, 25.9% meningiomas, 22.5% gliomas of various types, 11.2% sarcomas (of the vertebrae?), 5.8% extramedullary hemangiomas, 3.6% chordomas and 1% dermoids. Tumors of the spinal cord showed a slight preference for the lumbar region with 25.5% occurring there; 48.5% lay in the thoracic region, 19% in the cervical region, and 6% in the sacral region. In our material, meningiomas and neurinomas were about equal in incidence.

Sex distribution of patients with brain tumors

Sex distribution and the discovery of a clear sex predilection of certain tumor types has proved to be particularly noteworthy (Zülch, 1949; Borck and Zülch, 1951; 1952). See Table 3 and Figs. 20-22.

TABLE 3.   SEX AND AGE INCIDENCE OF VARIOUS BRAIN TUMORS

	Total	Med. age in years	Male	Med. age in years	Female	Med. age in years
1. Medulloblastomas	124	15.2	89	15.0	35	15.6
2. Spongioblastomas	203	16.5	93	17.8	110	15.6
a. *Cerebellar astrocytomas*	*137*	*16.5*	*59*	*18.3*	*78*	*15.1*
3. Oligodendrogliomas	202	36.6	114	36.5	88	36.7
4. Astrocytomas	240	36.0	146	36.3	94	35.5
5. Glioblastoma multiforme	417	45.8	287	45.4	136	46.9
a. *temporal*	*127*		*81*		*46*	
b. *frontal*	*121*	*46.7*	*87*	*47.1*	*34*	*43.5*
c. *parietal*	*75*		*51*		*24*	
d. *occipital*	*35*		*24*		*11*	
e. *brainstem and others*	*59*		*38*		*21*	
6. Ependymomas	151	22.0	82	22.4	69	21.4
7. Plexus papillomas	79	26.4	10	21.1	9	32.2
8. Pinealomas	13	27.6	10	25.0	3	36.7
9. Neurinomas	229	41.5	77	38.3	152	44.1
Spinal neurinomas (for comparison)	40		18		22	
11. Meningiomas	532	43.7	247	44.1	285	43.2
a. *frontal*	*186*		*94*		*92*	
b. *parietal*	*108*		*62*		*46*	
c. *temporal*	*109*		*43*		*66*	
12. Angioblastomas	54	39.4	37	38.5	17	41.5
19. Craniopharyngiomas	78	26.1	53	24.1	25	30.4
20. Pituitary adenomas	183	36.7	98	34.6	85	39.1
22. Epidermoids	42	32.6	30	33.8	12	29.7
23. Dermoids	4		3		1	
24. Teratomas	11		7		4	
27. Metastases	118	47.1	65	48.7	53	45.1

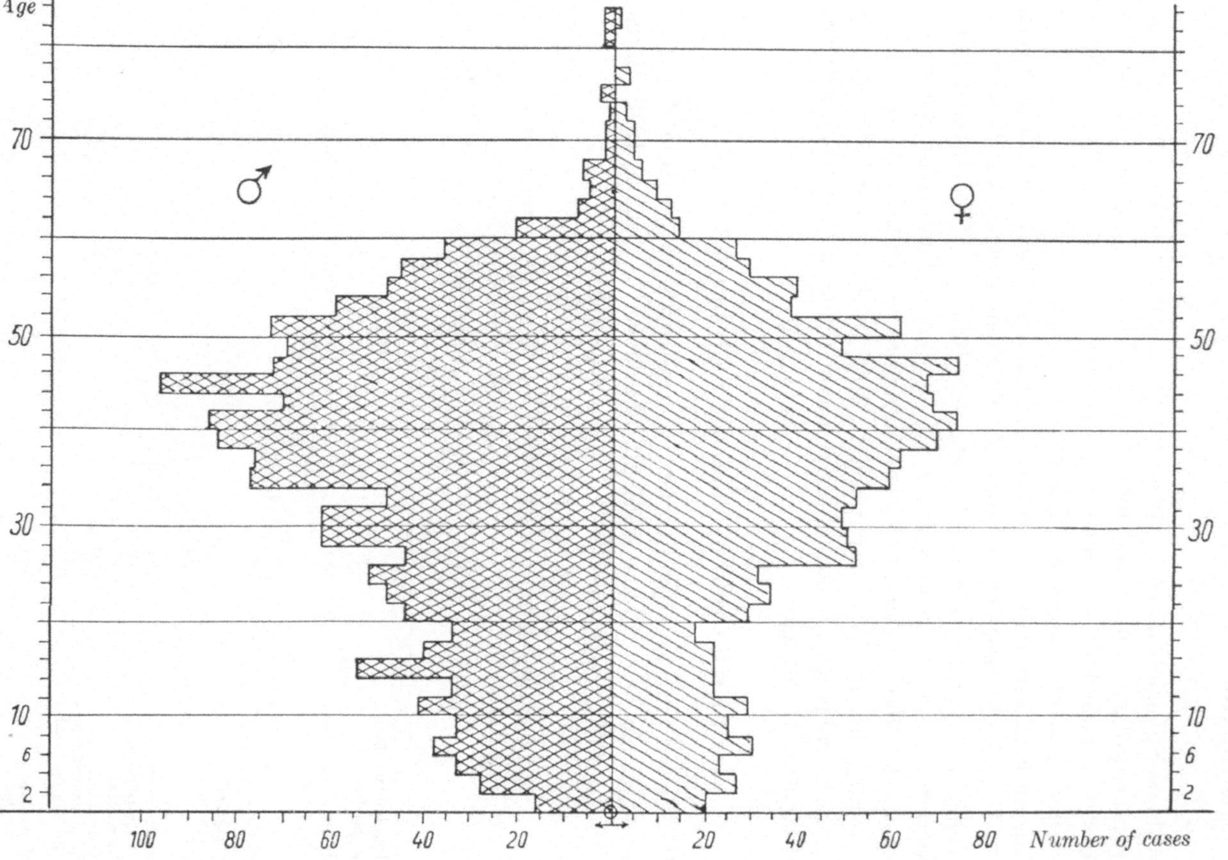

Fig. 20.   The distribution of brain tumors (total material included) according to sex and age (in 2-year groups). (Figs. 20–22 are taken from Zülch and Borck, Zbl. Neurochir. **12**, 93–97, 1952.)

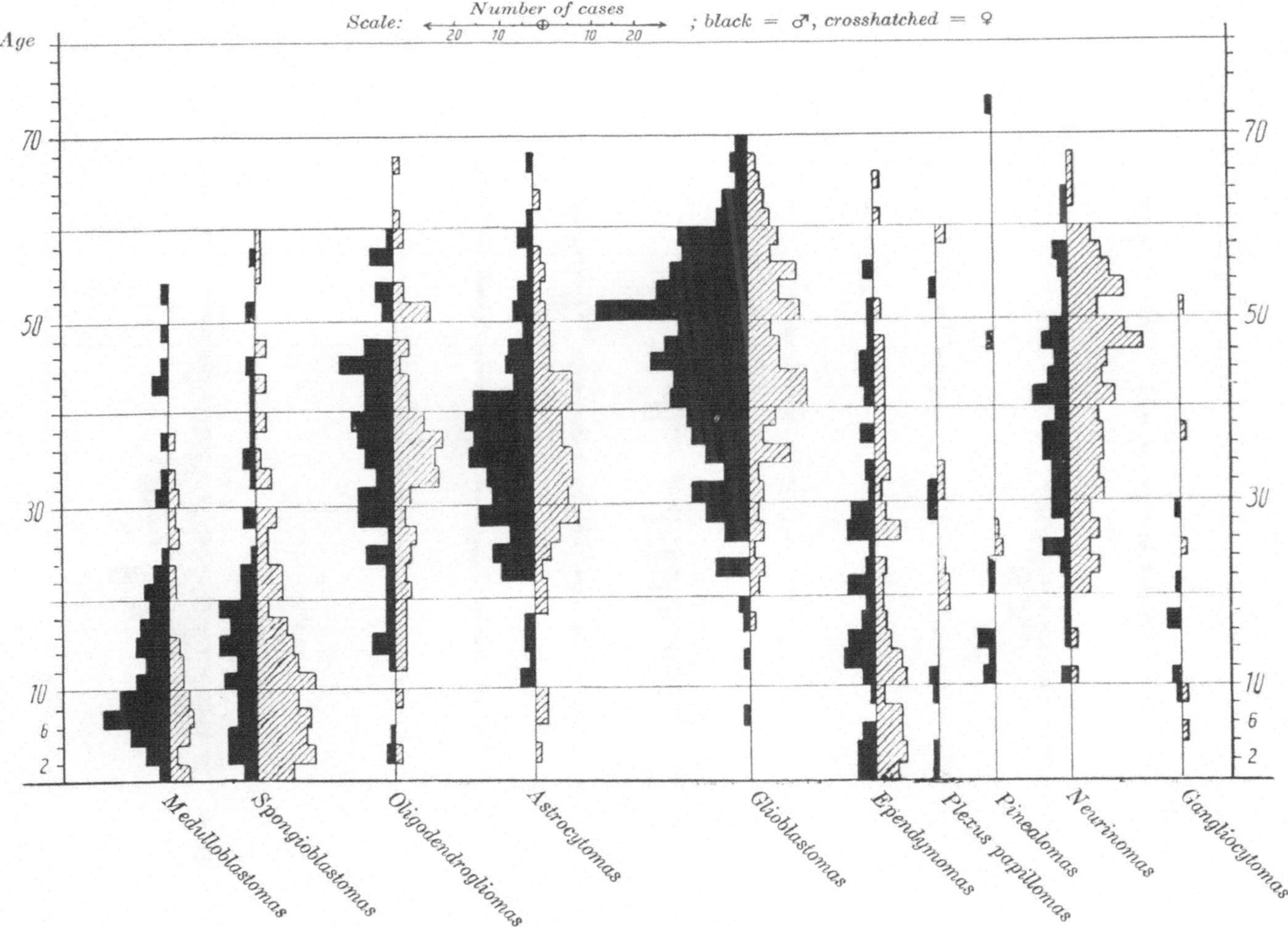

Fig. 21.
Distribution of different tumor types according to sex and age (in one-year groups).
(See Fig. 22.)

79

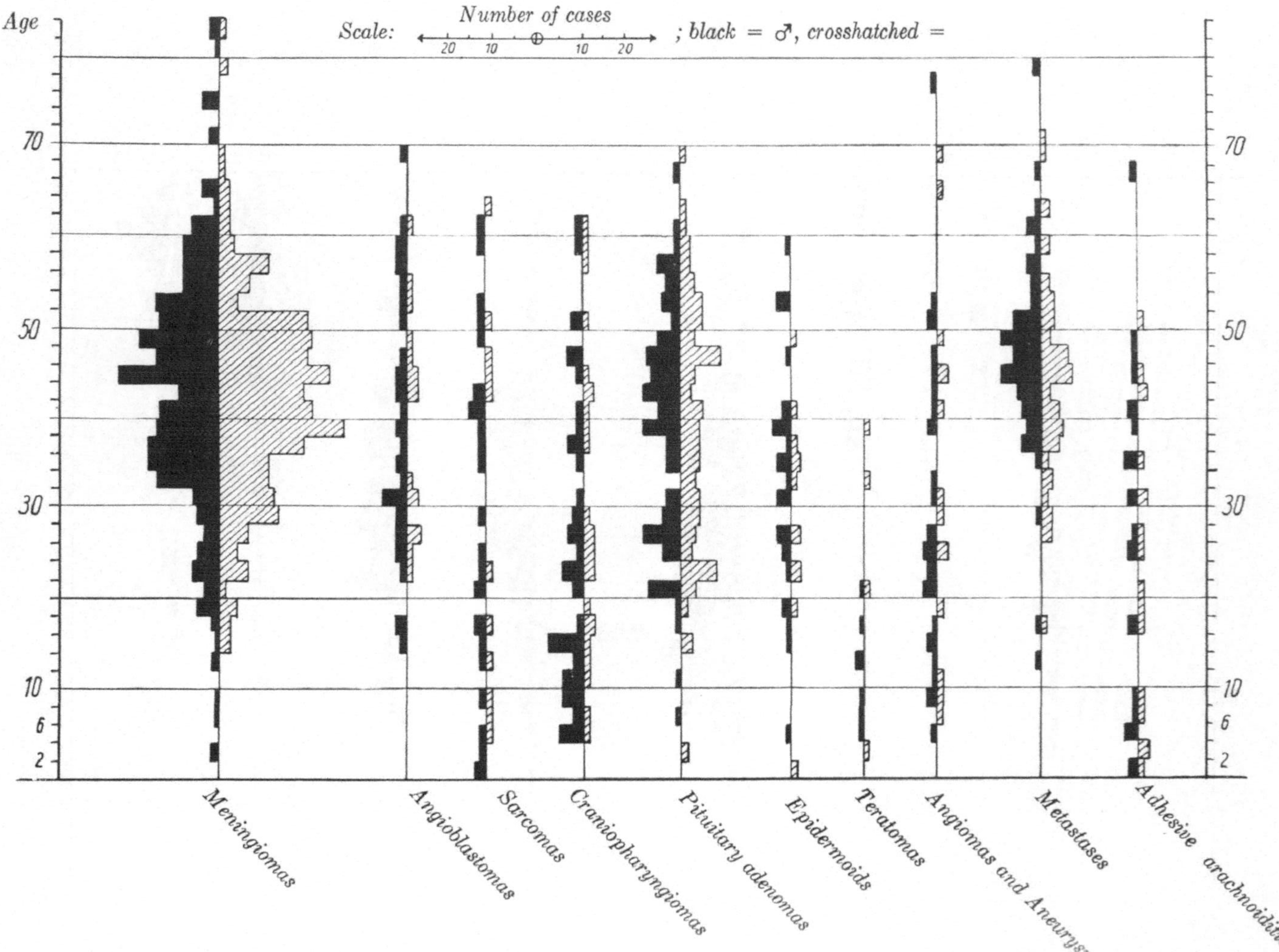

Fig. 22.
Distribution of different tumor types according to sex and age (in one-year groups).
(See Fig. 21.)

An analysis of our series has resulted in the general conclusion that there is a slight preponderance of males over females (55.62% to 44.38%, or approximately 11:9), which corresponds to results previously mentioned in the literature (Borck and Zülch, 1951). Moreover, certain brain tumors showed a particularly pronounced sex predilection. The preponderance of males was as follows:

Medulloblastomas	5:2	Angioblastomas	2:1
Oligodendrogliomas	9:7	Craniopharyngiomas	2:1
Astrocytomas	3:2	Epidermoids	5:2
Glioblastomas	2:1	Teratomas	7:4
Ependymomas	6:5	Angiomas and aneurysms	2:1
Pinealomas	3:1	Metastases	6:5

The preponderance of females was:

Spongioblastomas	11:9
Meningiomas	7:6
Neurinomas	2:1

It was of special interest that this general sex preponderance of patients with a given tumor was even more pronounced in a particular decade of life or at a particular site. Thus the male preponderance of craniopharyngiomas attained a ratio of 4:1 only within the first two decades of life. After the age of 40, females were four times more often affected by neurinomas as males (age 50) and even eight times more at the age of 55. In the meningiomas, females up to the age of 50 were more frequently affected (at a ratio of 3:2), whereas at the age of 60 matters became reversed and twice as many men were affected.

While females with meningiomas outnumbered males generally only 7:6, they were affected with chiasmal meningiomas twice as often as males and with cerebello-pontine angle meningiomas and spinal meningiomas four times as often (*see* also Lapresle, Netsky and Zimmerman).

Earlier statistics, e.g., those of Starr (1894), also revealed a preponderance of males in brain tumor patients at a ratio of 11:9; this preponderance, therefore, seems to be constant, and not as changing as it still is for bronchial carcinomas.

CHAPTER V

DESCRIPTION OF THE GROSS AND MICROSCOPIC APPEARANCE OF BRAIN TUMORS

Appearance to the naked eye

In the following presentation of the gross and histological structure of brain tumors, pure description takes precedence over interpretation. A need for a certain amount of caution in setting up hypotheses becomes apparent upon reading the older literature, since some of those contributions—for instance, the one concerning the problem of infiltrating vs. induced growth—are now useless. This is due largely to the fact that the findings themselves were left in the background and the arguments were overloaded with hypotheses. On the other hand, good descriptions of classical pathology still allow diagnoses of tumor types according to present classifications.

We must make every attempt not to confine ourselves to a study of the individual cell—an aspect that was, and still is, the guiding principle in many schools. Bailey in his later work on tumors has adopted the detailed study of the whole tissue, though it was he who had previously stressed the cell form so much. In Germany the tradition of the Nissl school—which has been responsible for the early and in this respect exemplary work of Olga Lotmar—prevented any such one-sided approach. Olga Lotmar presented tumors as case reports and then, one by one, dealt with nuclei, cells, architecture (syncytium), vessels, growth and fibers. The method that was customarily used in that school for the elucidation of a pathological process—emphasized particularly by Spielmeyer— was a study of serial sections with a variety of stains. Applied to the study of tumors, this technique resulted quite naturally in the consideration of the growth as an "organoid" whole. This explains why H. J. Scherer—a Spielmeyer follower—demanded a "complete" investigation.[1] Pathologists,

[1] Scherer unfortunately confined himself to a description of the connective tissue and the general architecture. He scarcely concerned himself with regressive processes and completely neglected such biological data as age incidence and site preference of tumors.

too, under the direction of Hueck and his pupils Essbach and Seifarth, pointed to the great necessity of an "organoid" concept of tumors.

A systematic tumor study alone can form the foundation for an accurate diagnosis. Such a study considers the age and sex of the patient, the site of the tumor, and its appearance to the naked eye—size, form, color, consistency, growth and relation to the brain and meninges. Histologically, we study cellularity, architecture, relation to the neighboring or infiltrated tissue, the appearance of the tumor cell, the rate of growth and viability of the cells, the intercellular substance, the stroma, and finally, regressive processes such as necrosis and necrobiosis (hyalinization, fatty degeneration, mucoid degeneration and cyst formation, calcification, and hemorrhages).

By comparing this information with the knowledge already accumulated we arrive at a diagnosis of the tumor type. Moreover, the most important points of *differential* diagnosis are already available since they are based on the morphological characteristics mentioned above. The prognosis is obtained from clinical knowledge of the behavior of this tumor type after radical operation (*See* Survival Periods, p. 122 ff.).

FORM, COLOR, AND CONSISTENCY

The form of a brain tumor depends very much on the manner of growth, described below. The shape of those tumors which grow by *expansion* is determined not only by their intrinsic growth properties, but also by the restrictions imposed on them by the surrounding tissue. Tumors of the ventricles, for instance, readily assume the latters' shape—those in the fourth ventricle take on the shape of a flattened pyramid, those in the third ventricle become round or pear-shaped, and in the lateral ventricles, elongated.

In the cerebello-pontine angle the *extracerebral* tumors are usually chestnut- or plum-shaped; in the spinal canal they assume the form of a kidney bean, or grow as long, finger-like tumors.

The meningiomas assume a hemispheral shape at the convexity and are round on the falx; if they grow into two intracranial fossae (tentorium) they are dumbbell-shaped; they are saddle-shaped along the sphenoid bone and occasionally spread out like a carpet. In addition to the main types of meningiomas with round, peaked, or flat growth, there are mixed forms in which a peaked projection of tumor emerges from a broad, flat base.

Little is known about the form of the *intracerebral* tumors. On cross sections oligodendrogliomas have a garland-like form since they spread along the gyri and expand them; the white matter at the center often undergoes cystic degeneration. The circumscribed astrocytomas assume by and large a spherical form and grow from the inside out. This tendency is particularly pronounced in the spongioblastomas which, although they infiltrate at the periphery, grow essentially by expansion. The intramedullary growths in the spinal cord usually assume the shape of a pencil and extend over many segments.

Color. The color of brain tumors depends on the main type of tissue present and on the amount of blood contained. The fibrous astrocytomas are white-yellow and glassy, both before and after fixation, during which they lose little but the slight coloration of their contained blood. The oligodendrogliomas, on the other hand, are rather pinkish, since they are relatively vascular and contain no fibers. Blood-vessel tumors, like angioblastomas, resemble a dark red cherry. Fatty degeneration of the tumor results in a yellow to ochre color (a patchy or striped pattern in neurinomas and glioblastomas). Hyalinization produces a grayish-translucency (neurinomas and meningiomas), mucoid degeneration a clear glassy appearance (chordomas). Old and fresh hemorrhages produce brown to dark or bright red colorations in glioblastomas. The cyst walls of spongioblastomas take on the dark brown color of hemosiderin.

Consistency. The consistency of brain tumors depends upon their content of cells, fibers, and blood vessels, as well as on the firmness of the invaded tissues. Cellular tumors poor in fibers—like medulloblastomas— are soft and granular like thick Cream of Wheat. On the other hand, relatively acellular tumors containing abundant fibers—like astrocytomas and spongioblastomas—are often as hard as cartilage.

These characteristics are quite apparent even on the cut surface: the astrocytomas, because of their sparcity of cells and abundance of fibers, have a smooth cut surface; oligodendrogliomas, which are cellular but have few fibers, have a "velvety" raw surface. Mucoid tumors, like some spongioblastomas, are correspondingly soft; tumors bearing many fibers— like the fibrous meningiomas—are elastic and firm. Depending on the amount of blood the vessels happen to contain, they feel springy or flabby. In certain meningiomas and craniopharyngiomas, and also in some regions of oligodendrogliomas, calcification can lead to hardening, even to the consistency of chalk.

Size and weight. The weight of tumors depends on their size. The largest tumor that was removed in our clinic was a true meningioma in an 11-year-old girl; it weighed 618 grams. In the literature a meningioma is reported which measured 18 x 14 x 9 cm, and weighed 1300 grams, including the bone (Kerschner[2]).

[2] Beitr. klin. Chir. **144,** 458, 1928.

Histological appearance

ARCHITECTURE AND CELL FORM

The historical development of the study of gliomas explains the serious confusion over problems of nomenclature. The neurosurgical-clinical group of investigators split off rather early from the anatomical-pathological group. The different works on tumors, therefore, contain varying terms and all-too-individual descriptions. Reviews of large series of tumors, as were possible in some American and European institutes, finally lead to considerable agreement in the oncological nomenclature.

The confusion of terms was at its worst in the description and naming of the tissue architecture. The evolution of a cell pattern must be clearly understood before giving it a name. By investigating the form and pattern of these architectural arrangements, the following classification can be employed (similar to that of H. J. Scherer):

Architectures of the first order. These are genuine tendencies toward pattern formation which are, so to speak, atavistic and so deeply rooted that they "break through" whenever growth is unhindered.[3]

We can distinguish a tendency for arrangement: in pseudorosettes, i.e., radiating around an imaginary center (Fig. 24c); in true rosettes, i.e., radiating around a minute true lumen (Fig. 24b)[4]; in ependymal tubules, i.e., the formation of epithelial tubules similar to the central canal with a large true lumen (Fig. 24a); in the form of palisades, phalanxes, files and rows, i.e., parallel cell arrangement in columns (Fig. 23c); onion-skin arrangement, i.e., in concentric cell layers around a center (Fig. 25c); in radial or crown-like patterns, i.e., radial arrangement around a blood vessel (Fig. 25a); in a satellite arrangement of the tumor cells around neurones, etc. Also some broad architectural features might be mentioned here—such as orientation in whorls or hooks (Fig. 23b) or in streams like a school of fish (Fig. 23a)[5].

[3] Because of limited space, the subject of origin of genuine architecture cannot be pursued. For further reference *see* the works of Lauche (1925); Krumbein; Gerlach (Wien. Klin. Wschr. **50**, 1535–1537, 1937); and others.

[4] We shall pass over the current debate on the occurrence of these "true rosettes" —apparently neuroepithelial-like structures—in retinoblastomas. We have presented the orthodox concept, although we consider it possible that these structures also develop secondarily. During mitosis or during regressive swelling of the cell, the swollen cell might be forced into the center of the pseudorosettes which are so common in these tumors. The so-called lumen would not be an empty space then, but merely the cytoplasm of a severely swollen cell whose nucleus, moreover, can be seen at the edge by focusing up and down.

[5] The architectural forms mentioned for particular types of tumors are, however, not always type-specific. It is a mistake to base classification on this one feature—like diagnosing a "neurinoma of the meninges" on the basis of palisading (*see* also Lauche, 1925; Krumbein).

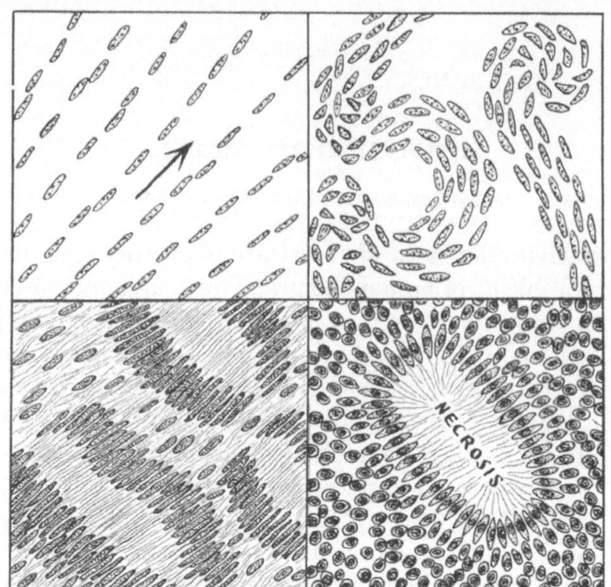

Fig. 23.   Arrangement of cells in patterns of: a) *top left:* streams like a school of fish; b) *top right:* whorls or loops; c) *bottom left:* palisades and rows; d) *bottom right:* pseudopalisades along the bands of necrosis. This last pattern does not depend on the intrinsic properties of cell growth but develops secondarily from regressive processes.

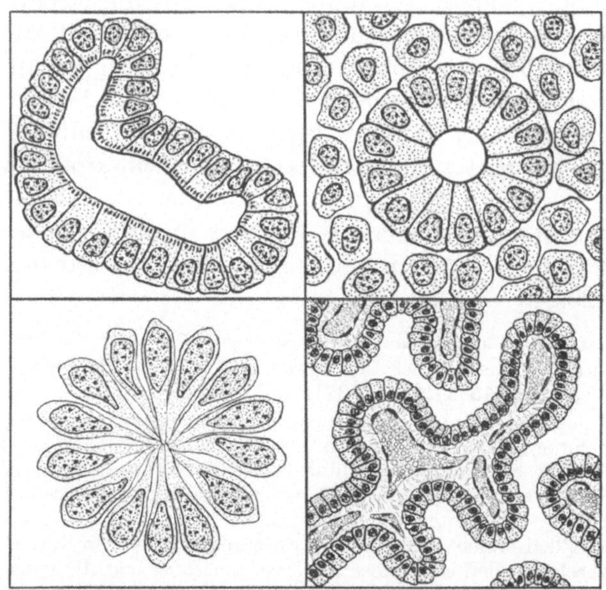

Fig. 24.   Arrangement of cells in: a) *top left:* ependymal tubules, i.e., large lumen similar to the central canal, lined by ependyma; b) *top right:* true rosettes, i.e., radial arrangement around the minute true lumen; c) *bottom left:* pseudorosettes, i.e., radial arrangement around an imaginary center; d) *bottom right:* papillae, i.e., fingerlike processes of stroma covered by epithelium.

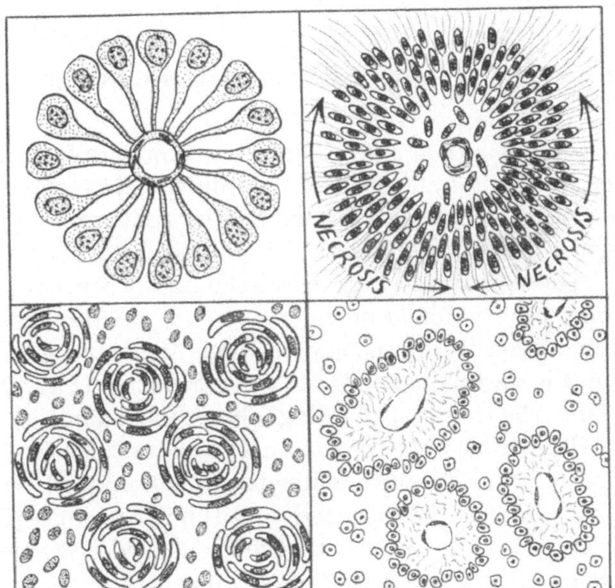

Fig. 25. Arrangement of cells in: a) *top left:* crownlike pattern, i.e., radially around a blood vessel to whose wall the cells are attached with their vascular feet; b) *top right:* perivascular cell cuffs, i.e., in a multicellular layer around the vessel, while the tissue further away from the vessel is destroyed by necrosis; c) *bottom left:* onionskin arrangements, i.e., concentric layers around an imaginary center; d) *bottom right:* pseudo-papillae, i.e., structures similar to papillae containing a vessel in the center and covered with one layer of cells. These structures develop "secondarily," i.e., through mucoid degeneration of the tissue between the vessels (See Fig. 33a).

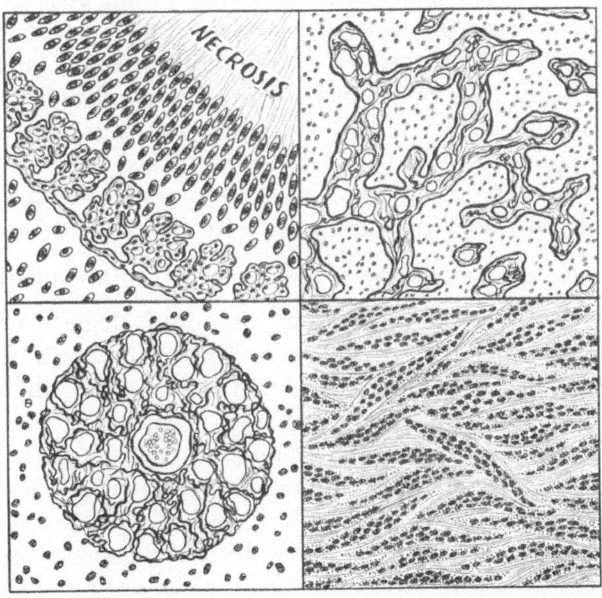

Fig. 26. Architecture of the stroma: a) *top left:* a barrier of blood vessels in the marginal zone of a necrotic area; b) *top right:* network of proliferating blood vessels in a glioblastoma; c) *bottom left:* perivascular proliferation around a large blood vessel in a glioblastoma; d) *bottom right:* feltwork of arachnoid infiltrated by the cells of a medulloblastoma. This stroma imposes a typical architectural pattern upon the tumor.

Architectures of the second order. These are secondary features and arise from the action upon the tumor of external influences, as for instance, from the orientating effect of the local tissue on the tumor cells (fibers of the corpus callosum or other commissures, U-fibers, meshwork of the arachnoid; *see* Fig. 26d). These features may arise secondarily from regressive processes. Examples may be found in the honey-comb picture resembling the oligodendroglioma seen in the spongioblastoma after mucoid degeneration (Fig. 33b), or in the neurinoma after fatty degeneration (Fig. 59c). Further examples include the pseudopalisading along the bands of necrosis in glioblastomas (Fig. 23d); the perivascular cell arrangement, after the same process, where the cells surrounding the nutrient vessels are preserved longest (Fig. 25d); or the pseudoependymal tubules in some plexus papillomas and hypophysial adenomas, where after mucoid degeneration of the supporting stroma only the covering epithelium persists.

Architectures of the third order. These formations arise during the course of reactive processes on the part of the body in response to regressive changes, as for instance in the case of endothelial proliferation of blood vessels at the border of large areas of necrosis (Fig. 26a).

This detailed discussion of architectural features was necessary because the use of such names as "rosettes" and "pseudorosettes" has resulted in great confusion. These terms have been employed interchangeably for the pseudorosettes of medulloblastomas, the ependymal tubules in ependymomas, the "true rosettes" in retinoblastomas, the perivascular arrangement of cells in glioblastomas, the pseudopapillae in spongioblastomas, and the radial pattern in ependymomas. Furthermore, it is necessary that true palisading in neurinomas be distinguished from other cell alignments, such as those along the border of a band of necrosis in glioblastomas. A clear grasp of this concept is a prerequisite for adequate understanding.

FORM AND STAINING PROPERTIES OF TUMOR CELLS

Universal staining, impregnation, or morphological characteristics peculiar to all tumor cells are not known. For a long time a disturbance in the nucleus-cytoplasm ratio was considered to be such a characteristic; the cell is supposed to lose in differentiation what it gains in intensity of growth. However, this applies only to certain malignant tumor cells which are completely dysplastic, like the elements of an anaplastic glioblastoma of the multiforme type, or the grotesque giant cells of the monstrocellular sarcoma. Other tumor cells are often markedly similar to the tissue of origin. Consequently, the differentiation between the tumor cells of the infiltrating neoplasm and those of the host tissue is sometimes difficult; it can become nearly impossible when it [comes to cells in the marginal zone of an astrocytoma, unless some local reactive astrocytes show up particularly well, due to their impregnation with the gold sublimate method. Certain tumor cells of astrocytomas and oligodendrogliomas cannot be differentiated from host tissue cells—a fact that is of great importance in the evaluation of tissue as well as needle biopsies. Tumor cells may be identical with the corresponding or analogous cells of the host tissue or with their developmental precursors (astrocytoma: astrocytes; craniopharyngioma: immature corium, etc.). Moreover, they can resemble regressive forms—for instance, the cells of the gigantocellular (gemistocytic) astrocytoma may be similar to normal astrocytes which have first actively proliferated and then undergone regressive ("ameboid") changes. Further difficulties are encountered in differentiating the perivascular accumulations of small "lymphoid" hyperchromatic cells—most likely tumor cells—in the marginal zones of pinealomas, oligodendrogliomas, and gangliocytomas from infiltrations of normal lymphocytes.

When a tumor engulfs the local host tissue as, for instance, the granule cell layer of the cerebellum, the host cells may be mistakenly described as "small, especially hyperchromatic tumor cells."

Furthermore, the numerous nuclear fragments of disintegrating medulloblastoma cells have often been mistaken for mitoses. Particularly striking was that error in a case of glioblastoma where the author, in addition to describing middle-sized spindle-shaped tumor cells, mentioned streams of "hyperchromatic small round cells" which were obviously fresh nuclear fragments along the border of necrosis.

The external cell form can be type-specific, like the star-shape of astrocytes, when stained by the gold sublimate method. This method may be looked upon as specific for astrocytes and other fiber-forming glia cells (e.g., the subependymal glia). Other methods, especially metallic impregnation, are in no way specific for neoplastic cells in general. Under no circumstances can oligodendroglia or even embryonic cells (such as "neuroblasts") be identified solely on the basis of supposedly selective metallic impregnation methods. Only the tumor cells of ependymomas seem to furnish a clue about their origin from ependymal cells in that blepharoplasts can be demonstrated with the Heidenhain or aniline-orange G stain, or with Hortega's fourth varient. However, they can be recognized only with oil immersion and must be distinguished from coarse formalin precipitates. The Rosenthal fibers are a type-specific characteristic of the cells of the subependymal glia, though only after the onset of regressive changes. Rosenthal fibers are also found in spongioblastomas; therefore we associate this tumor with the subependymal glia as its tissue of origin.

Certain tumor cells give evidence of internal secretion, such as those in the adenomas. The same has been assumed for the ganglion cells of the infundibular region (Driggs and Spatz; Bargmann *et al.*).

THE PROBLEM OF ISOMORPHISM

Hortega (1932, 1949) used to distinguish a tumor group ("isomorphic glioblastomas") on the basis of similarity of constituent cells. However, there is a great deal of overlapping, since these criteria are met by certain glioblastomas, as well as medulloblastomas and ependymomas. Above all, isomorphism provides no basis for a prognosis and should therefore not be used as a criterion for classification.

On the other hand, the study of giant cells and multinucleated cells in tumors is of particular importance, as the cells can arise primarily and secondarily. The latter process occurs especially in tumors of the astrocytoma and spongioblastoma series which have undergone mucoid degeneration. The cell nuclei then stick together and become hyperchromatic, and sometimes assume a "carpet-like" appearance. We also find considerable cellular dysplasias in rather benign meningiomas (type IV, 2 of Cushing and Eisenhardt—a transition-form between the endotheliomatous and the angiomatous subtype). These features arise in all likelihood through regressive changes and should not be interpreted as signs of malignancy (*see* Kernohan and Sayre; Marcos).

THE NUCLEUS OF THE CELL

Despite claims to the contrary (Schmincke, personal communication), the nucleus cannot be considered proof of the origin of the cell; it changes depending on the cell's vitality. Neuron-like vesicular nuclei with a distinct membrane and large nucleolus-like chromatin clumps appear during the rapid growth of astrocytes and fibroblasts, as well as in certain large cells of oligodendrogliomas and in many cancers. They can even be produced artificially if the tumor tissue, fixed in formol-ammonium-bromide, is later stained with Nissl's method. They stand out better than usual with Bouin or Susa fixation and by staining with cresyl violet. Recent studies of the nucleus (Casperson, Hydén; Bargmann) have shown that the nucleolus and the nuclear membrane are closely interdependent in their metabolism. It is erroneous to conclude, simply from the appearance of the nucleus, that a cell originates from the ganglion cell series. The form of the nucleus is subject to many external influences. Take a tumor growing in white matter, for instance: not only can the cell assume an elongated form—i.e., the astrocyte becomes "piloid"—but the nucleus, too, may be drawn out to a cigar-like shape. This point is particularly well illustrated in pathology by the growth of certain forms of sarcoma (Heine, 1931), and by the appearance of leukocytes when they infiltrate the cornea. The nuclei of the tumor cells usually resemble those of the corresponding normal tissue. The glioblastoma is especially atypical, since the nuclear mass here can be particularly large in proportion to the cell body. On the other hand, the cell body in monstrocellular sarcomas is occasionally quite voluminous in relation to the nucleus. The latter tumor shows particularly numerous atypical nuclear forms, which are described in the special section. The presence of inclusion bodies has been recognized in the literature (Russell, 1932) and has been found in malignant glioblastomas with impressive frequency; we have seen them especially in the monstrocellular sarcoma. Whether the assumption of the author, that this feature is a sign of this tumor's origin from a virus infection, is correct, will have to be left undecided (*see* also Krynauw and Jackson).

The cell body and nucleus can be altered, as has been mentioned before, by external influences. I should like to call attention to the action of electrical currents during the cutting and coagulation of brain and tumor tissue. The architecture can be artificially changed into loops, whorls, and streams; cells can be coagulated and can assume a hyperchromatic appearance (Zülch, 1940). Even the drying-out process leads to similarly severe changes near the surface of the tumor where the tissues may become condensed and hyperchromatic.

The appearance of tumor cells can also be considerably changed by X-ray therapy; for further details *see* p. 105.

THE STROMA

The mutual influence of parenchyma and stroma in tumors has been frequently studied. In the past decade it has again become a matter of considerable importance, while interest in the purely cytological analysis of tumors has diminished. Our modern conceptions are based particularly on the work of Schaltenbrand and Bailey, who have been unjustifiably criticized as having been carried away by "histogenetic trifles" (H. J. Scherer, 1933, 1935).

The original working hypothesis on the interpretation of blood vessels was that the degree of maturity of the blood vessels of the stroma rather paralleled that of the tumor cells. The more embryonic the cell type and the more malignant the tumor, the greater the amount of connective tissue, and the more diffuse its distribution throughout the tumor. Bailey and Schaltenbrand thought that, in brain tumors particularly, the tendency to respect glial barriers and the restriction of the connective tissue to the blood vessel walls was to be looked upon as evidence of comparative benignity. In the same way, the tumor cells' crossing of the glial membrane, i.e., the mixing of ectodermal and mesodermal elements or the invasion of the leptomeninges, could be considered characteristic of malignancy. This rule of thumb, however, has frequently been broken. For in oligodendrogliomas and in gangliocytomas of the temporal lobe—which are extremely benign—circumscribed tumor nodules and islands occur in the meninges.

Indeed in the spongioblastoma of the cerebellum this invasion leads to the formation of a surgically important "capsule." The same process in medulloblastomas, however, leads to widespread metastases via the cerebrospinal fluid. Here a hasty conclusion based on morphology would contradict biological behavior.

The same applies to statements of Schaltenbrand and Bailey that concern the mixing of the stroma with the tumor tissue in the form of diffuse inter-penetration. In medulloblastomas, the diffuse permeation by reticulin fibers has been taken as evidence of disruption of the glia-connective tissue barrier and therefore a sign of malignancy. The connective tissue in medulloblastomas, however, is as much confined to the blood vessels as it is in most other neuroepithelial tumors. In those portions where there *is* diffuse mixing of tumor cells and reticulin fibers we are dealing with remnants of the leptomeninges of the cerebellar folia which have been included in the tumor and diffusely spread. This can easily be recognized in the architecture (Zülch, 1940). (*See* also Figs. 28d, 30a.)

Even the assertions about the connective tissue in glioblastomas are not biologically unequivocal. If the presence of glomerulus-like vascular formations (Penfield, 1932) was to be accepted as a generally valid sign of malignancy, examination of other gliomas and paragliomas would quickly disclose some contradictions, since these loops and glomerulus-like formations occur in nearly all neuroepithelial tumors as a reaction to cystic degeneration or necrosis (Zülch, 1939). I have seen them develop even around a cyst in neurinomas, and since necrosis occurs mainly in malignant brain tumors, and cysts in benign ones, these formations lose their absolute biological value. We will have to assume that only the number and rate of growth of such formations, which are otherwise so similar, offers any basis for biological evaluation. In glioblastomas we must take into consideration the overall behavior of the blood vessels, which then reveals findings which are quite type-specific for malignant tumors. These formations are again not restricted to glioblastomas but can be observed in certain other malignant tumors. We shall discuss these structures more fully in our systematic description of the stroma. They must somehow be dependent on the metabolism of the malignant tumors—something which can be easily observed in the vicinity of small metastases of glioblastomas and other tumors (Zülch, 1948).

The structure of the stroma in various tumors

New methods for demonstrating blood vessels (staining of the red blood cells in the vessels in thick sections—Bertha, 1940, 1955; Wilke, 1943; Hardman, 1940; Sahs and Alexander; Luzzato; Essbach) have given us a better overall picture of the distribution of blood vessels in tumors than could be obtained with the usual stains in thin sections (Deery, 1932, 1934; Elsberg and Hare; Moniz; Scherer, 1933, 1935). These methods have complemented our own investigations on specimens cleared according to the method of Spalteholz, which have furnished good general survey material. Errors are apt to arise only in the case of thrombosed vessels, as in glioblastomas, where the erythrocytes can no longer be stained.

In astrocytomas of the hemispheres, we usually find only a few inconspicuous vessels, predominantly capillaries, which can scarcely be distinguished from the normal capillaries of the brain. An increased density of vessels can be seen more in the center of the tumor. The gigantocellular subtype is inclined, in our experience, toward the formation of repeatedly coiled, reduplicated vessels within the adventitial covering. The astroblastoma is distinguished by a dense, uniform vascular bed within its "pseudo-papillary" architecture. Its vessel walls are widened by the marked production of reticulin fibers, whereas the mesodermal cells proliferate only slightly. Astroblastomas occasionally advance along their growth zone by peculiar, finger-like buds which consist of a coil of vessels surrounded by tumor cells ("gliovascular system").

The ependymoma too has a dense regular vasculature like the astroblastoma. The blood vessels tend to show intimal proliferation all the way to complete occlusion (resulting in cyst formation). In spongioblastomas, there are regions with numerous, frequently coiled, blood vessels. Some spongioblastomas have such a high degree of vascularization that they have been considered as angiomatous mixed tumors (Bergstrand, 1937; Weiss). This applies especially to the sub-fornical region (Weiss) and to the outlet of the fourth ventricle, where our case No. 160 showed the presence of a tangle of vessels resembling a cavernoma. Both regions have their own special vascular architecture (Wislocki and Putnam).

In oligodendrogliomas, the vascular architecture is not characteristic; there are densely packed capillary networks in the zone of growth and also larger vessels with proliferation of their walls, all of which tend to show hyalinization and calcification. In neurinomas we often see small accumulations of vessels resembling cavernomas, particularly in the marginal zone. In medulloblastomas, the capillaries are not very numerous and only exceptionally show proliferation of their walls. Most interesting is the structure of the vessels in glioblastomas, where growth has taken place precipitously and the vessels are abnormally formed.

An attempt at systematic classification and description of vascular patterns is best achieved by introducing the following eight types (*see* also Udvarhelyi, Walter and Schiefer):

1. Large lacunar vessels of venous or arterial structure (according to the part of the vascular limb being studied). These are partly pre-existing

and partly new-formed vessels ("vascular fistulae, lacunae"), which ultimately grow as thick as a knitting needle and surround the tumor like a mantle (Fig. 46).

2. Dense, somewhat disordered capillary networks, which differ from the normal capillaries by a definite increase in reticulin fibers and a dilatation of their lumen (Fig. 26b).

3. Long vascular barriers of proliferating capillaries which frequently show the formation of loops and tangles. They also occur in single small groups, usually close to the necrotic areas (Fig. 26a).

4. Organized vascular systems reminiscent of cavernomas.

5. Glomeruli, either single or in systems, with definite, recognizable efferent and afferent limbs, especially close to areas of necrosis. The glomeruli, according to Scherer, lie at the border between areas of reactive and neoplastic proliferation.

6. Proliferation of the adventitia of pre-existing blood vessels, resulting in the growth of sprays and clusters of newly formed vascular loops around the central vessel (Fig. 26c).

7. Large recently thrombosed vessels.

8. Vessels disintegrating after endothelial proliferation or possibly as a late stage of thrombosis. Frequently large swarms of fibroblasts spread out from these foci (*see* also Deery, 1932, 1934).

The changes under type 1 are of great interest in the understanding of glioblastomas and account for the arteriographic findings. We have followed the development of these patterns in small metastatic glioblastomas (Zülch, 1948). The stimulus of the tumor tissue brings about proliferation of the neighboring capillaries, widens their lumen, subjects them and the veins to arterial pressure, and opens up arteriovenous shunts. In short, a jacket of dilated, aneurysmal "fistuli" (Tönnis, 1938)—consisting of lacunar or sinusoidal, ectatic vessels—develops around the tumor. They are most probably type-specific for the glioblastoma and are responsible for most of the arteriographic findings described by Tönnis (1938); Lorenz (1940); Schiefer and Udvarhelyi. The connective tissue of the glioblastoma remains confined to the blood vessels, with the exception of the diffuse swarms of fibroblasts mentioned above and in patches of scarring around necrosis.[6]

In the neoplastic regions of the growth zone there develops a stimulus which acts upon the vascular bed of the host tissue. These vessels subsequently become the stroma of the tumor. In this way the capillaries proliferate and undergo vasodilatation, leading to the capillary pattern

---

[6] Lack of space prevents a discussion of the recent accurate studies of the vascular pattern of meningiomas (Essbach).

described under type 2. The formation of necrosis in the tumor induces reparative reaction of the connective tissue in the marginal zone. A wall of connective tissue is thus erected from the neighboring capillary systems, which acts to limit and wall-off the tumor. Larger blood vessels are induced to form capillary buds. Under the influence of necrosis the lumen becomes enlarged, and the patterns described under type 3 develop.

Once the vessel is included in the tumor, the stimulus of the tumor tissue induces a proliferation of the wall which can lead to complete obliteration of the lumen (pattern in type 6), with consequent necrosis. In the center of the larger vessels there arises a peculiar proliferation of capillaries which is either primary or can be interpreted as due to re-canalization of thrombi. Such thrombi can also be seen in their fresh state (pattern of type 8).

When considering the stroma of the glioblastoma, it must be remembered that certain patterns—such as those described under type 5—are also present in brain metastases and other malignant tumors, e.g., sarcomas of bone (dos Santos). Consequently these two can be differentiated arteriographically only on the basis of the external shape of the tumor, as revealed by the surrounding vascular jacket. Differentiation between glioblastomas and metastases is an easy task if the latter are multiple. In 1911 Goldmann had already demonstrated similar changes in experimentally implanted tumors and human cancers of other organs.

It has to be stressed once again that the vascular proliferation adjacent to necrosis is not exclusively type-specific for glioblastoma, but can also occur around the cysts and small areas of necrosis of other neuroepithelial tumors.

A summary of our views on tumor blood vessels can be expressed as follows: architecture, quantity and form of the connective tissues of the blood vessels can be largely explained by their function as stroma; otherwise they arise as a consequence of regressive changes. The typical blood vessel pattern for each individual tumor type is known and will be discussed later together with other histological findings. Type-specific patterns of blood vessels are most apt to occur in glioblastomas where they can be employed in the differential diagnosis from astrocytoma.

Blood vessels, though, form only one component of the "organoid" total picture of the tumor. I could find no proof for the existence of the coordinated neoplastic growth of connective tissue and glia, in the sense of a gliosarcoma, even in those cases where the connective tissue predominated quantitatively. We see no need either for the introduction of a specific group of "angioplastic" gliomas.

The question of gliosarcomas with a coordinated participation of connective tissue was raised again by Spatz, who was instrumental in Hasenjäger's[7] publication of results that supported his theory. The results, however, do not seem convincing to me. Spatz also discusses the possibility of transitional forms between meningiomas and glioblastomas. (The description of the monstrocellular sarcomas or the fibrosarcomas of the dura may already have solved that problem.)

Growth

The growth of brain tumors can be described as expanding, infiltrating, or destructive, according to the custom of pathologists. All non-neuroectodermal tumors—with the exception of angioblastomas, sarcomas, and metastases—grow in brain tissue by expansion. Neuroepithelial tumors behave in different ways. Neurinomas, plexus papillomas and ependymomas grow by expansion, although a few examples of the latter force themselves into the host tissue by forming papillae (Zülch, 1940) and thus occasionally enclose islands of parenchyma. Spongioblastomas and pinealomas grow by infiltration in their marginal zone, but the bulk of the growth takes place "from within out," i.e., by expansion. This internal increase in volume is not very pronounced in circumscribed fibrillary astrocytomas and astroblastomas. The oligodendrogliomas and medulloblastomas grow predominantly by infiltration, but have considerable cell proliferation in the center and so possess an expanding component. Growth is purely diffuse only in diffuse astrocytomas and "diffuse gliomas."

Examples of destructive growth are glioblastomas, sarcomas, and metastases. Neuroepithelial tumors rarely invade the mesodermal tissue in a destructive or infiltrating manner. One exception is the subarachnoid space, into which nearly all neuroepithelial tumors (excluding the "peripheral" neurinomas) penetrate; the other, the perivascular space of the larger vessels (which is probably also permeated by C.S.F.) which the cells of glioblastomas infiltrate and into which the cells of oligodendrogliomas and gangliocytomas frequently spread in "lymphoid" form.

Certain neuroepithelial tumors stick to the dura but never infiltrate it (*see* pp. 97, 142). Only the meningiomas invade it, and the monstrocellular sarcoma permeates it occasionally with nodules. The meningiomas can grow into muscle after penetration of the bone (temporal muscle, for instance; my own observation).

The statements above are based on findings dealing with growth in the marginal zone. The question of whether "intracerebral tumors" grow by *infiltration* or by *induction* has not been worked out thoroughly since Storch. For *infiltrating* growth speak the peculiar "gliovascular" formations in the marginal zone of astroblastomas which seem to extend, finger-like, into the tissue, and the infiltration of the subarachnoid spaces by oligo-,

<hr>

[7] Zschr. Neurol. **161**, 153–159, 1938.

medullo-, ganglio-, and glioblastomas and even by the quite benign spongioblastoma. For *induced* growth speak the findings in monstrocellular sarcomas, where at some distance from the tumor single, obviously neoplastic,
cells begin to split off from the blood vessels (Zülch, 1953). Our observation
of smooth muscle cells in a medulloblastoma, with the cells swarming out
from the blood vessels, should also be mentioned here (Zülch, 1940).

Tissue culture, unfortunately, has not yet yielded any information
about the particular forms of growth of neuroepithelial tumors in brain.
These forms of growth are type-specific only to a degree. Thus we often
see a subpial accumulation of tumor cells and further extension under the
leptomeninges in medulloblastomas and glioblastomas. Only in oligodendrogliomas, however, is this subpial accumulation pronounced enough—with
the formation of tiny nodules and a marked increase of glial fibers—that
it can be used by the surgeon as a macroscopic characteristic. The oligodendrogliomas are frequently very sharply delineated from the neighboring
brain tissue; they can infiltrate the leptomeninges, expand them with
mushroom-like or nodular growths (*see* the classical case of Merzbacher
and Uyeda) and adhere to the dura, so that they may be easily mistaken
for a meningioma. They can grow in a patchy manner, which again brings
up the question of multicentric origin. They share with many gangliocytomas the tendency to form round-cell "lymphoid," probably neoplastic,
infiltrations around blood vessels of the marginal zone. However, this is all
that can be listed as somewhat specific for this tumor, since the oligodendrogliomas share the following growth characteristics with all densely
cellular tumors, particularly glioblastomas. For instance, the oligodendrogliomas follow all the fiber tracts—the U-fibers and commissures—but all
these can also be spared to a striking degree. The oligodendrogliomas are
often tumors of white matter which, growing from the deeper structures,
can spare the cortex for a long time. Nonetheless, one of their characteristics may be the diffuse distention of the cortex with disintegration of the
subjacent white matter. The role of the fiber tracts in determining the
form of tumors has been described above (*see* p. 88 ff.). This applies
somewhat to such structures as the lattice-work of the arachnoid, or
Bergmann's glia in the cerebellum, whose formative action brings about
rhythmic patterns like the cell columns of medulloblastomas (*see* Fig. 26d).
Not only the myelin sheaths but blood vessels, too, can exercise a formative
influence. Blood vessels furnish the means for spread of the so-called periadventitial sarcomas, diffuse sarcomatosis of the blood vessels (Fig. 75a)
and, to a lesser degree, for medulloblastomas. To be sure, perivascular
accumulations of cells around the border of oligodendrogliomas are also seen.

The external "infarct-like" appearance of certain glioblastomas and
metastases, as well as the similarity of their spread to that of purulent

encephalitis following brain wounds, indicates that a similar vascular factor plays a role in the spread of all these processes.

Special attention should be given to a description of tumor growth when it reaches the leptomeninges. Astrocytomas, oligodendrogliomas, glioblastomas, pinealomas and spongioblastomas can grow into the leptomeninges. Certain of these tumors, like medulloblastomas and to a lesser degree pinealomas and oligodendrogliomas, can even metastasize diffusely via the C.S.F., as can ependymomas after operation. The biological significance of these facts will be discussed on p. 116. H. H. Meyer occupied himself with these characteristics of certain gliomas and contrasted them with those of meningiomas. His concept of a separate entity, the "glioma of the meninges," remains problematical. Whenever medulloblastomas invade the leptomeninges they expand them slightly but continue with their rapid, unrestricted propagation. Spongioblastomas, though, expand the leptemeninges considerably and there is a marked formation of glial fibers in the arachnoid; blood vessels in this area become quite hyalinized. An oligodendroglioma greatly expands the subarachnoid space—like a mushroom or a balloon. In this region, it frequently attaches itself to the dura. The architecture of these three tumor types, upon breaking into the subarachnoid space, is type-specific.

The development of tumor cells, however, is still unknown, especially since even the question of whether the cells spread by *infiltration* or whether they are *induced* or transformed by some agent (*see* p. 96) has not yet been answered. The presence of Rosenthal's fibers in spongioblastomas far from the subependymal glia, even in the meninges, points more toward infiltration. Also unanswered is the question whether infiltration takes place at an undifferentiated stage, with differentiation occurring subsequently. Such undifferentiated stages could be the "lymphoid" cells in gangliocytomas, oligodendrogliomas and pinealomas (*see* also Kalm and Magun). We actually find around the blood vessels of gangliocytomas—in addition to "lymphoid" cells—small elements resembling nerve cells that appear capable of further maturation (Tönnis and Zülch 1939, Fig. 18). The spindle-shaped cell in the monstrocellular sarcoma is probably a precursor of the monster cell. As far as the medulloblastomas are concerned, though, I am inclined to reject the differentiation of cells into two different directions—ganglion and glial cells—and prefer to consider them as included local parenchyma.

Results of tissue culture

The behavior of tumor cells in tissue culture furnishes important information on the question of whether the growth of neuroepithelial neoplasms is infiltrating or induced.

Particularly instructive were the films made by Russell and her co-workers (1933, 1934), which showed type-specificity not only of the cells in their final stages of development but also in the patterns of movement during their growth. Oligodendroglioma and glioblastoma are clearly distinguishable, and the same is true for neurinoma and meningioma. The results of tissue culture are in favor of the *infiltrating* form of growth. The tumor cells appear to have regressed developmentally during their migration, but show considerable type-specificity in their movements. Finally, having reached their destination they appear to develop into their differentiated end-stage. The behavior of the stroma cannot be evaluated so easily, since the connective tissue cells, because of their ready adaptability, multiply quickly and thus obscure the picture.

Tissue cultures have now been carried out for nearly all brain tumors (Russell, 1933, 1934; Cox and Cranage; Canti, Bland, and Russell; Buckley; Murray; Fischer, 1946; Benedek and Juba, 1943; Lumsden; Costero and Pomerat). Using this method, a clear-cut differentiation of cell characteristics between neurinomas and fibroblastic meningiomas has been possible. The findings have likewise indicated a certain kinship between astrocytoma and glioblastoma multiforme.

Cytology of the cerebrospinal fluid in brain tumors

After breaking into the subarachnoid space, the neuroepithelial tumors may spread diffusely—as is usually the case with medulloblastomas but rarely with oligodendrogliomas—or they may form circumscribed metastases, e.g., ependymomas, plexus papillomas, astrocytomas, and oligodendrogliomas (*see* also Cairns and Russell). Glioblastomas, too, can metastasize along the cerebrospinal fluid pathways (Hasenjäger, 1939) and the monstrocellular sarcoma may spread diffusely in this fashion. We have seen diffuse metastases through the whole subarachnoid space following operation for plexus papillomas, ependymomas, and oligodendrogliomas.

But when is it permissible to assume, on the basis of C.S.F. findings, that a tumor adjacent to the ventricular system is present? This can be expected in cases similar to certain of ours, for instance, a case of diffuse metastasizing oligodendroglioma (E 33, Zülch, 1940), a case of monstrocellular sarcoma spread diffusely over the ependyma (case No. 881, Zülch, 1940; pp. 256–57), in sarcomatosis, and, most commonly, in the diffusely metastasizing medulloblastomas and carcinomas. A diagnosis of cell-type is possible in such cases by using smeared or embedded material from the centrifugate of the C.S.F. A secondary aseptic meningitis with corresponding pleocytosis is the usual consequence of operations for epidermoids, whose fatty acids constitute a strong irritant (Krieg, 1936; Verbiest, 1939). It can develop spontaneously following rupture of epidermoids, dermoids and teratomas (Gaupp).

Regressive processes

Regressive changes can make tumor tissue unrecognizable. However, in both type and extent they are quite characteristic for each of the various subtypes of neuroepithelial tumors. Knowledge of these processes is therefore both necessary and helpful in evaluating biopsies from altered tissues. Regressive changes, such as calcification and cyst formation, may permit localization of a tumor by X-ray or ventriculography (in case of puncture). Finally, they can be used in differential diagnosis, since the degenerative forms are, to a certain extent, type-specific.

NECROSIS

Necrosis arises through sudden vascular occlusion; it occurs mainly in glioblastomas where endothelial proliferation and thromboses are particularly numerous. It may be widespread or confined to small areas which appear in the form of streaks on histological section (Fig. 23d). If the vessel lumina are not completely blocked, wreaths of cells persist around the blood vessels, where they receive nourishment for a longer time. In addition to glioblastomas, necrosis occurs particularly in the small cell carcinoma of the bronchus and in the malignant retinoblastoma (Table 2; Fig. 25b). Smaller areas of necroses occur also in oligodendrogliomas, and less commonly in the ependymoma and spongioblastoma, where cyst formation predominates as in all comparatively benign gliomas. This observation is useful in formulating the rule of thumb that tissue destruction progresses slowly (necrobiosis) in the more benign neuroepithelial tumors, while it occurs suddenly with the formation of necrosis in malignant tumors. Only in medulloblastomas is such necrosis rare. Here the cells are more apt to disintegrate individually (by karyorrhexis) and to be scattered diffusely throughout the whole tumor.

Inflammatory infiltrates. Leukocytes appear around the border of necrosis in glioblastomas and in the stroma of metastases. Round cell infiltrates occur in many tumors (*see* pp. 89, 98), but their origin and significance is uncertain. Single plasma cells can be found in all mesodermal tumors. Superimposed infection from without may cause the whole tumor to putrify and be densely infiltrated with leukocytes (E 1522).

NECROBIOSIS, MUCOID DEGENERATION, CALCIFICATION, HYALINIZATION, AND FATTY DEGENERATION

Mucoid degeneration and liquefaction leading to cystic degeneration are particularly characteristic for certain brain tumors. Of the neuroepithelial tumors, the astrocytoma disintegrates through focal mucoid degeneration leading to the formation of large cysts, whereas the subtype astroblastoma forms a system of small cysts among the numerous preserved blood vessels. The oligodendroglioma also forms small cysts filled with mucoid material. The most pronounced disintegration is encountered in the spongioblastoma of the cerebellar vermis (the so-called cerebellar astrocytoma), where often—as in the case of angioblastomas—only small mural nodules are remaining (Fig. 32). The ependymoma of the cerebral hemisphere usually possesses one giant cyst. Cystic degeneration is uncommon in malignant glioblastomas and neurinomas, but when seen in the latter is most pronounced in the spinal form.

Cysts are almost never encountered within pinealomas and plexus papillomas; in the latter, however, a large cyst may sometimes lie next to the tumor, having developed, possibly, by transudation (secretion?). Smaller cysts can occur in meningiomas while larger ones are occasionally encountered in monstrocellular sarcomas (Fig. 73) and in metastases (Fig. 83). The cysts usually arise through mucoid degeneration and liquefaction, which often changes the basic tumor structure in a peculiar way: it makes the spongioblastoma at the beginning of cystic disintegration look rather similar to the oligodendroglioma (Fig. 33b). In addition to this mucoid disintegration of the tumor tissue, transudation plays a large role in the maintenance of the cyst contents and in the refilling, after therapeutic puncture, of certain tumors, for instance the angioblastoma. It is amazing, though, how long large tumor cysts which have been emptied can continue to remain empty[8].

In craniopharyngiomas, mucoid degeneration leads to cyst formation, producing either small networks of cysts or giant solitary cysts with only a small mural tumor. Solitary cysts following liquefaction of the tissue frequently develop in chromophobe adenomas of the pituitary. Mucoid degeneration may be recognized particularly by its metachromatic properties in the cresyl violet stain. The presence of so-called mast-cells in connective tissue tumors has the same significance. We found this commonly in the vascular connective tissue of angioblastomas and less frequently in meningiomas.

This discussion so far has dealt only with the origin of cysts within the tumors themselves. In the brain, however, the macroscopic concept "cyst" includes also the following processes, arranged according to pathogenesis:

I. Intracerebral ("brain cysts")[9]

    a) parasitic cysts

[8] Bucy and Gustavson reported symptom-free periods of 12 years following puncture (Cushing's case No. 5) ,7 years (case No. 7), and 7½ years (case No. 17); all were cystic astrocytomas of the cerebellum. The most remarkable case is that of Bucy (1946) (case No. 30) in which therapeutic puncture of the cyst resulted in a symptom-free period of 15 years.

[9] *See* also Lemke; Drew and Grant.

    b) brain cysts following vascular occlusion (birth trauma, poren-
cephaly, embolism and thrombosis)

    c) post-traumatic

    d) within a tumor

II. Extracerebral (arachnoid cysts)

    e) as a result of neighboring inflammation

    f) following an old meningitis

    g) from a congenital malformation

The content of the cysts is quite variable. The cyst fluid of craniopharyngiomas resembles brown-black motor oil, in which small crystals of
cholesterin are dispersed. The contents of arachnoidal cysts which develop
from congenital malformations are milky (*see* p. 247).

Spinal-cord tumors often contain large pencil-shaped cavitations. In
the literature tumor growth and cyst growth have often been looked upon
as essentially parallel processes. In my opinion, however, cyst formation
is a regressive process within the tumor. Cysts in spinal ependymomas,
spongioblastomas, and angioblastomas therefore correspond to the large
cysts within the same tumors of the hemispheres and cerebellum.

Calcification. Calcification is often sufficiently advanced to be demonstrable on X-ray in oligodendrogliomas, less often in ependymomas of the
hemispheres, plexus papillomas, gangliocytomas, and spongioblastomas of
the cerebellum. Of the extracerebral tumors, most of the craniopharyngiomas are calcified, as are a portion of the teratomas and dermoids, and
certain meningiomas.

Histologically, calcification occurs in very different parts of the tissue.
In oligodendrogliomas, the tumor vessels themselves, or the capillary
system of the neighboring cortex, calcify (similar to Sturge-Weber's disease), or calcifications appear free in the tissue. A similar pattern of calcification can also occur in spongioblastomas, gangliocytomas, and ependymomas. In meningiomas, the best known form of calcification is the
psammoma body—the final stage of calcium incrustation of hyalinized,
onion-skin patterned cell balls (Figs. 25c, 66a); also encountered are
pencil-shaped calcifications or, more rarely, calcification of individual
capillaries. Calcium deposits are very frequent in craniopharyngiomas
where the "keratoid" parts are involved; lastly, they occur in teratoids
and dermoids. It practically never occurs in angioblastomas and neurinomas, and is a rarity in pituitary adenomas and glioblastomas. If calcification is seen in the latter, the possibility of malignant degeneration of an
oligodendroglioma must be considered. The circumstances under which
calcification occurs, and the role of pseudocalcium and calcium (Bochnik)
have not yet been studied. A diffuse dusting of the tissue with tiny calcium

specks—for instance, in the wall of capillaries—is often the precursor of massive calcification.

Hyalinization. Connective tissue tumors, such as meningiomas, undergo hyalin degeneration in large areas. In neuroepithelial tumors, such as spongioblastomas and oligodendrogliomas, blood vessels often show hyalin changes; the larger vessels in glioblastomas can also be hyalinized. A similar degeneration occurs in neurinomas where whole sections appear "hyalin-like" (even though neuroepithelial cells do not form hyalin in the strict sense of the word). X-ray irradiation also leads to "hyalin-like" changes in the vessel walls.

Fatty degeneration. Slow necrobiotic deterioration of the tumor tissue usually leads to diffuse fatty degeneration, of which neurinomas can be considered the best example. The characteristic yellow color in glioblastomas, and particularly the ochre-yellow streaks along the border of necroses, are signs of locally advancing degeneration by fatty change. Here, close to the necrosis, a zone of macrophages is formed—not infrequently in the form of rod cells—which rapidly accumulate fat and are often transformed into round, compound granular corpuscles. In this way the tumor cells still show the normal potentialities of some types of glia or their tissue of origin—they can proliferate and form compound granular corpuscles, etc. However, gradual fatty degeneration of larger portions of the tumor—with partial vascular occlusion—also occurs in glioblastomas. It is interesting that fatty degeneration almost never occurs in medulloblastomas with their meager vascular supply. Moreover, astrocytomas and oligodendrogliomas only show scattered individual compound granular corpuscles. The latter are uncommon in meningiomas where, if they do occur, they lie in the center of the islands in the endothelial type, and are diffusely scattered in the fibromatous type. They are seldom seen in craniopharyngiomas and are completely absent from pituitary adenomas. On the other hand, the interstitial cells of angioblastomas often show abundant fatty degeneration with the presence of birefringent lipids (fatty infiltration?). In neurinomas, fatty degeneration, together with "hyalin changes" and liquefaction, brings about the loose architecture of type B. Through the transformation of the tumor cells into round, fat-filled elements with centrally-placed pyknotic nuclei, there develops in paraffin-embedded tissue a histological picture startlingly similar to the honey-comb pattern of the oligodendrogliomas (Fig. 59c).

HEMORRHAGES

Massive hemorrhages (glioma apoplecticum) occur in oligodendrogliomas and glioblastomas—less often in pituitary adenomas—where hemorrhages of different ages are often found beside one another; they can result in the death of the patient. Massive hemorrhages can be explained by the pathological structure of the vessels: in oligodendrogliomas, through hyalinization and complete calcification; in glioblastomas, through their precipitous growth and hyalinization. The pressure differences following ventriculography or the consequences of arteriography may easily induce a fatal hemorrhage. In markedly calcified oligodendrogliomas caution should be used in the use of these diagnostic methods, particularly since they are superfluous because of the ease with which such calcified tumors can be demonstrated roentgenologically. Small hemorrhages are encountered in other tumors as well. Thus, the black-brown color of eosinophilic pituitary adenomas, for example, and the red-brown discoloration of the cyst wall in spongioblastomas point to frequent hemorrhages.

OTHER REGRESSIVE PROCESSES

The cells of the gigantocellular astrocytomas are similar to astrocytes which have first passed through a progressive and then a regressive phase (the nuclei are pyknotic and lie peripherally). They resemble some forms of amoeboid change. Since the gemistocytic astrocytes of this subtype lie in the central portion of the tumor, and normal cells grow in the marginal zone, it seems not impossible that the large cells arise from the smaller cell type through some particular kind of regressive process. In spongioblastomas we find the well-recognized degeneration forms of the Rosenthal fibers. These have been described repeatedly in the literature and have been used as support and foundation for certain theories about syringomyelia (Bielschowsky, 1920; Tannenberg). They have been interpreted in a number of different ways: as malformed myelin sheaths (Bielschowsky, 1920; Hallervorden, 1952), derivatives of axis cylinders (Tannenberg; Jung), derivatives of blood pigment, and heme bodies (Liber).[10] We agree with the view expressed by Verhoeff and Hortega (1944) that the Rosenthal fibers are the result of alterations in the glial cells themselves.[11] (See below).

Our own extensive but as yet unpublished studies with various staining methods showed that Rosenthal's fibers occur almost exclusively among the cells of the subependymal glia. We are apparently dealing with a special degeneration form of the fibrous part of these cells arising through swelling (*see* also Zülch, 1940). In our material, the formation of Rosenthal's fibers was confined to spongioblastomas and to the reaction of the subependymal glia in other types of tumors which lie near the ventricle—

[10] The changes described by McLean (1936) and Verhoeff as cytoid bodies, particularly in pathology of the eye, correspond only partly to Rosenthal fibers.

[11] *See* GRCEVIC, N., and P. O. YATES: Rosenthal fibres in tumours of the central nervous system. J. Pathol. and Bacteriol. **73**, 467–472, 1957; also DIEZEL, P. B., Dt. Z. Nervenheilkd. 1957, in press.

ependymomas, angioblastomas, etc. Moreover, they occur diffusely (Hallervorden, 1952) in von Recklinghausen's disease.

In cylindromatous epitheliomas, the center of the cell columns and streams undergoes liquefaction with the formation of the well-recognized "cylinder" (*see* p. 223). Since it would require too much space to mention all the minor alterations of tumor cells, only those artificial changes will be mentioned which occur through autolysis in the saline solution in the trap of the surgical aspirator. In epithelial tumors like the pituitary adenomas, these alterations can lead to cell swelling, with a high degree of dissociation of the tissue which can make it unrecognizable. Allowing the tissue to remain in physiological saline for any period of time should be avoided. Cell alterations due to electrical current and drying have been mentioned on p. 91.

Changes due to X-ray radiation

X-ray radiation, today, still represents a special form of tumor treatment. The sensitivity of various tumor types to X-ray has been studied in a large number of investigations. We know that fast-growing tumors, such as medulloblastomas and glioblastomas, can be arrested to a considerable degree, but that they always recur, which means that the tumor tissue is not destroyed. The other neuroepithelial tumors have only slight X-ray sensitivity—the most sensitive, probably, being the cellular and fast-growing oligodendrogliomas. Ependymomas and astrocytomas are also supposed to be X-ray sensitive. The pituitary adenomas are quite radiosensitive and X-ray radiation is for many authors the therapy of choice in cases devoid of chiasmal or pressure symptoms.

The changes in the tumor cells were particularly striking in a case of an intensively irradiated monstrocellular sarcoma, a tumor that tends to show various abnormalities anyway. Here, all the tumor cells were transformed into medium-sized and large, round elements with large nuclei, whereas the tissue originally was made up of spindle or monster cells (Zülch, 1940).

In oligodendrogliomas and astrocytomas we have seen the well-recognized, marked enlargement of vessels with widening of the wall (hyalin-like change) and narrowing of the lumen (for example E 537).

According to present opinions, X-rays act on the parenchyma primarily by destroying the blood vessels (Scholz, 1938; Kalbfleisch). In general, the number of fibers increases, the cell population decreases, and the connective tissues proliferate. The tumor cells finally alter their structure and often become dysplastic, multinucleated, and hyperchromatic, developing giant forms—in short, they lose the normal nucleus-cytoplasm ratio (*see* also Zeman, 1949, 1950). New work of Arnold, Bailey *et al.* has reopened this question. With the aid of the betatron, the authors were able to carry out more exact measurements at the site of action than had been previously possible. It was shown that in acute experiments with very large doses, a circumscribed area of brain necrosis could be produced in the path of the beam. Moreover, they observed that the delayed X-ray necrosis after six to nine months does not develop from vascular lesions but apparently arises from primary parenchymal injury in the form of a selective necrosis of the white matter. Several of our own observations on human material support this concept to some degree; what actually occurs probably lies somewhere between these two concepts. I have observed the following (*see* Zülch, 1956):

1. An oligodendroglioma of the temporal lobe with complete cystic degeneration of the regional white matter after intensive irradiation (this condition was erroneously described in the first German edition of this book as a "withering" of the tumor itself).

2. An olfactory groove meningioma in a young woman with a glassy-atrophic transformation of the white matter of the whole surrounding region.

However, since even small doses produced injury in animal experiments, I feel that the whole question of X-ray dosage requires re-investigation.

From reports in the literature (Fischer and Holfelder; Scholz and Hsü; Markiewicz; Kalbfleisch; Pennybacker and Russell; Eicke, 1952; Zeman, *et al.*) it has also been shown that the "late necrosis" can resemble a glioblastoma externally (*see* figures in Scholz and Hsü); this has also been supported by some of our own observations. Another important point is that these necroses are obviously not necessarily complete at the end of the first year, but often appear, for the first time, only after several years have elapsed and thus are partly a chronic, progressive process. This was the situation in the above mentioned case 2, where after five years certain regions still showed progressive necrosis. Finally, the case of Eicke shows that after particularly heavy radiation not only the white matter but also the cortex can undergo necrotic changes (similar to the findings of Arnold and Bailey), and be transformed into a collagenous scar. In conclusion, since in many cases such delayed necrosis occurred after customary X-ray doses of 6,000–8,000 r, brain tissue cannot be considered completely radiation-resistant. Some of the so-called therapeutic results of irradiation can be ascribed to the action of an actual "internal" decompression produced by degeneration of the white matter.

CHAPTER VI

TUMOR AND BRAIN

Reaction of the surrounding tissue

The reactions of the surrounding brain can be divided into two types: first, direct changes in the morphological and physico-chemical structure of the surrounding brain tissues, and second, displacement and changes in the form of the brain produced by purely mechanical factors (which themselves can lead to changes of the first type, as a result of constriction, herniation, circulatory inadequacy or stasis).

The immediately adjacent brain reacts differently to the tumor, depending on its type of growth. Infiltrating gliomas, like astrocytomas or oligodendrogliomas, may elicit no reaction at all, with the tumor tissue merging imperceptibly with the uninvolved brain. In oligodendrogliomas, zones of calcified capillaries occasionally overlie the tumor in the neighboring gyri (Zülch, 1941; Döring, 1939). Reactive astrocytes are occasionally seen here as well as in the border zone of gangliocytomas (Zülch and Tönnis, 1939); they also occur between the papillae of the growth zone of ependymomas (Zülch, 1940) or they surround metastatic carcinomas (Casper). The numerous vascular changes associated with glioblastomas have been described in the discussion of stroma. The findings in the surrounding tissue some distance away from the monstrocellular sarcoma are quite surprising: here, far within the normal brain, the neoplastic cells begin to detach themselves from the capillaries (Zülch, 1953).

Phagocytic activity is observed particularly around glioblastomas, where rod cells occur at the margin of the necrosis and microglia proliferate (Penfield, 1927). In malignant tumors especially, numerous vascular lesions have been observed at some distance from the tumor (small foci of demyelinization—Bodechtel and Döring). The astrocytes, too, are thought to proliferate at some distance from the tumor.

Changes in the fluid-content and the consistency of the tissue (*brain edema* and *swelling*) are particularly prominent in malignant tumors, such as glioblastomas, metastases, and monstrocellular sarcomas. As long as there are no hemorrhages, the *swelling* of the white matter in the immediate vicinity of the tumor, of the lobe, or even the whole hemisphere, is most prominent (Zülch, 1953). This increase in volume can cause great difficulty with the clinical localization of small metastases. Moreover, the *brain swelling* produces an increase in volume which, adding to the volume of the tumor, can lead to a marked shift of the intracranial structures and to symptoms of herniation (*see* below). On the other hand, we have observed *brain edema* only in the vicinity of hemorrhages into the tumor and in the case of brain abscesses. In both "open" and "closed" brain abscesses the increase in fluid can be so marked that the hemisphere is virtually "drowned" (Zülch, 1943). *Brain edema* is very prominent after operation and trauma. It is accompanied in part by a slight degree of primary *brain swelling*, and in part by brain swelling secondary to the edema.

Brain edema and brain swelling

Our knowledge about the morphology and pathogenesis of *brain swelling* and *edema* is as yet incomplete. However, it seems certain that these two conditions are different and that they can exist either separately, together, or one after the other.

Brain swelling alone is apparently more common in the white matter (Fig. 27); brain edema alone is more frequently observed in the cortex.

The best way to differentiate the two macroscopically is still by the pathologists' general rule of thumb: in brain edema, the fluid runs out of the cut surface and the blood in the vessels smears; in brain swelling, however, the cut surface is dry and sticky, and the cross sections of the vessels remain visible. Opinions about the consistency differ, but I would express the difference as follows: in brain edema the tissue is rather elastic; in the more advanced cases rubbery, with protein-rich edema fluid; and after longer duration, doughy and pulpy. In brain swelling I found the tissue firm and sticky; later, when more advanced, both doughy and sticky.

Even the histological differences between brain swelling and brain edema can—to a degree—be described today. In brain swelling we find a finely vesicular distention of the myelin sheaths, an enlargement of the oligodendroglia similar to acute swelling, and disintegration of astrocytes with clasmatodendrosis. On Masson trichrome staining, no fluid can be found in the interstitial tissues (Zülch, 1943, pp. 11–12). Recent work of our own has indicated that brain swelling, as Reichardt suspected, occurs particularly in acute catatonia, and that sudden death can be attributed to brain stem compression. The first changes seem to take place in the myelin sheaths. The interfascicular oligodendroglia often respond with mitotic proliferation. The predilection of these alterations for white matter is quite obvious.

On the other hand, in brain edema we see with Masson's stain an accumulation of fluid in the interstitial tissue, at first most markedly around

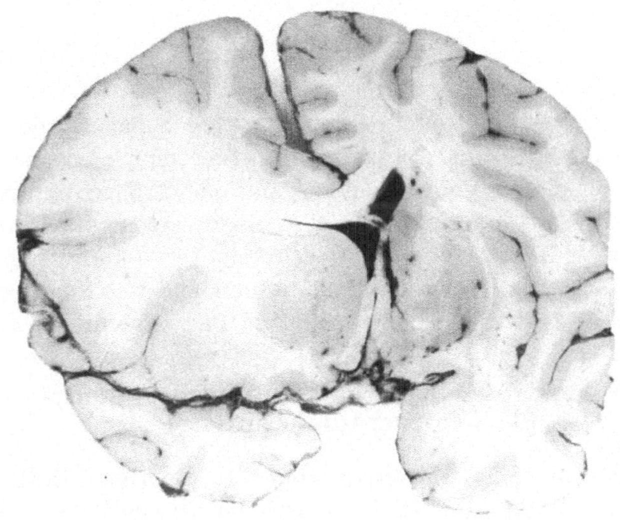

Fig. 27.   Marked swelling of the left frontoparietal white matter with high degree of displacement to the opposite side. A case of parietal glioblastoma.

the vessels, and furthermore a widening of the perivascular and pericellular spaces, particularly after any embedding which produces shrinkage (paraffin). Moreover, the parenchyma and stroma undergo secondary changes: the astrocytes undergo clasmatodendrosis, the oligodendroglia show mucoid swelling; in edema secondary to inflammation, the microglia begin to proliferate and the vessel walls swell and may disintegrate. In this way, the changes secondary to edema are similar to the end-stages of primary swelling, so that the manner of their development can be elucidated only by study of certain rather fine histological details (Zülch, 1943). Both processes lead to the same end result: marked abnormality of the parenchyma, occasionally advancing locally to a necrosis (Jacob's "oedema-necrosis").

Changes in the brain tissue surrounding extracerebral tumors are variable.

In tumors like meningiomas, which grow purely by expansion, the displacement of the surrounding tissues, as a consequence of the tumor's slow growth and small volume, is so slight that it is completely reversible. In the larger extracerebral tumors we nearly always find local circulation disturbances with demyelinization of the surrounding tissue, edema and necrosis. Similarly, pressure atrophy and softening of the adjacent pons can occur in acoustic nerve tumors. The brain often reacts to epidermoids with a pronounced surrounding encephalitis, caused apparently by the fatty acids and cholesterin (Mahoney; Verbiest, 1939). A marked degree of marginal gliosis occurs not infrequently in craniopharyngiomas; it forms a layer of several millimeters that can hardly be differentiated histologically from a true spongioblastoma.

However, very slowly progressing atrophic changes, too, can take place in the adjacent brain. An example is the cerebellar cortical atrophy described in a case of racemose angioma and one of Paget's disease of the skull, or rather in the marginal zone of spongioblastomas. The increase in volume of the white matter around different brain tumors in different locations has been studied with the planimeter and was found greatest in the parietal white matter, smallest in that of the temporal lobe (Häussler).

Mechanical distortions and displacements
of intracranial contents

The increase of volume resulting from the tumor growth leads to displacement of the neighboring brain. This is not the only space-consuming process, for brain edema and brain swelling associated with malignant tumors—especially small metastases—provide a much greater increase in volume than the actual bulk of the tumor itself. In addition there occur circulatory disturbances with hyperaemia, and alterations in the cerebrospinal fluid pathways which lead to obstruction and local hydrocephalus of individual ventricles (hydrocephalus of the ipsilateral inferior horn, or the ventricle of the opposite side).

All these processes take up space and cause the displacement of the brain. For a long time it was difficult to interpret such displacements, and for a while they were assumed to be "hernias" (Meyer, 1920). Later, however, Spatz (1937) correctly related them to the cisterns. To him they represented a local brain swelling of those parts of the brain that ordinarily lie in the cisterns or next to them. The studies of Tönnis (1938), and Riessner and Zülch revealed, however, that these "intracisternal brain swellings" were only part of a larger displacement of the brain tissue. They are, so to speak, the "indicator" of the direction of these processes, where the more advanced portions of the shifting brain suffer the more severe distortions as they are caught against the dural folds and thus become more apparent. For the cisterns are usually so located that they protect the brain from the sharp dural and bony edges by their fluid cushion, and therefore allow a certain mobility of the brain parts lying in or around them.

Thus, the falx is covered by the interhemispheric cistern, the tentorium by the cisterna ambiens and basalis, and the sphenoid ridge by the cistern of the lateral fissure—all protecting the brain from direct contact.

The filling of the cisterns with brain, following local rise in pressure, is therefore not due to local swelling but is part of a displacement of the brain, produced primarily mechanically; it serves to compensate for the increase in volume by the space-occupying lesion.

Since we are not dealing with local brain swelling, the expression "intra-cisternal brain swelling" (Spatz and Hasenjäger) is inappropriate. Also Ostertag's (1935, 1941) term "cisternal tamponade," although meaningful in itself, is unfortunate. We have adopted the most common expressions "herniation into the cisterns" or "internal brain hernia," which indicates correctly the displacement of brain into pre-existing spaces.

The direction of the displacement of the brain is determined by the partitioning of the intracranial cavity, by the attachment of the brain at its base, and by the stresses and strains set up within the brain due to the fiber tracts and blood vessels (Kautzky and Zülch). The falx is a considerable barrier to lateral displacements; however, it can itself be displaced by space-occupying lesions and its free edge pushed to one side. The parts lying under the falx in the frontal region are easily movable, since the cisterna interhemispherica[1] there (i.e., the space between the corpus callosum and the lower edge of the falx) is quite deep. It is shallow in the posterior third and therefore makes displacement difficult. Lateral movements can occur in the parietal region only when the corpus callosum and adjacent convolutions have first been pushed downwards (meningiomas). In the occipital region, on the contrary, the falx prevents nearly any lateral displacement. (However, the falx can bulge a little.) The base of the third ventricle is held in place by the pituitary stalk, so that lateral displacements are possible only between the inferior edge of the falx and the infundibulum.

The tentorium, too, forms quite a firm barrier to displacement. But it has been shown by ventriculography that even the tentorium may yield to local pressure by a tumor, i.e., tumors of the acoustic nerve. A moderate amount of sagittal displacement is possible along the long axis of brain stem from the medulla to the region of the quadrigeminal plate. This can be important, particularly in the symptomatology of brain stem compression (*axial* displacement of the brain stem). The displacement begins when the brain yields locally to the pressure of the growing tumor. As this happens, the adjacent portions of the ventricles are deformed and the reserve space of the neighboring cisterns and overlying sulci is used up and filled with brain tissue. The shift of the brain often goes beyond the midline of the cisterns and indents the corresponding portion of the opposite hemisphere. The local increase in pressure does not confine itself to the homolateral hemisphere but extends into the opposite hemisphere by displacement of tissue between the edge of the falx and the base; that way the reserve space available there can also be filled. Finally, the pressure is transferred from the structures above the tentorium to those beneath it

[1] We are using for the main cisterns the names introduced by Spatz (Spatz and Hasenjäger).

(axial displacement), leading to herniation of the cerebellar tonsils into the foramen magnum. In tumors of the posterior fossa, upward displacement through the incisura tentorii is possible. Thus, there exist well-recognized patterns of displacement due to space-occupying processes in various locations (Riessner and Zülch). This forms the basis for localization by ventriculography or arteriography. An accurate analysis of a ventriculogram or arteriogram can be carried out only by those who are thoroughly familiar with these rules of displacement (Kautzky and Zülch). The change in those regions of brain adjacent to the cisterns is only a small—though visually very impressive—part of the whole process but it shows the *direction* of the displacement particularly well.

The forms of internal herniation (Riessner and Zülch). A thorough knowledge of the individual types of herniation into the cisterns is important for the anatomists. Displacements in the *cisterna interhemispherica* occur mainly in the anterior portion; in the posterior portion they occur with any magnitude only following processes located dorsally which have first displaced the corpus callosum downward (Fig. 17, No. 52). The arteries of the median fissure (the pericallosal and calloso-marginal arteries), which lie one over the other, will be displaced separately since the former lies in moveable tissue close to the corpus callosum, while the latter may be held in place by the falx. If the increase in volume of the two hemispheres is equal—hydrocephalus of the lateral ventricles—lateral displacement is absent. The corpus callosum will be pressed up from below against the falx, whose lower edge causes a sharp pressure groove which can lead to virtual transection of the corpus callosum.

In the *cisterna ambiens* portions of the adjacent temporal lobe gyri will be pressed downwards through the incisura tentorii, displacing the midbrain to the opposite side—temporal or tentorial pressure cone. This can be demonstrated arteriographically by the position of the posterior cerebral artery[2]. Hemorrhagic infarcts in the medial part of the occipital pole may develop as a result (Moore and Stern). Conversely, the superior vermis can be pressed through the incisura into the supratentorial region from the posterior fossa (displacement from below upward). This somewhat pyramidal-shaped part of the cerebellum can squeeze the midbrain and the quadrigeminal region and bring about considerable morphological alterations[3]. The posterior part of the third ventricle will be displaced upwards and anteriorly (kinking or "horse-tail" form of the aqueduct).

[2] *See* K. J. Zülch, *Roentgendiagnostik beim Krampfanfall.* Verh. 57th Internists' Congress, Wiesbaden, 1950.

[3] Clinical symptoms from these centers occur in the form of attacks of decerebrate rigidity (acute syndrome of the quadrigeminal plate), which have been misinterpreted previously as "cerebellar fits." Moreover, the same symptomatology can arise through displacement from above downwards with tentorial pressure cone, e.g., through large tumors of the cerebral hemispheres (Riessner and Zülch).

Parts of the hippocampus and especially the uncus are pressed into the *basal cisterns*, forcing the peduncle toward the other side and compressing the third nerve. In the case of an extreme generalized increase of volume of one hemisphere, the brain can be pressed simultaneously into the cisterna interhemispherica, ambiens and basalis; the different parts join one another in a ringlike form: the so-called "circular herniation" into the cisterns.

The changes in the *cisterna chiasmatica* have so far received little attention but are probably important in the arteriographic alterations of the proximal portion of the anterior cerebral artery. The base of the gyrus rectus is pressed posteriorly and medially into the space around the anterior angle of the chiasm.

In the region of the *cisterna of the Sylvian fissure* (c. lateralis), the caudal portions of the orbital gyri are displaced into the middle fossa over the sharp edge of the sphenoid ridge, or, in reverse, the gyri of the temporal lobe slide into the anterior fossa.

The direction is indicated by the position of the middle cerebral artery or the vessels of the Sylvian group which are displaced at the same time. Arteriographic evaluation of this process is still lacking (Kautzky and Zülch).

The best-known of all the changes occurring around the cisterns is the cerebellar pressure cone—herniation into the *cisterna magna*. In young patients, because of the compliance of the bony canal, the wedge-shaped invasion by the tonsils can reach grotesque proportions (most of the Arnold-Chiari malformation?). Occasionally, with great pressure of the tonsillar cone on the medulla, there develops caudally a knobby enlargement of the medulla oblongata which pushes the tonsils downward before it as it descends (Riessner and Zülch).

We have subdivided the cerebellar pressure cone into three stages according to severity:

1. Definite mark of a pressure groove on the tonsils
2. Definite displacement of the tonsils
3. Displacement of an elongated tonsillar cone (Fig. 71)

Since the three principal arteries of the brain lie in the three large cisterns (anterior c. art.—cisterna interhemispherica; middle c. art.—cisterna lateralis; posterior c. art.—cisterna ambiens), a pronounced displacement of the brain into the cisterns (herniation) can cause infarct-like lesions at certain preferential sites, especially if additional factors such as edema and swelling impair the circulation (e.g., at the calcarine region from herniation into the cisterna ambiens). In the case of chronic, generalized increased pressure tiny herniations of the brain force themselves into small dehiscences of the dura (mostly at the base) or into the burr holes used for ventricular puncture.

Manifestations of brain herniation

Herniation of important portions of the brain into the two most prominent physiological bottlenecks—incisura tentorii and foramen magnum—gives rise to certain clinical signs (temporal pressure cone; tonsillar pressure cone). Constriction of the midbrain develops at the incisura, most often in space-occupying lesions of the temporal and temporo-parietal regions or the posterior fossa (with displacement from below upward). Constriction of the medulla oblongata at the foramen magnum develops preferentially following space-occupying lesions of the frontal lobes, the posterior fossa, or after generalized increased intracranial pressure (e.g., non-communicating hydrocephalus of the lateral and third ventricles). In instances of compression from herniation into the cisterna ambiens, the opposite border of the midbrain may be pressed against the tentorial edge and sustain an indentation with subsequent hemorrhagic softening (Kernohan's tentorial notch; ipsilateral pyramidal syndrome). In addition to these compressions of the midbrain from without, due to herniation of portions of the brain into the incisura, compressions may also occur from within in tumors of the quadrigeminal plate; in this case the tumor pushes against the surrounding midbrain "like a cork in the neck of a bottle."

Obstructive hydrocephalus. An obstruction in the cerebrospinal fluid pathways occurring anywhere from the choroid plexus to the arachnoidal granulations results in the development of an obstructive hydrocephalus (Dandy, 1921) of the ventricles lying behind the block. The constant pressure on the brain tissue produces atrophy which can be demonstrated by the perivascular deposition of fat. However, all cases of hydrocephalus are completely reversible at the beginning and partly so later on. This can be explained by the initial expansion of the ventricles and the "inflation" of the brain—an expansion that takes place at the cost of the subarachnoid space; the sulci disappear with the increase in intracranial pressure. If the increased pressure disappears, the enlargement of the ventricles vanishes and the subarachnoid space is re-established. If the hydrocephalus persists it is no longer reversible, and the brain is compressed into a thin mantle—most drastically exemplified by the paper-thin third ventricular floor.

In addition to these well-recognized processes, mention should be made of certain particular hydrodynamic mechanisms which have recently been discussed (Zülch, 1950). In occlusion of the aqueduct, the suprapineal recess can expand to the size of a chestnut; it pushes its way under the tentorium against the superior cerebellar vermis. The brain substance may perforate at various places, most frequently on the medial wall of the trigonum of the lateral ventricle, and the cerebrospinal fluid escape through the opening and form a subarachnoid cyst the size of a chestnut. This cyst may extend into the cisterna ambiens in the direction of the anterior lobe of the cerebellum. It does not succeed in re-establishing a connection between the ventricles and the subarachnoid space or result in a spontaneous cure; this has to be accomplished surgically (ventriculo-cisternostomy).

CHAPTER VII

PROGNOSIS

Metastasis of brain tumors

In spite of reports to the contrary, a true metastasis to other organs of most groups of "brain tumors" has not been established. Acceptable descriptions, particularly for neuroepithelial tumors, are lacking. In my opinion metastases seem to have been demonstrated only in a few pinealomas, and as a great rarity in medulloblastomas of the cerebellum. On the other hand, cases of "artificial" metastasis by contamination at the time of operation have been reported. Examples of these include the oligodendroglioma of the galea (Martin) and the glioblastoma of the subcutaneous tissue (Tarlov and Davidoff). However, the metastases only "vegetated" like a tissue culture and underwent no appreciable "autonomous" growth. The cases of apparently spontaneous metastasis of glioblastomas are still a matter of controversy (a frontoparietal glioblastoma with metastasis to the lungs and tracheobronchial lymph nodes, Mittelbach).

Mittelbach's case was the subject of some doubt when it was first presented at the German Pathological Congress in 1934 and despite a renewed defense in 1935 was not accepted. The detailed description which appeared later pointed more to the glioblastoma's being a small-cell bronchogenic carcinoma with cerebral metastases.

Only the two peripheral representatives of the medulloblastoma group. (retinoblastoma and sympathoblastoma) form frequent exceptions to the rule. They metastasize to bone, lymph nodes, and liver.

On the other hand, medulloblastomas of the cerebellum metastasize outside of the central nervous system only rarely. In 1955, I reported (*see* Zentralbl. f. Neurochir. **16**, 44, 1956) two cases of typical medulloblastomas; the first of these, in an eight-year-old boy, metastasized to the vertebral column and pelvis; the second, in a 12-year-old girl, metastasized to the skin of the thigh. Because of these observations, Wohlwill's (1930) report (metastasis of a medulloblastoma to the lymph nodes of the neck) will have to be considered the first report of such a case. A case of ours reported earlier (E 323, a 20-year-old patient of Prof. Brütt) did not have a medulloblastoma, but must be assumed to have suffered from meningeal sarcomatosis. At first I had made a diagnosis of medulloblastoma on the basis of a small fragment of tissue in which only the leptomeninges were infiltrated with tumor, but the possibility of sarcomatosis was left open. Two years later, after intensive X-ray therapy, a tumor nodule developed in the neck close to the hairline. Three years postoperatively, the patient died of a recurrence. At autopsy a fist-sized mass of tumor was found which extended from the operative site into the neck musculature and was attached to the superficial lymph nodes. Histologically, a diagnosis of sarcomatosis of the meninges was verified (*see* p. 205). Immature gangliocytomas of the sympathetics, too, can occasionally metastasize to other organs. Metastases into the *brain*, however, are very rare in sympathoblastomas.

An explanation for this peculiar behavior has not yet been forthcoming. Perhaps certain internal pressure relationships are responsible, since, for example, in the medulloblastoma group the two *peripheral* representatives —the retinoblastoma and sympathicoblastoma—metastasize to tissues of different embryonic origin, while their histologically identical *centrally-occurring* cousins—the pinealoma and medulloblastoma of the cerebellum —spread only within the central nervous system.

Spontaneous metastases *within the central nervous system* probably occur only by way of the cerebrospinal fluid, and spread via the blood stream would not explain the topographical pattern. There are near and distant metastases. The tendency to metastasize is a basic characteristic of some tumor groups, such as the malignant medulloblastomas, where a seeding either with or against the cerebrospinal fluid current can occur as far as one meter away. The gross appearance is that of a diffuse spread like frosting, or in the form of plaques, or circumscribed nodules (Bailey and Cushing, 1925; Bodechtel and Schüler; Mittelbach; Zülch, 1940). A similar diffuse spread is seen in diffuse sarcomatosis of the meninges which is hard to differentiate from medulloblastoma on inspection (case No. 980, Zülch, 1940, p. 363).

In medulloblastomas there is a diffuse spread of cells into the cerebrospinal fluid once the tumor has broken into the subarachnoid space or the ventricles.

In other gliomas and paragliomas dissemination is more focal and less widespread (astrocytomas: Cairns and Russell. Oligodendrogliomas: Cairns and Russell; Bailey and Bucy, 1929; Martin, 1931; Greenfield and Robertson; Zülch, 1941[1]. Ependymomas: Cairns and Russell; Ostertag, 1941; Tarlov and Davidoff; Zülch, 1940. Plexus papillomas: van Wagenen, 1930; Ostertag, 1941; Töppich; Zülch, 1956. Pinealomas: Berblinger, 1930,

---

[1] Bodechtel and Schüler's case No. 5 was probably also an oligodendroglioma.

1944; Groff; Dias; Alajouanine *et al.*, 1937; Zülch, 1956; Werner, 1939. Glioblastomas: Cairns and Russell; Hasenjäger, 1938[2]).

With the exception of astrocytomas, we have seen such spontaneous metastases of neuroepithelial tumors many times with each tumor subtype in our collection. We think, with Cairns and Russell, that they are even more frequent than has been assumed up to now. These authors found metastases eight times in 22 consecutive cases of neuroepithelial tumors in which the spinal cord was sectioned. If the spinal cord were sectioned regularly, metastases would probably be found more frequently in the region of the cauda equina, where all the residue collects, and along the dorsal columns. Ostertag (1941) reports that he observed such metastases in 20% of the cases.

Our own case of an astrocytoma-like glioma of the cerebellum, which showed mucoid degeneration and had spread diffusely via the cerebrospinal fluid, must be considered a great rarity (case No. 306, three years old). The tumor did not have the typical appearance of a spongioblastoma but more that of the protoplasmic astrocytoma of the cerebral hemispheres.

Polmeteer and Kernohan recently reviewed their own material between 1922–1942 and found 42 cases of a spread of neuroectodermal tumors to the meninges. They found metastases in twenty medulloblastomas, six glioblastomas, five ependymomas, five oligodendrogliomas, three astrocytomas, two retinoblastomas and one pinealoma.

As the macroscopic findings indicate, the formation of metastases can also be recognized in the air study (Learmonth and Camp). We have observed spontaneous metastases of non-neuroepithelial tumors via the cerebrospinal fluid only in monstrocellular sarcomas.

Other cases cited in the literature are either inadequately described or inconclusive, or must be rejected altogether.

Kalm (1950) has recently described a case of metastasis in a 46-year-old patient with sarcomatous degeneration of a tentorial meningioma. In this case there was a diffuse spread within the meninges overlying the dorsal columns and at the root entry-zones which could be detected microscopically but was not apparent to the unaided eye. I studied the histological sections personally and can fully confirm his statements.

On the other hand, Schmincke (1925) described multiple dural tumors as "implantation metastases" of bilateral cerebello-pontine angle tumors. In all probability, these were fibroblastic meningiomas in a case of von Recklinghausen's disease.

[2] Our own case (No. 961) of a 51-year-old man who had undergone a decompressive operation showed an enormous brain fungus. A section through the midbrain revealed an obstruction of the aqueduct by a gray-brown metastasis the size of a cherry pit. A similar metastasis was present in the roof of the fourth ventricle between the dentate nucleus and the tonsil.

Beside *spontaneous* metastases via the cerebrospinal fluid, there are *artificial* ones which follow operation and have particularly grave consequences. A diffuse dissemination occurs over the whole subarachnoid space and ventricular system, with an obstruction at the narrow points and a rapidly fatal outcome. Such diffuse dissemination has been described especially for oligodendrogliomas (Bailey and Bucy, 1929; Zülch, 1941) and for ependymomas (Müller[3]; Zülch, 1940). This lethal effect of the cerebrospinal fluid block can result either from artificial metastases or those that come about spontaneously as in medulloblastomas. However, a general effect of those metastases in the sense of a toxic tumor cachexia (Fischer-Wasels, 1927) is as rare from the metastases of brain tumors as it is from the primary brain tumor itself. Where it arises, it can be explained by the impairment of the endocrine functions of the invaded brain (e.g., metastases of pinealomas to the infundibulum).

The route of metastases. The only recognized route of metastases of brain tumors is via the cerebrospinal fluid (apart from the above-mentioned exceptions). The spread of the metastases shows that, in addition to the known direction of the cerebrospinal fluid current, counter-currents must occur (seeding of medulloblastomas in the third ventricle, infundibulum, and lateral ventricles). In general, metastases quite understandably select the distal parts of the cauda equina or the dense meshwork of the arachnoid in the region of the posterior columns (similar to meningitis). The following are some isolated observations of possible importance to this problem: in our case No. 366 (Zülch, 1940) a pinhead-sized metastasis of a medulloblastoma developed actually beneath the ependyma. On the other hand, in an ependymoma (Zülch, 1940) the seeding occurred over the ependyma, and the blood vessels of the tumor's stroma apparently had arisen from the shed-off tumor fragment itself. In the same case a spread of neuroepithelial neoplasm had occurred in the *outer* layer of arachnoid of the cisterna magna (Zülch, 1940). Finally, in the case of Hasenjäger, the spread of daughter tumors in a glioblastoma which lay adjacent to the ventricle occurred at defects in the ependyma and the tumor cells did not extend into the subependymal tissues (in contrast to the medulloblastoma). According to the view of this author, the blood vessels did not arise from the subependymal tissues purely in the capacity of stroma, but either grew out of this layer as a consequence of a neoplastic stimulus or arose from the shed-off tumor fragment itself.

In the discussion of the so-called multiple gliomas it was pointed out that the question has not yet been settled in a number of cases whether we are dealing with an unrecognized form of metastasis or multifocal origin. Reference was made to four of our own cases of glioblastoma occurring in

[3] Zbl. f. Neurochir. 5, 199–206, 1940.

both the second and third frontal convolutions and in the occipital lobe. In these a direct connection by means of cellular bridges could not be demonstrated and because of their superficial position, metastasis via the cerebrospinal fluid was seriously considered. Still less clear was the case of a monstrocellular sarcoma in a 40-year-old patient (case No. 829) in which there was a plum-sized tumor on one side between the lenticular nucleus and internal capsule, while on the other side a similar cherry-sized nodule was situated in the white matter of the hemisphere, again without demonstrable connection by cellular bridges.

The situation is quite different with the *mesodermal* intracranial tumors. Here blood-born metastasis has been verified in single cases. Winkelman *et al.* have reviewed all the cases in the literature. Pompeu and Pinto and I (1954) have described a case of a meningioma with a 22-year history in which death ultimately occurred from metastases (particularly in the lungs, where the metastases weighed 1760 grams). I have also seen cases of metastases in monstrocellular sarcomas: case E 870 of a 53-year-old patient (metastasis in lungs and liver) and case E 1639 (cardiac metastases).

Recurrence after operation

All brain tumors recur after incomplete removal. Where growth is slow, as in the spongioblastoma of the cerebellum, the interval can be unusually long and may exceed a decade (cases of Bailey and Bucy, and Cushing's have been mentioned in the section on Regressive Changes and Mucoid and Cystic Degeneration, p. 101 ff.). This possibility should always be taken into consideration in evaluating the therapeutic effects of operation or X-ray therapy. Only in exceptional cases are there tumors whose growth at some time during the patient's life seems to become dormant, the tumor "withering" away to some extent (our case No. 197 of a 69-year-old woman with a spongioblastoma of the fourth ventricle; *see* also picture 19 in Schaltenbrand, 1938).

Among patients with intracerebral neuroepithelial tumors, those with spongioblastomas can be permanently cured after total extirpation—if the tumor's position makes this feasible. This is also possible in ependymomas of the ventricle and spinal cord, and in certain fibrillary astrocytomas. This may perhaps also be achieved in oligodendrogliomas where an extensive lobectomy can be undertaken early. Otherwise, oligodendrogliomas—which often grow invasively—and astrocytomas usually recur in three to five years or later. Glioblastomas and medulloblastomas recur without exception even after apparently total extirpation and X-ray therapy. All apparent exceptions to this rule were later shown to have been an error of classification.[4]

[4] Bucy mentioned this in 1946 in regard to Cushing's patient with a 12-year sur-

Among the intracerebral mesodermal growths, the angioblastoma has a good prognosis (permanent cure after total extirpation), and all forms of sarcoma have a bad one. The prognosis of sarcoma is similar to that of glioblastoma and slightly better only in isolated cases (*see* pp. 117, 204 ff.).

The results are better in the extracerebral tumors. Here we see permanent cures as a rule after complete removal of meningiomas (where the site of attachment to bone and dura has been removed as well), neurinomas (total removal is difficult), and craniopharyngiomas (total removal is possible only in those with a suprasellar or pre-chiasmatic location—Tönnis, 1949). Cure is also possible in pituitary adenomas.

The recurrence, just like the primary tumor, can undergo de-differentiation. To be sure, considerable caution concerning this statement is justified (*see* Histological de-differentiation, below) but such a process has been demonstrated in our cases of ependymomas (Zülch, 1940), and was mentioned as a possibility in oligodendrogliomas (Zülch, 1941).

Histological de-differentiation

Our prognosis depends heavily on whether a tumor maintains its histological identity or changes its morphological and biological character in response to internal or external influences. Making a prognosis on the basis of histological findings presupposes that the tumor is morphologically so uniform that its *general* biological character can be predicted with certainty by studying only a *portion* of it.

Brain tumors can be morphologically different in different regions. They may have various architectures and cell types from their very outset: thus the monstrocellular sarcoma may consist simultaneously of 1) uniform spindle cell regions arranged in streams and 2) pleomorphic monstrocellular portions. In oligodendrogliomas, too, up to three cell types may be present simultaneously, which have in common nothing but a certain architectural arrangement (*see* p. 144). In spite of this, the histological picture in both these tumors is so type-specific in each region that the experienced examiner can generally make the diagnosis from any single histological pattern. Apitz has described the parallel situation in renal carcinomas very clearly (*see* p. 19).

Beside these "normal" variations in form, there are a large number of alterations that follow regressive changes and the reactive processes which ensue. These are described in the corresponding chapters in the general part and special part under Differential diagnosis. It must be emphasized again that the experienced pathologist can make a diagnosis from the

---

vival after removal of a medulloblastoma. Re-examination demonstrated that the tumor was really a leptomeningeal sarcoma (Bucy, 1946, p. 223).

degenerated portions as well, something which is important in the rapid diagnosis of tumors during operation.

At this point we must ask ourselves whether the histological structure and the biological behavior can vary not only in *different* parts of a tumor studied at the *same* time but also in the *same* tumor examined at *different* stages of its development. This question must be answered in the affirmative and has been stressed particularly for astrocytomas (Teltscharow and Zülch), and oligodendrogliomas (Zülch, 1941).[5]

Thus Globus (1931) reported the transformation of benign into malignant tumors; of these the best is case No. 3; case No. 6 is very probable, but some of his other cases cannot meet the criteria mentioned. Mistakes arise when, in the first examination, the marginal zone of the tumor is studied and, in the second, its center portion. This criticism cannot be applied to our own case of astrocytoma mentioned above, since at autopsy it showed both firm, benign, fibrillary portions and soft, malignant, necrotic ones.

The studies of W. Müller (1933) are—in certain instances—also liable to this criticism, since he regards the picture as seen in different excised portions as different stages of development. These histological pictures quite typically co-exist in the same tumor as a result of degenerative changes in a biologically uniform astrocytoma—something that can be readily appreciated in sections through the whole tumor. Scheinker (1938) also describes similar cases.

In summary, we must accept the possibility of de-differentiation in astrocytomas, oligodendrogliomas and ependymomas—in the latter two particularly after operation. How frequently this occurs we do not know. In astrocytomas it plays a significant role: of 55 cases investigated by us, using large sections through the whole tumor, six belonged to the group of malignant astrocytomas which prompted us to introduce them as a subgroup.

Biological evaluation (degree of malignancy)

An evaluation of brain tumors according to the current rules of pathology would be unsatisfactory for our purposes, since malignancy cannot be judged on the basis of histology alone but is dependent upon a number of characteristics. According to Hamperl a fundamental change in approach can now also be observed in pathology. The cranial cavity, however, is governed by a set of special rules, described in detail above (p. 110 ff.). There, due to the rigidity of the "water-tight" cavity, the pressure rela-

---

[5] Such a claim can be made with assurance, however, only when all the antecedent and secondary regressive deviations from the normal picture are known and taken fully into consideration.

tionships are so unique that we can say—without any exaggeration—that in the long run *every* unoperated brain tumor is "malignant" and fatal so far as the patient is concerned. It is necessary, therefore, to distinguish between two forms of malignancy in brain tumors: a "primary" one related to the type of tissue growth, and a "secondary" one related to its location.

The malignancy of brain tumors may then be expressed in two groups of characteristics:

1. *Biological*
    Intrinsic growth properties
2. *Clinical*
    Actual volume of the tumor
    Reaction of the surrounding tissue—brain edema and swelling
    Relationship to the cerebrospinal pathways—occlusive hydro-
        cephalus
    Relation to vital centers—irritative and deficiency symptoms

These characteristics can be considered together in a simplified way by classifying the tumors according to site, type, and age of incidence (*see* p. 58 ff.).

The following indications have until now served as:

Evidence of relative malignancy

Gross morphology: Infiltrating and destructive growth, without regard for organ boundaries; rapid growth; tendency toward metastasis and recurrence despite total removal.

Histology: Pleomorphism with disordered arrangement, deficient maturation of the cells, disturbance in the ratio between nucleus and cytoplasm and particularly multinucleation, the formation of giant cells, and disproportionate size of nucleoli; rapid growth with numerous and atypical mitoses, short life-span of the cells, either with diffuse cell disintegration or rapidly proceeding regressive processes like necrosis; incomplete and disorganized arrangement of the stroma, particularly of the vasculature.

Signs of relative benignity

Gross morphology: Expanding growth respecting organ boundaries, formation of a capsule, and absence of metastases; recurrence only following incomplete removal.

Histology: Regular cellular structure, slow growth (without mitoses), low cell density with maturation of structures (formation of fibers, etc.), and orderly, normally arranged stroma, especially blood vessels.

We could now investigate each brain tumor according to these criteria, but we would quickly see that the above-mentioned characteristics can scarcely serve as a rule of thumb for a biological evaluation. For instance, if we compare the medulloblastomas and the oligodendrogliomas, we find that they are both equally cellular. The medulloblastoma is rather more isomorphic than the oligodendroglioma which frequently shows quite pleomorphic regions. The number of mitotic figures can be quite considerable in oligodendrogliomas, even those with a long clinical history, and both tumors show infiltrating growth. In spite of all this, there is a fundamental difference in their biological value; the medulloblastoma is highly malignant, the oligodendroglioma relatively benign. Moreover, the principle developed originally by Bailey—the parallelism between a higher degree of histogenetic development and benignity of a tumor—has not turned out to be completely valid. There are malignant ganglion cell tumors with complete maturity of cells (*see* Tönnis and Zülch, 1939, case No. 36); the spongioblastomas, which according to their position in the histogenetic scale are apparently immature, are mostly benign (quite apart from their often unfavorable location) and represent the most benign of known gliomas in the cerebellum. The "immature" astroblastomas, furthermore, are much more benign than the "mature" protoplasmic astrocytomas, etc.

From all this it appears that the only possible means of biological evaluation of brain tumors is a statistical determination of the average post-operative survival period of patients with various tumors.[6] This approach has been successfully used by Bailey and Cushing, to whom we are indebted for Table 4.

TABLE 4. AVERAGE SURVIVAL PERIOD OF DIFFERENT HISTOLOGICAL TUMOR TYPES

1. Medulloepithelioma	8	months
2. Pineoblastoma	12	months
3. Spongioblastoma multiforme	12	months
4. Medulloblastoma	17	months
5. Pinealoma	18	months
6. Ependymoblastoma	19	months
7. Neuroblastoma	25	months
8. Astroblastoma	28+	months
9. Ependymoma	32+	months
10. Spongioblastoma unipolare	46+	months
11. Oligodendroglioma	66+	months
12. Astrocytoma protoplasmaticum	67+	months
13. Astrocytoma fibrillare	86+	months

[6] As Hamperl (1937) has put it so clearly: "The prognosis of a given tumor type cannot be determined only on the basis of anatomico-histological study but has to be considered together with the clinical symptomatology and history of all cases. To decide about each tumor type in a particular location one must first take into consideration all tumor types which occur at that given site. Once this has been done, a prognosis of a particular case can be made, based on its anatomico-histological picture. The fact that the histologist is unable to decide with assurance about the benignity of a tumor type from morphological observations alone may, at first, be an unpleasant realization for him but it prevents him from attaching too much importance to certain details".

In individual cases, however, even these figures could be inadequate, as long as the tumor site had not been taken into consideration. A small inoperable spongioblastoma of the aqueduct could not be evaluated according to the average survival period of this tumor type. On the other hand, the average survival period of a group with as benign a prognosis as the cerebellar spongioblastomas (so-called astrocytomas) has been lowered so by the inclusion of inoperable cases (spongioblastoma of the chiasm, for example) that a new "biological" way of grouping them was necessary: a grouping by location, age group, and tissue type.

Cushing (1931) described the first clinically useful entities: the astrocytomas (spongioblastomas) and medulloblastomas of the cerebellum in children. We have set up new groups: the ependymomas of the cerebral hemispheres in children, the gangliocytomas of the basal temporal lobe in the second and third decades, the oligodendrogliomas of the thalamus (in children) and of the second and third frontal convolution (in middle age), and the ependymomas of the foramen of Monro in middle age (Zülch and Schmid, 1955). In preparation for the ultimate classification of tumors along these lines we have presented the charts of age-curves and of sites of preference of these and other groups (*see* pp. 58–81). The goal of an ultimate classification and biological evaluation of *all* brain tumors is in sight, but will be achieved only by the combined contributions of the clinic and pathological laboratory. Until then we must still be guided by the results of Cushing and his co-workers and by the results of other neurosurgical clinics whose statistics have been made available.

TABLE 5.   POSTOPERATIVE SURVIVAL OF FIVE YEARS OR MORE

Type of Tumor	No. of Patients	Approx. per cent of 476 survivors	Tumor type as per cent of 2,023 cases
Astrocytomas, cerebellar	39	8.0	4.5
Astrocytomas, cerebral and pontine	24	5.0	8.0
Spongioblastoma polare	11	2.0	1.6
Oligodendrogliomas	6	1.2	1.3
Ependymomas	7	1.4	1.3
Medulloblastomas	6	1.2	4.3
Plexus papillomas	4	0.8	0.6
Pituitary adenomas	152	30.0	17.8
Meningiomas	119	24.0	13.4
Acoustic neurinomas	77	15.0	8.7
Craniopharyngiomas	24	5.0	4.6
Epidermoids and dermoids	7	1.4	0.7
Total:	476		

The application of this kind of statistical approach to brain tumors appears to have begun with Lebert, who, in 1851, compared the survival period of patients with intracranial "fibroblastic" tumors to that of patients with intracranial carcinomas and found the latter shorter by several years.

The statistical analysis of large series began with the follow-up studies of Cushing's clinical material—subjected to uniform operative technique and histological evaluation—by his earlier co-workers van Wagenen (1934), Cairns (1936), Henderson, Eisenhardt (1935), and Davidoff (1940). I have not reproduced this statistical data, since it has in the meantime been expanded by a number of contributions from larger clinics (Olivecrona, Tönnis, *et al.*). An outstanding supplement to these data are the findings of Eisenhardt (1935) which are organized according to post-operative survival periods of five years or more (*see* Table 5).

Using these data, we can summarize the *average life expectancy after* "*radical removal*" *of the principal brain tumors*[6] *as follows:*

Extracerebral group

Neurinomas	Cure (reoperation possibly necessary)
Meningiomas	Cure
Pituitary adenomas	Cure (X-ray therapy sometimes required)
Epidermoids and dermoids	Cure
Teratomas	Cure

Intracerebral group

Benign tumors

Angioblastomas	Cure
Spongioblastomas	Site often contraindicates operation; cure with tumors of the optic nerve, mid-line cerebellum (so-called "cerebellar astrocytoma") and occasionally spinal cord

Relatively benign tumors

Circumscribed fibrillary astrocytomas	Improvement for many years; often cure
Oligodendrogliomas	Improvement, three to five years; recurrence usual; cure?

[6] The clinical terms "cure" or "improvement" are used here in a *pathological* sense and are based on permanent or temporary arrest of tumor growth. Improvement, therefore, means that the clinical condition after the immediate post-operative period was characterized by temporary arrest of progression; cure, that this state was maintained permanently.

Ependymomas	According to site: single cures in fourth ventricle and lateral ventricle (?); recurrence in two to five years in ependymoma of the cerebral hemispheres in children
Plexus papillomas	Cure possible; prolonged survival known, danger of implantation metastases
Pinealomas	Radical operation nearly impossible; recurrence likely; after relief of C. S. F. block, prolonged remission
Gangliocytomas	Varies according to site and type; cure or improvement over many years possible with those of temporolateral site

Malignant tumors

Medulloblastomas	Improvement up to 15 months or longer with intensive X-ray therapy; always ultimately fatal (recurrence, metastasis)
Glioblastomas	Improvement 6–12 months, possibly longer with intensive X-ray therapy; always ultimately fatal

CHAPTER VIII

NEUROEPITHELIAL TUMORS: THE MEDULLOBLASTOMAS

1. MEDULLOBLASTOMAS

Cerebellar medulloblastomas

(*Synonyms: Glioma sarcomatodes, isomorphic glioblastoma, neuroblastoma, granuloblastoma, embryonic neurogliocytoma, neurospongioma, spheroblastoma. Also a large part of the tumors previously described as "meningeal sarcomas" belong here.*)

HISTORICAL NOTE AND DEFINITION

The medulloblastomas were first described as an entity in 1924 by Bailey and Cushing under the name of "spongioblastoma cerebelli," though pathologists had previously known them as glioma sarcomatodes, meningeal sarcoma, and "diffuse sarcomatosis of the meninges." The first name was given up in 1925 in favor of the present one in order to eliminate confusion with the "spongioblastoma multiforme." Cushing's study outlines the symptomatology and the biological behavior of the medulloblastomas. Detailed anatomical descriptions are to be found in the contributions of Masson and Dreyfuss; Marburg (1931); Nishii; Wohlwill (1930); Roussy, Oberling and Raileanu; Ringertz (1955); Kershman; Raaf and Kernohan; Spitz, Shenkin and Grant; Stevenson and Echlin; Del Rio Hortega (1932); Ringertz and Tola; and Zülch (1940). At present, we look upon the medulloblastoma as a neuroepithelial tumor; Nishii's idea that it is a sarcoma seems unjustified. The medulloblastomas of the cerebral hemispheres have, upon close investigation, turned out to be tumors of another type.

INCIDENCE AND SITE

The medulloblastomas are well known as malignant cerebellar tumors of childhood and adolescence. The peak of incidence falls between the ages of 7–12 (Fig. 3). However, occasional cases occur up to the fourth decade as well. They make up 20% of all brain tumors of childhood and ado-

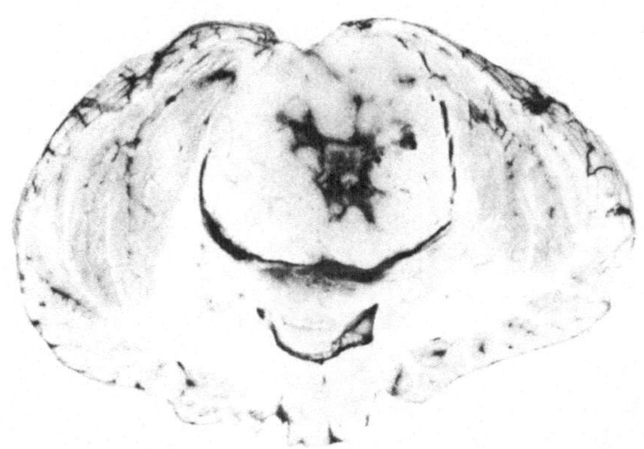

Fig. 28. Large medulloblastoma of the midline of the cerebellum with slight necrosis of the center. The tumor is sharply demarcated from the surrounding tissue. (Case 1020)

lescence, but only 0.8% of tumors occurring after 20 years of age. In our series they comprised 4%, in Cushing's series, 4.3%, and in Ringertz' 6.5% of the total. In a series of McK. Craig, Keith, and Kernohan, they formed 20.1% of brain tumors in children. Of a collection of 1,792 gliomas of various authors, 10% belonged to the medulloblastoma group. According to Cushing, boys are affected three times more frequently than girls. Out of a series of 4,000, we had 159 patients with medulloblastomas which could be investigated statistically; of these, 114 were males and 47 females. The youngest patient was six months old, the oldest 53 years. The average age in Ingraham's series of cerebellar medulloblastomas was 7.5, in Ringertz' 13.8 years. Of special interest is Cushing's experience with identical twins with medulloblastomas (*see* Leavitt). I know of a similar observation (*see* p. 40). There are also single cases in identical twins.

Medulloblastomas may reach the size of a tangerine and lie mainly in the inferior cerebellar vermis, into which they spread from the roof of the fourth ventricle (Fig. 17, Nos. 1 and 2; Fig. 28). From here they expand in all directions but only infrequently do they lie with their main portion in one hemisphere. The fourth ventricle, filled with the tumor projecting from above, is usually enlarged, and the vermis is compressed into a thin lamella on the upper surface of the tumor. With further growth, tongues of tumor may push between the cerebellar tonsils into the cisterna magna, as happens in the ependymoma. Medulloblastomas also occur, though rarely, in the pons.

APPEARANCE TO THE NAKED EYE

Grossly, the medulloblastomas often appear well circumscribed (Fig. 28); however, at their margin they grow diffusely into the surrounding tissue (Fig. 29). The cerebellar folia with their leptomeninges are thus

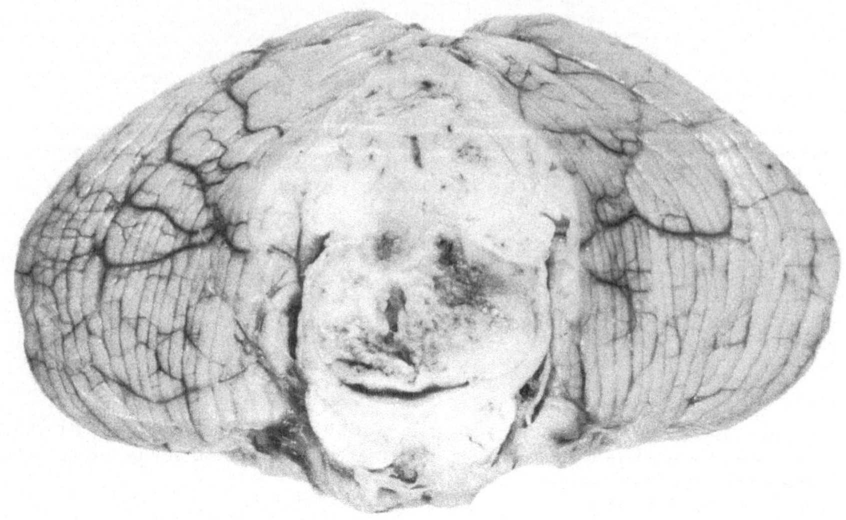

Fig. 29.   Medulloblastoma of the pineal gland (pineoblastoma) with extension into the cerebellar vermis and beginning infiltration of cerebellar folia. (Case 1078)

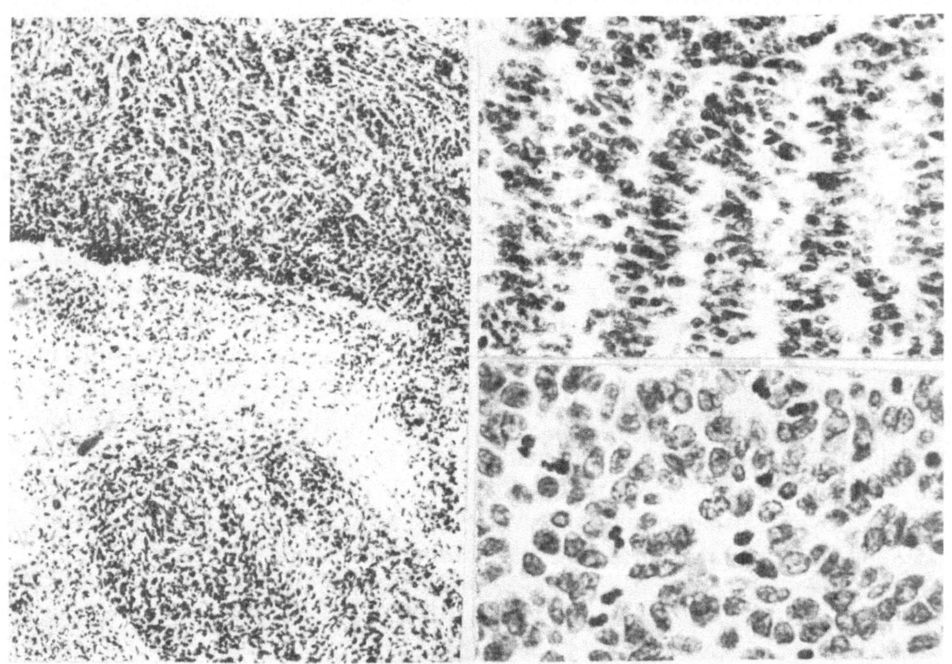

Fig. 30.   a) *left:* Spread of a medulloblastoma into a cerebellar folium and the overlying leptomeninges. Note the presence of one Purkinje cell and the infiltration of the tumor into the white matter, the subpial region and massive spread in the arachnoid. (x78, Nissl stain); b) *top right:* Parallel (comb-like) arrangement of cells in a medulloblastoma. (x272, Nissl stain); c) *bottom right:* Typical cell arrangement in a medulloblastoma with pseudorosettes and many mitoses. (x230, Nissl stain).

130

engulfed in the tumor mass. Medulloblastomas are grayish-pink, since they are not very vascular; their consistency is soft and granular (like thick Cream of Wheat), and firmer only when a lot of connective tissue has been included. Occasionally, they can appear partly encapsulated, as, for instance, when one wall is formed by the roof of the ventricle.

HISTOLOGICAL APPEARANCE

Histologically, medulloblastomas consist of closely-packed, isomorphic, elongated cells with round or oval nuclei, or of beet- or carrot-shaped cells which show an orderly arrangement often in concentric patterns (pseudo-rosettes, *see* Figs. 26c, 30c) or clustering in islands. True rosettes do not occur (*see* pp. 85, 88). Occasionally the nuclei are rather vesicular and neurone-like, a fact that might have been responsible for the opinion of Hortega (1932) and others that they were neuroblasts. The rate of growth is very rapid; numerous typical mitoses can be found, even though many cells have only a short life-span (disintegration of nuclei). The remnants of degenerated nuclei must be distinguished from mitoses which often stain lighter. The elongated tumor cells have to be differentiated from the dark, round, granule cells of the invaded cerebellum. I consider the ganglion cells and astrocytes, which occasionally occur in the tumors, as remnants of the pre-existing infiltrated tissue. Medulloblastomas show little tendency toward degeneration; small areas of necrosis or fatty degeneration occur only occasionally, and then usually in the center of the tumor. Calcification and cyst formation are very rare. The blood vessels are predominantly capillaries and are infrequent; the tumor cells form neither glial nor reticulin fibers. The reticulin fiber network which may be present comes from the engulfed leptomeninges.

Hemorrhages do not occur in this tumor. There are rare cases in which striated or smooth muscle cells are present (Marinesco and Goldstein; Zülch, 1941). In their growth, the tumor cells prefer to follow the blood vessels, resulting in spotty, perivascular spread in the marginal zone. On breaking into the leptomeninges, the tumor assumes a different architecture: the cells arrange themselves into single rows between the arachnoidal meshes (Fig. 26). From there the cells proliferate beneath the pia and spread into the neighboring cerebellar folia. Upon reaching the open subarachnoid space, they can be carried either with or against the C.S.F. current, and seed out in the form of buttons, plaques, nodules, or a diffuse spread like frosting (aqueduct, infundibulum, floor of the lateral ventricles, dorsal surface of the spinal cord, cauda equina, or the leptomeninges over the hemispheres, where the tumor molds itself into the sulci and cisterns). The tendency to metastasize is marked and nearly inevitable, despite

X-ray therapy, if the patients live long enough. The incidence of metastases is given in the literature as 20–47.6%.

Recurrence after operation is almost inevitable. The survival period averages 8–15 months after the onset of symptoms. Survival is apt to exceed this period only after operation or X-ray radiation. A survival period of several years has been mentioned in the literature; however, the likely possibility of a histological misdiagnosis should be considered in all these cases (*see* footnote, p. 120). I have observed three cases of metastasis to other organs of cerebellar medulloblastomas, two of which were cases of my own, the third a referral by Dr. Bachman, Berlin.

DIFFERENTIAL DIAGNOSIS

The medulloblastoma can be differentiated from the spongioblastoma of the cerebellum (so-called cerebellar astrocytoma) with the naked eye. The spongioblastoma has a good capsule and peels off from the surrounding brain tissue; it is firm and elastic. Histologically, it possesses glial fibers and is relatively acellular, showing the formation of Rosenthal's fibers. Mitoses and perivascular infiltration in the marginal zone always speak in favor of medulloblastoma. The ependymoma of the fourth ventricle is harder, smoother, and more nodular, and can be separated easily from the overlying brain. It generally grows from the floor of the fourth ventricle, and though it has a similar cellularity, can be differentiated histologically on the basis of its characteristic architecture: spaces free of nuclei around the vessels, and a lack of mitoses.[1] The angioblastoma usually lies in the cerebellar hemispheres, is vascular, often has large cysts, and generally occurs in an older age group; it can be easily differentiated histologically. True sarcomatosis of the leptomeninges sometimes cannot be distinguished locally from metastases of a medulloblastoma to the subarachnoid space. In sarcomatosis, however, larger circumscribed tumors are absent.

The rapid growth of the medulloblastoma explains its short clinical history; spinal metastases account for the early signs of posterior column and cauda equina involvement (loss of reflexes, root pain in the distribution of the cauda, etc.). The clinical symptomatology is a combination of the cerebellar symptoms and symptoms of generalized increased intracranial pressure from aqueduct block. As this tumor more often lies in the midline, symptoms of the vermis and anterior lobe predominate.

The retino-, pineo-, and sympathoblastomas

We group the tumors of early infancy and childhood of the retina, pineal region (Fig. 29), sympathetic trunk, and adrenals with the medullo-

---

[1] Mitoses in cerebellar ependymomas are exceptional but they are commonly observed in ependymomas of the cerebral hemispheres.

blastomas; these are histologically very similar to the cerebellar medullo-blastomas and biologically very malignant. Their tendency to metastasize is still more pronounced; the tumors of the eye and adrenals directly invade tissue of a different embryonic origin (mesoderm) or metastasize to it—retinoblastoma particularly to the bones and lymph nodes, and sym-pathoblastoma to the bones, lymph nodes, and liver. The pineoblastoma does not metastasize except via the C.S.F.

These four forms have similarly undifferentiated cells. Pseudo-rosettes occur with corresponding frequency and the different medulloblastomas can be so similar in architecture that even an experienced pathologist may not be able to tell one from the other without knowing the organ from which each came. The retinoblastoma alone has a histologically specific trait, namely the formation of "true" rosettes (Fig. 24b), whose origin is still imperfectly understood. They do not occur in the metastases of this tumor. Moreover, the number of mitoses here is very great and the bulk of the tumor undergoes necrosis as a result of poor vascularization (cuffs of cells remain around the vessels, however; *see* Fig. 25b).

CHAPTER IX

NEUROEPITHELIAL TUMORS: THE GLIOMAS

2. THE POLAR SPONGIOBLASTOMAS (INCLUDING THE SO-CALLED CEREBELLAR ASTROCYTOMAS)

(Synonyms: Gliomyxoma, myxosarcoma, fusicellular oligodendrocytoma, "central neurinoma," gliome muqueux.)

HISTORICAL NOTE AND DEFINITION

The term spongioblastoma appears to have been first used by Kauffman and reappears later in the writings of Ribbert (1918), and Globus and Strauss (1935). At first, however, this name was applied to ependymoma-like tumors (Ribbert) or to medulloblastomas (Bailey and Cushing, 1924). The present conception is based on the classification by Bailey and Cushing of 1926. Spongioblastomas are poorly defined as a group; best known is the basal group in the region of the hypothalamus and chiasm, and in the pons. We now include the so-called cerebellar astrocytomas with them. In our opinion, the "central neurinomas" of the literature also belong to the spongioblastoma group. Finally, it must be emphasized that the spongioblastoma in our classification is a clearly defined, benign group with specific characteristics. It has nothing to do with the spongioblastoma multiforme of the older nomenclature (Ostertag et al.; Stochdorph, Grill et al.), and cannot be diagnosed simply in any case of a spindle cell tumor which appears to consist of "spongioblasts." Spongioblastoma, according to the definition of Russell (1955), is a malignant tumor which does not produce fibers.

Further references: Bailey and Eisenhardt (1932); Bergstrand (1932, 1937); Bucy (1942); Bucy and Gustafson (1939); Busch and Christensen (1937); Echols, Hare and Wolf; Hausmann and Stevenson; Josephy; Loisel; Martin and Cushing; Opalski; Pilcher; Ringertz and Nordenstam; Russell and Bland (1934).

INCIDENCE AND SITE

The spongioblastomas occur predominantly in the young, and they are the principal tumor of the chiasmal region in childhood and adolescence.

Our youngest patient was eight months old, the oldest 60 years. The peak of incidence lies between three and seven years (Figs. 4, 5).[1] These tumors form 7.1% of the total of all our material and 24.1% of tumors of childhood and adolescence. One hundred and thirty-four of our cases (series of 4,000) were males and 158 females. Of Cushing's series, 6.1% were spongioblastomas.

The bulk of spongioblastomas lie over the chiasmal region, in the chiasm itself, or in the optic nerves. They may fill the third ventricle (Fig. 31) and extend through the foramen of Monro into the lateral ventricle. But rather rarely do they grow on the lateral wall of the lateral ventricle (like the ependymomas of the cerebral hemispheres), though they can reach the size of a fist. They grow to the size of a pea in the aqueduct, the size of a walnut in the quadrigeminal plate, and the size of a plum in the fourth ventricle. Most often, they attain the size of a walnut or tangerine in the cerebellum (*see* Fig. 32) as so-called "cerebellar astrocytomas" (*see* below). Finally they grow as thick as a pencil or larger in the central portion of the posterior columns of the cord.

APPEARANCE TO THE NAKED EYE

The spongioblastomas are well-circumscribed tumors of variable size (Fig. 17, Nos. 3–6; Figs. 31, 32), grayish-pink and translucent, and have a tough, elastic or occasionally mucoid consistency. Often they degenerate into small or large cysts; occasionally there are small hemorrhages in the tumor tissue, or the cyst walls show brownish discoloration. Spongioblastomas grow mainly by expansion, although they infiltrate at the margin. They have a tendency for local invasion of the meninges.

HISTOLOGICAL APPEARANCE

The spongioblastomas are moderately cellular tumors with cells orientated in streams and whorls (*see* Figs. 34a, 23a) something like a neurinoma; there are, however, no true palisades. The tumor cells are uniform, elongated or worm-shaped, and bipolar (Fig. 34a); there are also some with one long and many short processes (astrocyte-like, *see* Fig. 33c). The streams and whorls of cells interdigitate or join in parallel or wavy bands, or form other patterns. The cell processes can be wound like corkscrews, or gathered together like a braid of hair. They form numerous glial fibers[2] and have oval or elongated nuclei with a moderate amount of

---

[1] Though the age curves are drawn separately for the spongioblastoma of the cerebellum and for the other spongioblastomas, the two curves are practically identical.

[2] In spongioblastomas we regularly find Rosenthal's fibers (*see* Regressive Processes, p. 104). These seem to be a typical degenerative form of the glial fibers of the subependymal glia. In addition to preference of these fibers for a subependymal location and the marked morphological resemblance between the subependymal glia (Opalski) and the tumor cells, the finding of Rosenthal's fibers seems to point toward the fact that spongioblastomas originate from the subependymal glia (*see* also pp. 23, 104).

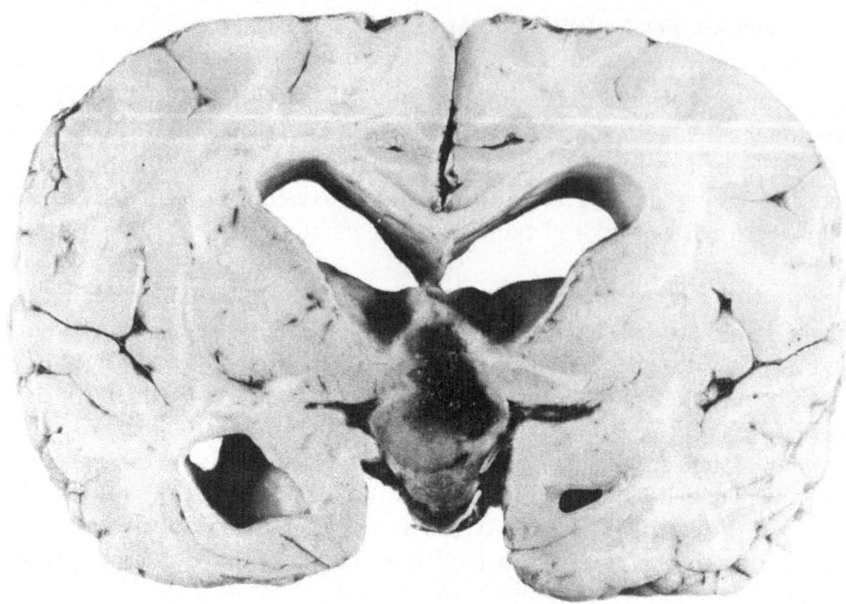

Fig. 31. Coronal section showing a spongioblastoma of the chiasm (hypothalamus). The whole third ventricle is filled with tumor which protrudes through both foramina of Monro. The chiasm has been compressed into a thin band under the tumor. Note the enlargement of lateral ventricles. (Case 1091)

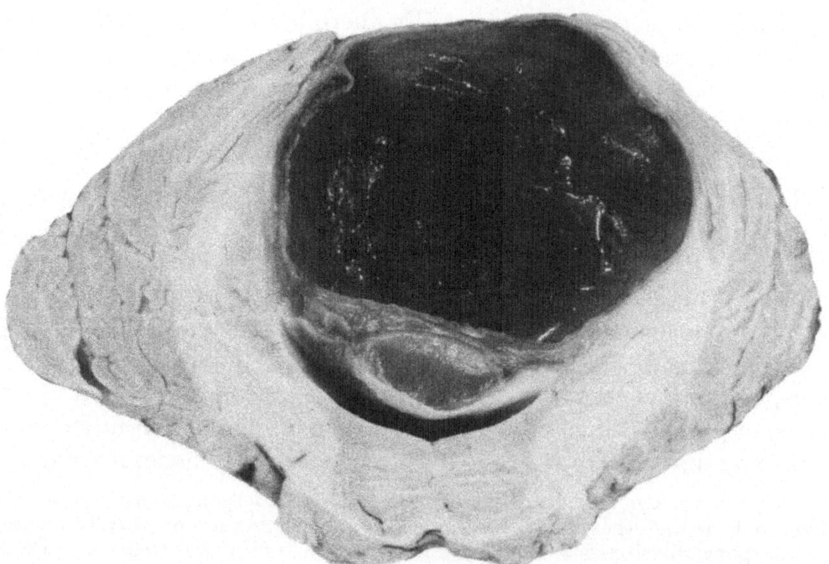

Fig. 32. Huge cystic spongioblastoma of the midline of the cerebellum (so-called cerebellar astrocytoma). The solid portion of the tumor is seen in the lower part of the cyst. (Case 1592)

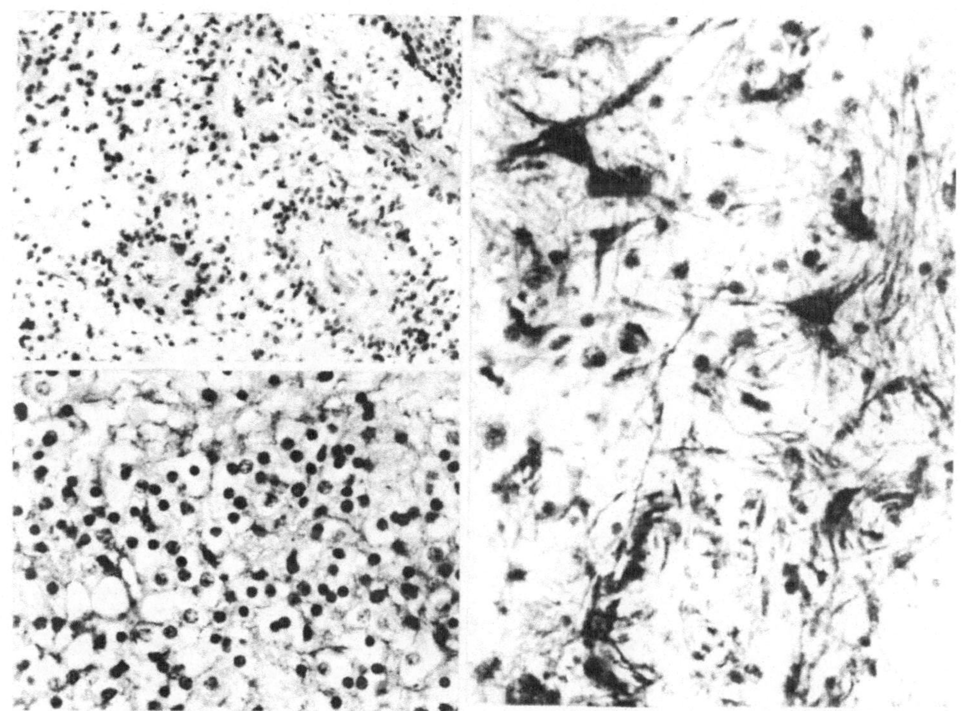

Fig. 33. Spongioblastoma. a) *top left:* Mucoid degeneration with the formation of cysts. This can lead to the development of papilla-like structures around the blood vessels (pseudopapillae). (x100, Nissl stain); b) *bottom left:* A honeycomb architecture resembling oligodendroglioma, which develops in a spongioblastoma through regressive processes, particularly through mucoid degeneration. (x270, Nissl stain); c) *right:* Cell types of a spongioblastoma as seen on metallic impregnation: the elongated, spindle-shaped cells (similar to spongioblasts), and other cells resembling astrocytes and astroblasts. (x300, gold sublimate impregnation)

chromatin. Mitoses do not occur, and growth is very slow. The vessels are usually infrequent, but sometimes clustered together like an angioma; often they develop reactively in the form of vascular coils along the margin of a cyst or an area of mucoid degeneration. Blood vessel coils also develop within the tumor inside the adventitial spaces.[3] They have a marked tendency toward hyalinization. Beginning with mucoid changes of the tumor cells, the whole tumor can undergo mucoid degeneration and cyst formation (Figs. 32, 33a). Cuffs of cells persist around the blood vessels because of better nourishment and may cause a pseudo-papillary architecture, similar to that of an ependymoma (Figs 33a, 25d). Fatty degeneration is hardly ever seen, calcification occasionally in the tumor proper, or in

[3] At those places which are normally very vascular—pituitary stalk, area postrema, and subfornical region—the spongioblastomas may manifest extreme vascularity ("mixed angioglial tumors"). Around the chiasm and third ventricle they have been termed "infundibulomas" (Globus, 1942).

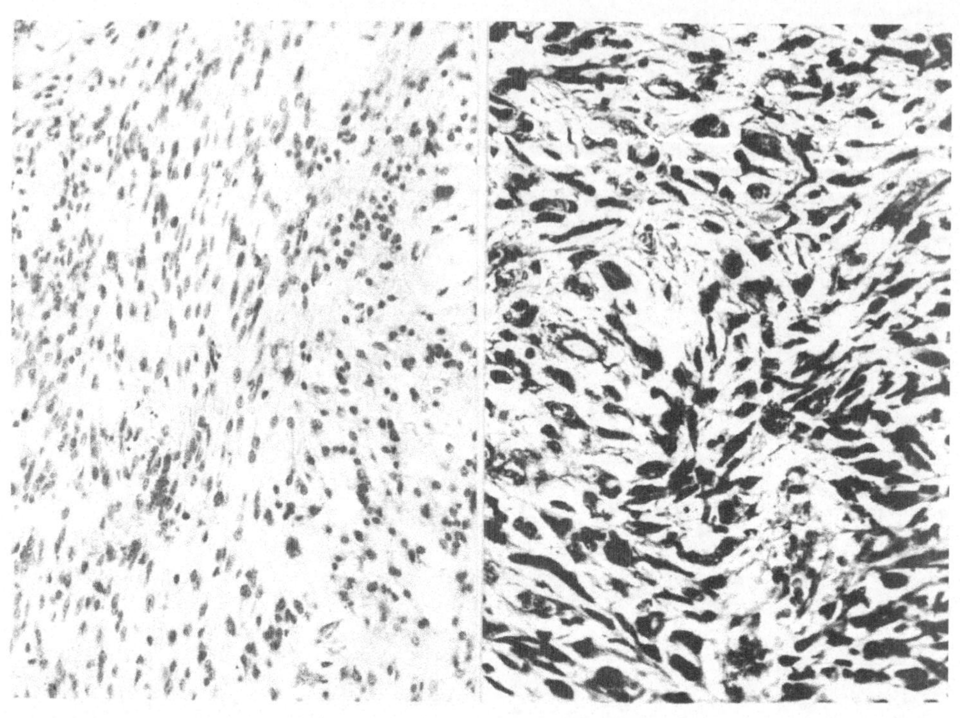

Fig. 34. a) *left:* Typical architecture of a spongioblastoma: elongated cells with spindle-shaped nuclei are arranged in streams. (x120, Nissl stain); b) *right:* Atypical architecture of an oligodendroglioma: elongated, spindle-shaped nuclei and also short, plump ones lie "bare" in a meshwork formed by minute vacuoles. (x170, H. & E. stain)

the surrounding brain tissue. Metastases do not occur. When the location is favorable, total removal usually assures a cure.

DIFFERENTIAL DIAGNOSIS

Parts that show mucoid vacuolization of the tumor cells may histologically be mistaken for an oligodendroglioma (Fig. 33b), with which the spongioblastoma shows a certain kinship. The demonstration of Rosenthal's fibers always favors the diagnosis of spongioblastoma. A good correlation between growth of the tumor and the clinical syndromes is not available. "Gliomas of the chiasm" and the "optic nerve gliomas" are nearly always spongioblastomas and are often accompanied by anomalies of pigmentation or other manifestations of incomplete von Recklinghausen's disease. The gliomas of this disease are almost always spongioblastomas.

The spongioblastomas of the optic nerve

(*See* also the contributions of Bürki; Lundberg; Martin and Cushing; Rettelbach and Schutzbach; Verhoeff.)

Spongioblastomas can occur in the optic nerve either in its orbital portion alone, on both sides of the optic foramen in the shape of an hour-

138

glass, or predominantly in the chiasm. In the last case the chiasm is pressed into a flat band at the base of the tumor (Fig. 17, No. 3; Fig. 31). By virtue of the definite parallel arrangement of the nerve fibers of the optic pathways, the architecture and cell form of the tumor are forced to orient themselves longitudinally (*see* Architecture, p. 85 ff.). The spongioblastomas expand the arachnoid sheath of the optic nerve by their infiltration. Depending on their site, these tumors are surgically accessible either through the orbit or by a combined intracranial-orbital approach (Tönnis, 1950). Usually they occur as a part of the picture of von Recklinghausen's neurofibromatosis.

Spongioblastomas of the cerebellum (the so-called cerebellar astrocytomas)

(*Synonyms: Gliocytoma embryonale and glioneuroblastoma of Bergstrand; they form most of the cases of the so-called "piloid" astrocytomas of Penfield, 1927.*)

HISTORICAL NOTE AND DEFINITION

This important glioma type was described a long time ago by Fedor Krause, Landau (1911), and especially by Hildebrandt, but it has become well-known only since Bailey and Cushing's work (1926). We are indebted to Bergstrand (1932, 1937); Bucy and Gustavson; Ringertz and Nordenstam; and Zülch (1940, 1956) for special studies of this tumor. The so-called cerebellar astrocytoma seems so strikingly similar to the spongioblastoma that we have included it in that group, especially since Bergstrand has demonstrated its special position. There are, of course, astrocyte-like cell forms in these tumors but the majority are spongioblast-like. Moreover, architecture, behavior, and the presence of Rosenthal fibers indicate that this tumor belongs to the spongioblastomas. It does not seem logical to split a group as clinically and biologically uniform as the so-called cerebellar astrocytomas into astrocytomas and spongioblastomas of the cerebellum, as has been done by some authors.

INCIDENCE AND SITE

The cerebellar spongioblastomas show an incidence peak between 8–15 years (Fig. 5) and are thus essentially tumors of childhood and adolescence. The youngest patient successfully operated upon was eight months old. Of our 4,000 intracranial tumors, 187 were spongioblastomas of the cerebellum, i.e., 4.7%; 81 were males and 106 females. Their incidence in Cushing's series was 5%. They formed about one third of the cerebellar gliomas in Kernohan's series (1952).

They lie in the cerebellar midline but frequently expand into one or the other hemisphere.

The spongioblastomas of the cerebellum generally lie in the vermis, reach the size of a plum or a hen's egg, are well demarcated from the cerebellum, and can be separated from the cerebellar folia—where the correct plane of dissection can easily be found—like peeling an onion. Because of the manner in which they grow into the leptomeninges, they act as if they were encapsulated (Fig. 17, No. 5, 6; Fig. 32). The cysts, which are present in most cases, may exceed the size of the tumor many times and extend far into the cerebellar hemisphere; their walls often show brown pigmentation from hemorrhages. The consistency of the tumor is firm, or tough and elastic; only rarely is it softer, due to mucoid degeneration—and even then can it be distinguished from the medulloblastoma because of the latter's granular, soft structure.

The cerebellar forms have the typical structure of spongioblastomas; in rare instances they are calcified, as can be shown on X-ray. Not infrequently there are remnants of previous hemorrhages in the form of macrophages loaded with hemosiderin; the tendency to form Rosenthal fibers is particularly pronounced. The architecture of the perivascular cell cuffs can lead to confusion with ependymomas, especially when liquefaction of the tissue and separation of the cell clusters is advanced. Cerebellar spongioblastomas are biologically the most benign gliomas known. There are no recurrences following complete removal. The slowness of growth is well-demonstrated by the fact that occasionally a single evacuation of the cyst may leave the patient symptom-free for years (*see* footnote 1, p. 101).

The cases usually have a long history. Because of the obstructive hydrocephalus, they generally begin with signs of a general increase of intracranial pressure, with very little in the way of localizing signs from the vermis. Compared with medulloblastomas, however, symptoms of involvement of the cerebellar hemispheres are more common.

After prolonged growth without decompression, the tumor can extend rostrally and lead to compression of the collicular region. This results in the so-called cerebellar fits which indicate imminent danger to life.

Meningeal gliosis—astrocytosis of the cerebellar arachnoid

Schmincke (1924, 1925) and Oberling (1922, 1943) have described cases of spongioblastomas of the cerebellum and optic nerve in which the extension into the meninges exceeded that of the primary tumor. We have seen no cases in which such an additional classification would be necessary. Only one case of a diffuse spread into the meninges and beneath the pia could justifiably have been called a gliomatosis. However, most of that tumor had undergone mucoid degeneration and rather resembled a protoplasmic astrocytoma. It remained unclassified. O. T. Bailey (1936), Walker (1941), and Abbott and Glass (1955) have described leptomeningeal gliomas related to the astrocytoma group. They are derived from glial rests of the type described by Wolbach.

A kind of spongioblastoma is sometimes observed to arise from the nasal region (E. W. Davis, 1942; M. B. Schmidt: *Gliomas of the Nose.* 1900.)

3. THE OLIGODENDROGLIOMAS

(Synonyms: "Diffuse glioma," round cell sarcoma, sarcoma angiolithicum, gliome à *petites cellules rondes, oligodendroblastoma, and oligodendrocytoma.)*

HISTORICAL NOTE AND DEFINITION

The oligodendrogliomas, as a tumor type, were first predicted in 1924 by Bailey (Bailey and Hiller), and then described in 1926 with Cushing and in 1929 with Bucy. A large number of typical descriptions have appeared since then, though with little success as to defining the limits of this group, where atypical cases are more controversial. The differing percentages of oligodendrogliomas in the material of Cushing (1932), Foerster and Gagel (1938), Bailey (*see* Környey, 1937), Kernohan (1955), and in our own, demonstrates how the definition of this group varies, though the figures are gradually becoming more comparable. We have made an attempt, therefore, in 1941 and 1955, to define this group anew. H. J. Scherer (de Buscher and Scherer) also tried to delineate the oligodendrogliomas and astrocytomas. Numerous cases published can·still be recognized as oligodendrogliomas: Merzbacher and Uyeda; Landau; Bielschowsky (1914); Orzechowski and Kuligowski; Bodechtel; Scheinker (1938); Donat and others.
The fusiform oligodendrogliomas of Roussy and Oberling (1932), Hortega (1932), as well as Busch and Christensen (1937), correspond to our spongioblastomas.

Further references: Earnest, Kernohan, and McK. Craig; Greenfield and Robertson; Horrax and Wu; Környey (1937); Kwan and Alpers; Martin (1931); Reymond and Ringertz.

INCIDENCE AND SITE

The oligodendrogliomas are tumors of the middle decades with the peak of incidence falling between 35 and 40 years (Fig. 7). Only the oligodendrogliomas of the thalamus show a preference for the younger age group.

Our youngest patient with an oligodendroglioma was three, the oldest 68. The figures on incidence vary between the 1.3% of Cushing's, 1.6% of Gagel's, (Foerster), 5% of Kernohan's, and 7.8% of our own series. The average percentage of the different authors taken together is 3.1. Among the spinal tumors, Kernohan found 4.1% oligodendrogliomas. In our series of 4,000 cases, 174 were males and 138 females.

It has been possible to work out different subgroups of oligodendrogliomas according to their typical location. They lie especially frequently at the base of the second and third frontal convolutions (frontolateral). They may reach the size of an egg and invade the convolutions back above the Sylvian fissure and the underlying white matter (Fig. 17, No. 7; Fig. 35). The same subtype may lie more caudally, in the parietal gyri (parieto-lateral oligodendroglioma—Fig. 17, No. 8) but here it spreads subcortically or extends into the first temporal convolution. There are also parasagittal oligodendrogliomas located either in the frontal gyri bordering the sagittal fissure (fronto-medial oligodendroglioma)—Fig. 17, No. 9, Fig. 36, in the rostral corpus callosum and septum, or in the splenium of the corpus callosum (Fig. 17, No. 11). In the temporal lobe they infiltrate the gyri of the temporal pole (temporal oligodendrogliomas, Fig. 17, No. 10), from which place they can extend into the frontobasal or temporomedial (hippocampal) regions. In the occipital lobes they lie medially or occupy all of the cortex. A favorite location (although nearly always in children) is the thalamus (Fig. 17, No. 12), which may be expanded to the size of a small fist ("oligodendrogliomas of the brain stem") and from which place the tumors may extend on into the neighboring midbrain. Finally, oligodendrogliomas occur in the spinal cord and, apparently very seldom, in the cerebellum (one case of our own). In this last location they must not be confused with spongioblastomas undergoing mucoid degeneration. This is important, because regressive changes in spongioblastomas may give rise to architectural patterns confusingly similar to oligodendrogliomas. Conversely, oligodendrogliomas can contain spindle-cell "spongioblastic" portions.

APPEARANCE TO THE NAKED EYE

The oligodendrogliomas can often be specifically identified by their surface and manner of spread. They expand the cortex diffusely, making it appear hypertrophic (Figs. 35, 36), while the underlying white matter shows large and small mucoid cysts and necrosis. Small nodules sometimes occur in the cortex and can be recognized by the palpating finger or the eye of the surgeon. When the tumor breaks through the leptomeninges, it forms large lumps that project beyond the surface like bluish-red mushrooms. These types of oligodendrogliomas tend to adhere to the dura and

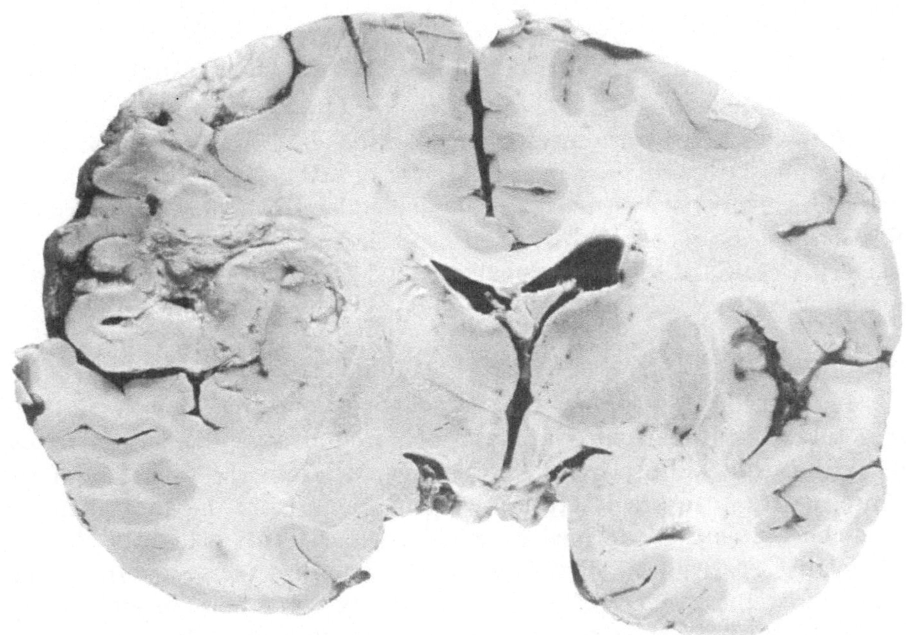

Fig. 35. Frontolateral oligodendroglioma at the foot of the third frontal convolution. The convolutions are infiltrated by the tumor, forming a garland-like pattern. Small cysts are formed in the depths of the white matter. Displacement to the opposite side. (Case 55)

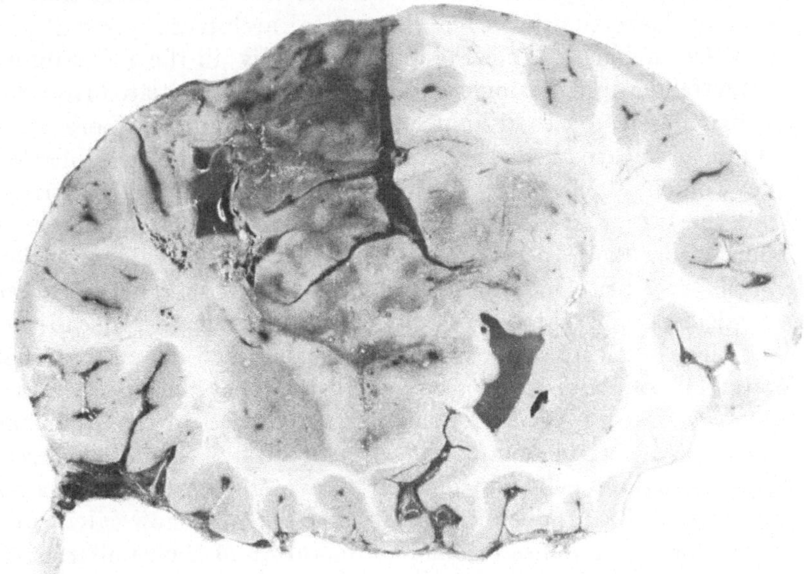

Fig. 36. Frontomedial oligodendroglioma growing along the convolutions of the longitudinal fissure. Through the infiltration of the corpus callosum and the septum, the tumor has spread to the opposite hemisphere. The convolutions are enlarged; in the depths there are small cysts. (Case 169)

are often first taken for a meningioma. To the surgeon, they appear either firm or moderately so, gray-red or the color of raw meat, friable or calcified, and occasionally necrotic in small parts. Oligodendrogliomas, after formalin fixation, can be recognized by their cross section which is gray-pink and velvety. Occasionally, large or small calcified granules can be felt that make a grating sound when cut with the knife.

HISTOLOGICAL APPEARANCE

In its typical portions, the oligodendroglioma has a very uniform structure: closely-packed, chromatin-rich, round cells, similar to normal oligodendroglia, diffusely infiltrate the cortex from the direction of the white matter. The architecture is very characteristic: the bare nuclei lie in a delicate network formed by small compartments of lightly stained, vacuolated spaces (so-called honeycomb structure, see Fig. 37a). This characteristic, however, often shows up only after paraffin embedding. The cells may even show a certain resemblance to plant cells. In occasional regions they may be more spindle-shaped (Fig. 34b), although the above described vacuolated pattern is still strongly suggested. In addition there are parts that contain carpets of large cells (Fig. 33c) which show considerable similarity to plump astrocytes and can be impregnated with gold sublimate. Here too, however, the typical architecture is still recognizable and the nucleus is typical of oligodendroglia: in the gold sublimate and other metallic impregnations, the cells can be differentiated from those of the astroglial series by their light, unimpregnated nuclei. There are also giant and multinucleated cells of all varieties but without any indication of malignancy (Zülch, 1955; 1956). The blood vessels are liberally distributed throughout the tumor, mostly as dense capillary networks in the growth zone. Their walls tend to undergo hyalinization. Typical networks of vascular coils may arise around small areas of necrosis. The vessel walls are often calcified, and patches of calcification also lie free in the tumor tissue. The blood vessels break easily, so that small and large hemorrhages are not rare. The oligodendrogliomas have a tendency to undergo mucoid and cystic degeneration in either small or large areas. On the other hand, fatty degeneration is uncommon. The remnants of engulfed cerebral parenchyma—ganglion cells, myelinated fibers, glia—persist for a long time. The adjacent brain, even if it is tumor-free, may show calcification, mostly in the form of a dense calcium encrustation of the capillaries. The oligodendrogliomas are often sharply separated from the surrounding brain. They proliferate into the arachnoid and distend it with mushroom-like growths, and from there grow onto the pachymeninges (see p. 96 ff.). In the marginal zone, there are often vessels showing small, round-cell infiltrations, possibly tumor cells. The rate of growth of these tumors is

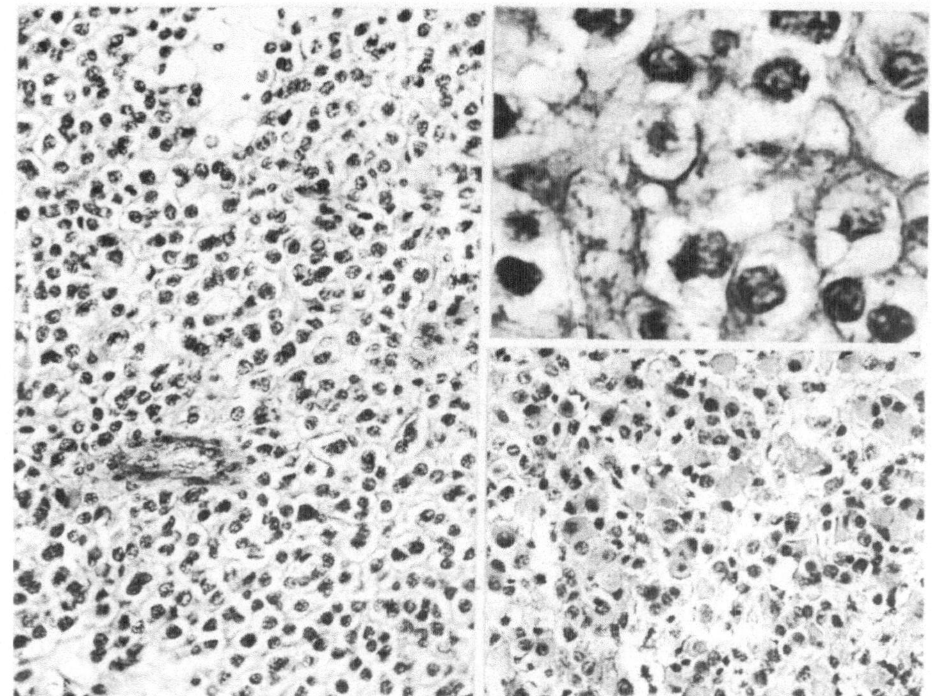

Fig. 37. a) *left:* A typical appearance of an oligodendroglioma in paraffin-embedded material; dark, bare nuclei lying in small vacuoles (honeycomb structure); in many vacuoles more than one nucleus is present. A small cyst has formed in one region (x160, H. & E. stain); b) *top right:* Higher magnification of Fig. (a). (x635); c) *bottom right:* Atypical appearance of an oligodendroglioma: cells with chromatin-rich, round nuclei and abundant cytoplasm lie in a similar net of vacuoles. (x140, H. & E. stain of paraffin material).

quite variable and typical mitoses are often seen. The tumor cells can accumulate around nerve cells (satellitosis).

METASTASIS AND RECURRENCE

Spontaneous metastasis via the cerebrospinal fluid does occur. Recurrences are frequent even after extensive removal as the oligodendrogliomas often grow in multiple foci, i.e., in many centers connected by thin bridges of neoplastic cells. Thus wide resection of whole lobes gives the best results. After some operations, a diffuse seeding throughout the whole cerebral and spinal C.S.F. space has occurred.

DIFFERENTIAL DIAGNOSIS

Differentiation between typical circumscribed astrocytomas and oligodendrogliomas is easy macroscopically. However, when oligodendrogliomas adhere to the pachymeninges, they are often confused with meningiomas.

We have already referred to the variability of the histological picture in oligodendrogliomas. The mixed forms should be searched for typical architectures, using either one large or several smaller sections. The differentiation from an *astrocytoma* which has undergone mucoid degeneration may frequently be accomplished by using the following rule of thumb: in relation to the delicate cystic network which is found in both tumors, the nuclei in the astrocytoma lie at the intersections, whereas those in the oligodendroglioma lie within the network's small compartments. In its large-cell portion too, the oligodendroglioma is similar to the astrocytoma. However, in the oligodendroglioma the nuclei have a vacuolated halo and remain recognizable as a light spot in the gold sublimate preparation. Calcification cannot serve as the *sine qua non* of the oligodendroglioma since, in our experience, only a small percentage (20%) of these tumors show calcification histologically, but its presence always speaks in favor of such a diagnosis. I must admit that the histological differential diagnosis between the oligodendroglioma and astrocytoma may be among the most troublesome ones. Distinguishing this tumor from the *glioblastoma* can also be difficult. The great amount of necrosis, the high degree of blood vessel reaction, the abundant proliferation, and particularly the occurrence of lacunar and sinusoidal vascular configurations, as well as the variegated appearance grossly and histologically are all in favor of the *glioblastoma*. Large hemorrhages can occur in both tumors. Study of only a small part of the tumor can make the differentiation from the *spongioblastoma* undergoing mucoid degeneration (*see* p. 138) extremely difficult; otherwise its typical architecture will always provide the key (note also the Rosenthal fibers). In addition, the vacuolated periphery of the cells and the greater cell density in the oligodendroglioma should be taken into account. According to our rule of thumb, the oligodendroglioma is a cellular tumor poor in fibers, whereas the spongioblastoma is poor in cells but rich in fibers *see* Fig. 34). Confusion with the acoustic neurinomas—because of the architectural similarity with regions showing fatty degeneration—or with chordomas should not occur. Finally, *ependymomas*—particularly those in the region of the foramen of Monro—may show an architecture very similar to that of the oligodendroglioma, especially if the wide nucleus-free halos around the blood vessels of the ependymoma are not apparent. The complete uniformity of ependymomas, however, the absence of honeycomb architecture, and the presence of blepharoplasts here provide the key for the identification of these tumors.

Relationships between tumor growth and the clinical picture. The diffuse permeation by the tumor of the otherwise preserved cortex seems to cause frequent focal seizures; the not infrequent massive hemorrhages into the tumor, particularly after such neurosurgical procedures as ventriculography or arteriography, can be explained by the hyalinization of the blood vessels and their pronounced calcification. Because of only moderate demands for space and little tendency to brain swelling, increased intra-cranial pressure occurs late.

Prognosis. Oligodendrogliomas belong to the comparatively benign gliomas; extensive operative removal may result in improvement for a period of three to five years, and under certain circumstances complete lobectomy may bring about a cure.

4. THE ASTROCYTOMAS

(*Synonyms: Glioma durum, spider-cell glioma, "Pinselzellgliom," star-cell glioma, astroma, amoeboid-cell glioma.*)

HISTORICAL NOTE AND DEFINITION

The astrocytomas were first described by Virchow (1863–1865) as the "glioma durum" and were among the first gliomas to be recognized. Other terms include the spider-cell glioma of Simon, astroma of v. Lenhossék, amoeboid giant-cell glioma of O. Lotmar, the fibrillary and protoplasmic astrocytomas, and astroblastomas of Bailey and Cushing (1926), the fibrillary, afibrillary and giganto-cellular astrocytoma of Roussy and Oberling (1932), and the piloid, gemistocytic and diffuse astrocytomas of Penfield (1932). H. J. Scherer (1933, 1935; de Buscher and Scherer) published a series of studies on astrocytomas (*see* also Historical Development of Classification). The history of astrocytoma study reflects that of gliomas in general.

The "astroblastomas" have been incorporated into the astrocytomas as a subgroup because their appearance, growth, content of glial fibers, and cell type seem to point to that group. Their biological behavior, too, corresponds to that of the astrocytomas (*see* also pp. 24–25). The astroblastomas are a group that can be described precisely in terms of their architecture and cell type, and are relatively benign in character. However, to diagnose any glioma (particularly a glioblastoma) in which a few astroblast-like cells occur as an astroblastoma is by no means justified. This particular misinterpretation is frequently encountered in the literature.

The so-called cerebellar astrocytomas are described with the spongio-blastomas, to which they belong according to their localization, appearance, growth, cell-type and biological behavior (*see* p. 23, 139). As regards the "subependymal astrocytomas" (astrocytome sousépendymaire), *see* ventricular tumors in Tuberous Sclerosis (pp. 44, 169).

The third group of glioblastomas described by Busch and Christensen (1947) belongs rather to the large-cell astrocytomas. Kernohan (1949) grouped astrocytomas (as grades 1 and 2) together with glioblastomas (as grades 3 and 4).

Further references: Alpers and Rowe; Bailey and Bucy (1930); Bergstrand (1932, 1933); Foerster and Gagel (1939); H. J. Scherer (1933, 1935); de Buscher and Scherer; Teltscharow and Zülch; Waggoner and Löwenberg (1937, 1939).

INCIDENCE AND SITE

Astrocytomas occur predominantly in middle age, where the peak of incidence falls rather precisely around 35 years (Fig. 6). Our youngest patient was four years old, the oldest 67. 166 of our series of 4,000 cases were males, and 117 were females. The astrocytoma, as above defined, comprised 7.1% of our material; in Cushing's series 9.8% of cases were either astrocytomas of the cerebral hemispheres, or astroblastomas.

From other series of cases, the pertinent figures have to be derived, since the so-called cerebellar astrocytomas were included.

The astrocytomas lie predominantly over the convexity of the brain and we recognize the following types: frontodorsal astrocytomas of the first and second frontal convolutions that grow deep in the direction of the anterior horn, often containing a large cyst (Fig. 18, No. 2, and Fig. 17, Nos. 13–16); frontomedial astrocytomas that extend into the white matter from the frontal pole along the first frontal convolution and the medial gyri, often infiltrating and expanding the septum (Fig. 18, No. 12; Fig. 17, Nos. 14, 17); frontolateral astrocytomas in the laterobasal convolutions directly under the third frontal gyrus, with spread into the frontal white matter and an occasional formation of a large cyst (Fig. 18, No. 6; Fig. 17, Nos. 15, 18)—a finger-like extension usually reaches into the white matter of the insula; diffuse frontal astrocytomas of the whole frontal white matter (Fig. 17, No. 22) that may grow through the corpus callosum to the opposite side. The astroblastoma is often encountered in the frontal portion of the cingulate gyrus (Fig. 17, No. 19). There are, furthermore, astrocytomas of the temporal poles (Fig. 17, No. 21) that grow occipitalward through the white matter or penetrate into the basal region of the frontal lobes and medially into the basal ganglia; parietolateral astrocytomas (Fig. 17, No. 20; Figs. 38, 39), precentral or postcentral, with spread in the direction of the ventricular wall, and frequently with large cysts; parasagittal tumors, often reaching the mesial surface of the brain (parietomedial astrocytomas); astrocytomas of the thalamus, often bilateral (Fig. 17, No. 23); astrocytomas of the midbrain; the pons (Fig. 17, No. 24, Fig. 40) and the spinal cord. A break-down, according to regions, of our 52 cases—studied by large sections—showed that frontal astrocytomas were most common (26 cases), followed by temporal (16) and centroparietal astrocytomas (10), with only sporadic occurrences in other regions.

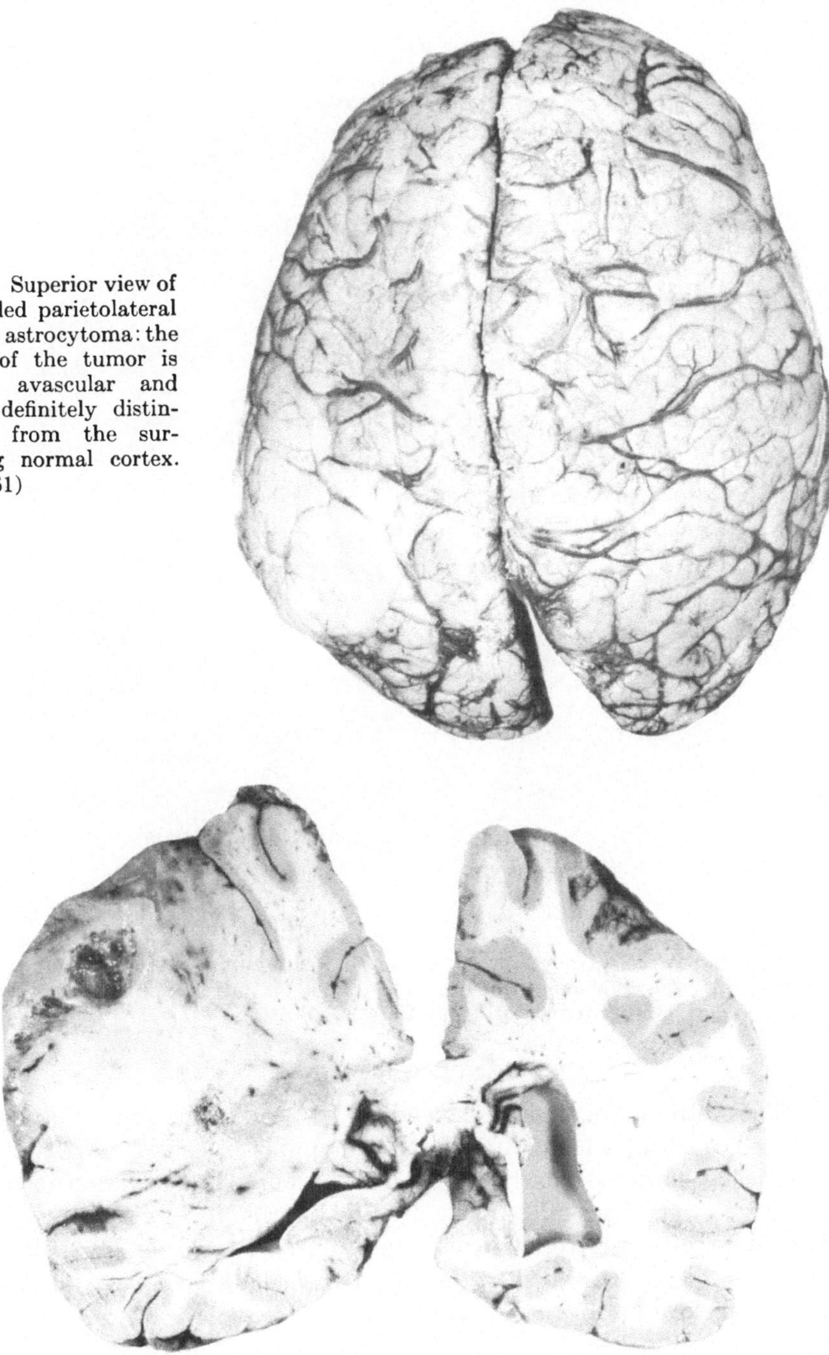

Fig. 38. Superior view of a left-sided parietolateral fibrillary astrocytoma: the surface of the tumor is whitish, avascular and can be definitely distinguished from the surrounding normal cortex. (Case 261)

Fig. 39. Cross-section through a right parietolateral astrocytoma. The tumor reaches from the surface to the wall of the trigonum where it has degenerated, forming a meshwork of small cysts. (Case 497)

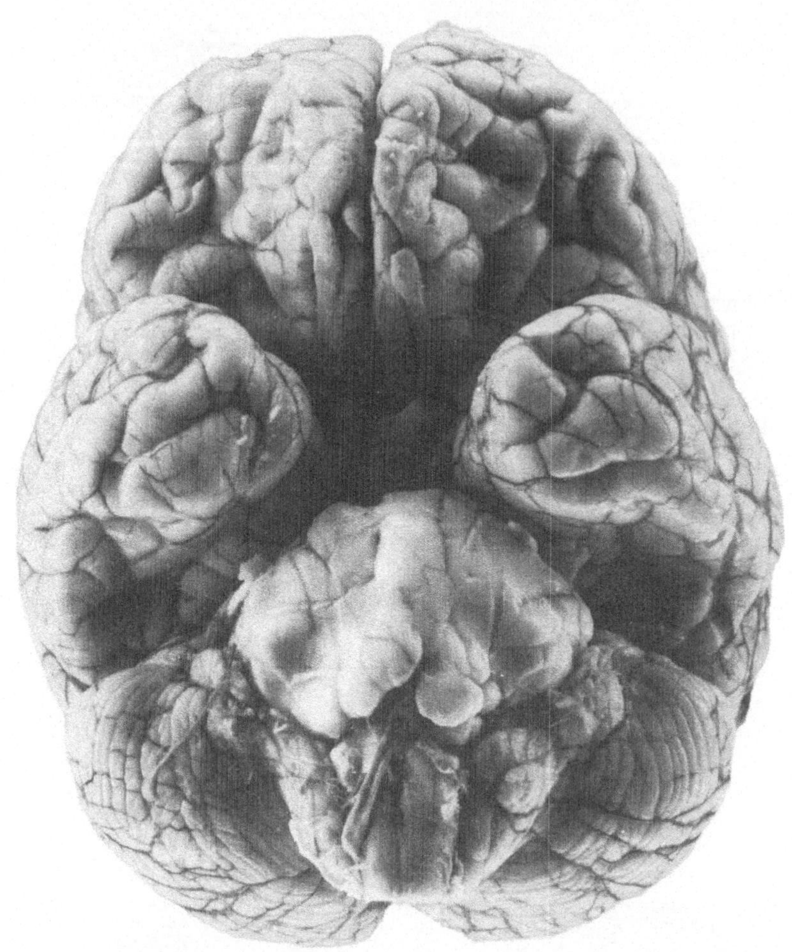

Fig. 40. Large astrocytoma of the pons, extending in a lobulated fashion over the surface. Bilateral cerebellar pressure cone. Signs of increased intracranial pressure (flattened gyri, obliterated sulci). (Case 270)

APPEARANCE TO THE NAKED EYE

The astrocytomas are—depending on their subtype—sharply circumscribed, firm, whitish tumors, cartilaginous in consistency, that grow superficially either diffusely or like a mushroom. Degeneration into small and large cysts often takes place in their depths, in which case their consistency is softer. Astroblastomas can often be recognized by their degeneration into small uniform cysts, i.e., their spongy cut surface. Astrocytomas vary from apple to chestnut size.

HISTOLOGICAL APPEARANCE

At present we distinguish four histological subtypes: fibrillary, protoplasmic, and gigantocellular astrocytomas, and the so-called astro-

150

blastomas[4]. Of these types the fibrillary forms are the most common, the protoplasmic the least, while the gigantocellular astrocytomas and the astroblastomas occur in about equal numbers and fall in the middle. The gigantocellular forms occur particularly often in the frontal lobes, the protoplasmic in the temporal lobes, and the fibrillary in both with about the same frequency. The astroblastomas are distributed about equally over all regions.

The astrocytomas usually consist mainly of one of the recognized astrocyte types, but really pure forms are rare. The gigantocellular astrocytomas may possibly develop from fibrillary and protoplasmic types through degeneration. The circumscribed astrocytomas grow infiltratingly at their margin, but there is considerable cell proliferation in their center, "from within out," so that they grow by expansion as well. The rarer diffuse forms permeate the brain substance uniformly and expand it only little, so that at first they can be distinguished from brain swelling only by their consistency.

The cells of astrocytomas generally have middle-sized, round, or kidney-shaped nuclei centrally placed with a moderate amount of chromatin (Fig. 41a). Only in the gigantocellular types are the nuclei hyperchromatic (pyknotic) and eccentrically located (Fig. 42b). The cellularity of the astrocytomas is not great, the cells are uniformly distributed, and mitoses—an indication of rapid growth—are extremely rare. The cell body is of variable size: hardly visible (Fig. 41a), medium sized or large as in giant cells (Fig. 42b). The name of each subtype is determined by the predominating cell type.

The fibrillary types, the astroblastomas, and a portion of the gigantocellular astrocytomas form abundant glial fibers, giving the tumor its firm consistency (Fig. 41b, c). The astroblastomas show a unique architecture (Fig. 42a), i.e., the astroblastomatous cells are arranged radially around the numerous, uniformly-spaced blood vessels. This characteristic is most obvious at the growth zone where finger-like vascular buds, wrapped in a mantle of tumor cells, grow out of the tumor.

Blood vessels are rare in the fibrillary types and consist of capillaries only (Fig. 41a). The astroblastomas have a uniform network of blood vessels whose walls show fibrous thickening, a characteristic feature of the architecture of this tumor (Fig. 42a); coiled, tortuous, "reduplicated" vessels occur in the gigantocellular types. All astrocytomas, with the exception of the diffuse type, tend towards mucoid transformation with resulting cyst formation; the fibrillary and gigantocellular astrocytomas form large solitary cysts, while in astroblastomas the tissue between the

[4] We hope in the future to be able to divide the astrocytomas consistently into these subgroups: large-and small-cell fibrillary, and large-and small-cell afibrillary types.

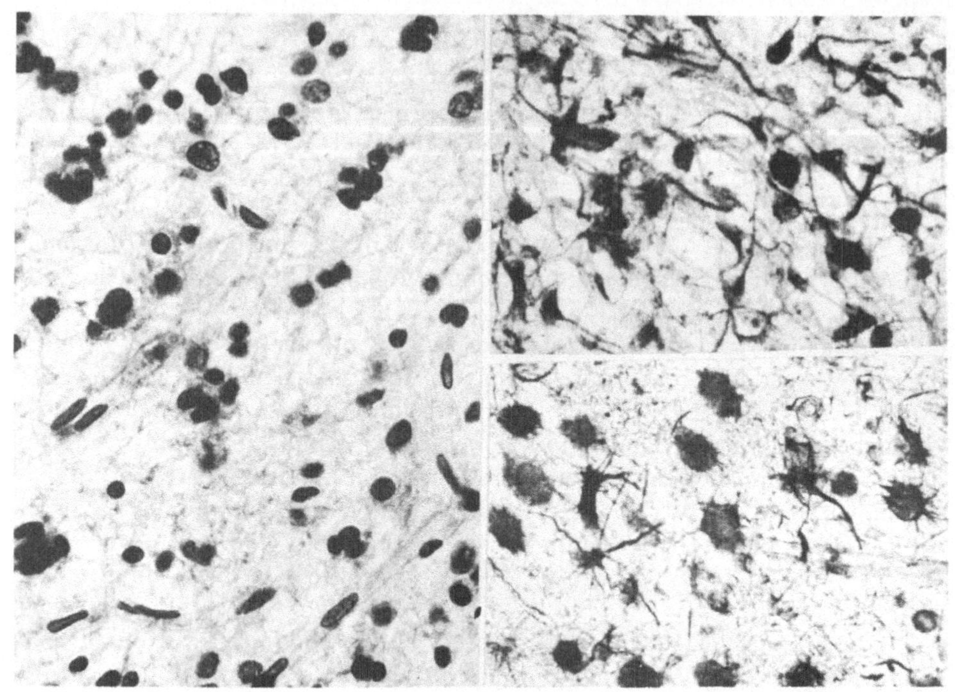

Fig. 41. a) *left:* Typical appearance of a fibrillary astrocytoma in chromatic stain: astrocytic nuclei are single or grouped in small clusters; in the ground substance there is fine network of fibers. The blood vessels are normal capillaries. (x270, Nissl stain); b) *top right:* and c) *bottom right:* Tumor cells of astrocytoma on metallic impregnation. Small and large and occasionally plump cells with starlike processes. A few vascular feet going to capillaries are seen. (x250, gold sublimate impregnation)

persisting blood vessels tends to degenerate into a network of tiny cysts. Calcification is rare, necrosis is almost always absent; hemorrhages into the tumor substance are unknown. The presence of fat is limited to single gitter cells, found mostly around the blood vessels. The four types previously described may occasionally merge. Further variation in tissue type is rare. However, a not inconsiderable group of cases (about 10% of the tumors studied by us) show malignant propensities, often even a gradual transformation into glioblastoma. The incidence rate increases with the increased use in investigations of cross sections of the entire tumor (astrocytoma malignum).

In one of our autopsy cases is was possible to demonstrate the coexistence of a circumscribed, firm astrocytoma, the size of a small fist, and, next to it, of its diffuse spread—obviously having occurred later—into the whole brain. While the histological picture in the circumscribed firm part was that of a benign acellular fibrous astrocytoma, the picture in the regions of diffuse spread—where necrosis was present as well—was clearly

152

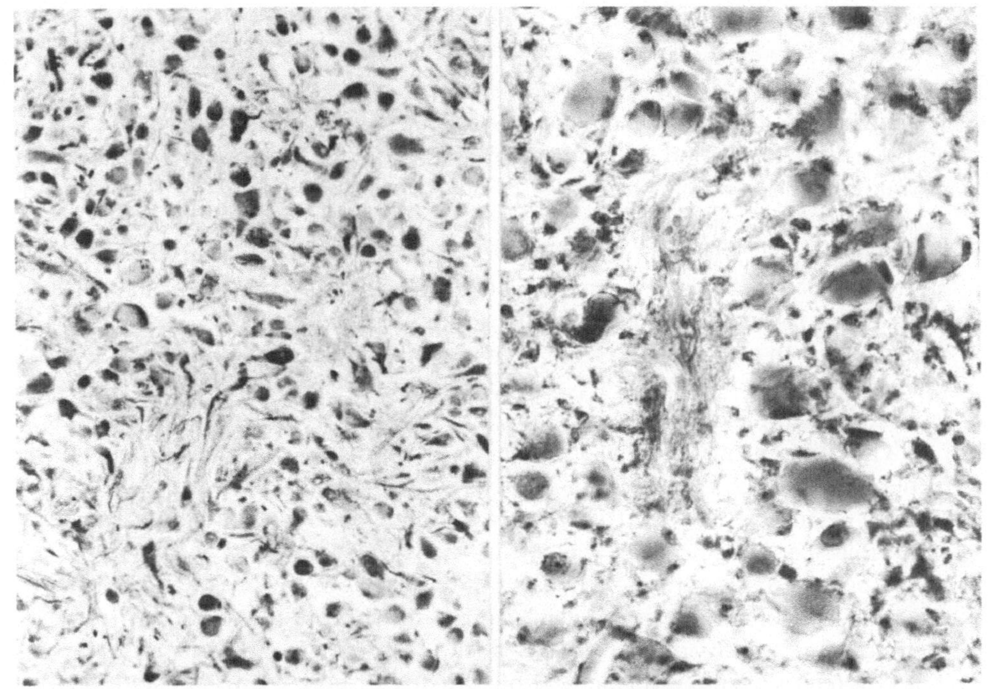

Fig. 42. a) *left:* Cell types of a subtype of astrocytoma, which has been earlier designated as "astroblastoma," are arranged radially or tangentially on the blood vessels. (x100, gold sublimate impregnation); b) *right:* Gigantocellular astrocytoma. Large cells contain pyknotic, often eccentric nuclei. (x112, Nissl stain)

that of a gigantocellular pleomorphic glioblastoma, with marked involvement of the blood vessels (*see* Teltscharow and Zülch, 1948).

DIFFERENTIAL DIAGNOSIS

A demonstration of glioblastoma characteristics is important for the recognition of "malignant" astrocytomas.

At operation, numerous large fistulous vessels filled with arterial blood (Tönnis, 1938), and numerous areas of necrosis in its depths speak in favor of glioblastoma. In the autopsy specimen, glioblastoma is characterized by its variegated appearance with hemorrhages, necrosis, and fatty degeneration, as well as by engorged blood vessels in the marginal zone of the tumor and its immediate vicinity. Histologically, the following count in favor of a glioblastoma: 1) cellularity, multinucleation, pleomorphism, disorganized pattern, lack of glial fiber formation, mitoses and other signs of rapid growth; 2) wild proliferation of the vascular stroma and formation of vascular loops and aggregates—glomeruli—sinusoidal spaces, and thrombosis; 3) frequent dissolution of the parenchyma and tumor substance by necrosis, bounded by barriers of blood vessels and gitter cells and, 4) absence of calcification.

In favor of the astrocytoma is 1) sparcity of cells, orderly cell structure and pattern, formation of glial fibers, absence of mitoses and of an abnormal nucleus-cytoplasm ratio; 2) no, or only a slight degeneration of the invaded tissue (which takes place by cyst formation, if at all); 3) few blood vessels with uniform structure and distribution, without evidence of proliferation, and 4) absence of necrosis and fatty degeneration, with a tendency towards mucoid degeneration and cyst formation. In order to differentiate an astrocytoma from a simple gliosis on a biopsy, the use of the Holzer stain may be recommended; this shows a very acellular fibrous feltwork in the simple gliosis—something that does not usually occur in tumors.

The differentiation from oligodendroglioma, too, occasionally presents difficulties, though this decision is not so important at operation since both tumors belong to the "relatively benign gliomas." Oligodendrogliomas can sometimes be recognized by the cortical nodules (which can be either seen or palpated), astrocytomas by their circumscribed firmness. Moreover, oligodendrogliomas not infrequently grow mushroom-like into the leptomeninges and are attached to the dura, thus resembling meningiomas. They frequently undergo calcification which can be recognized roentgenologically or by the palpating finger or an instrument. After fixation the surface of oligodendrogliomas is velvety, finely granulated, and grayishpink; that of astrocytomas is smoother, glassy, lardy and yellowish. The cortex in astrocytoma is expanded in a spherical fashion, while in oligodendroglioma individual convolutions are invaded, and look hypertrophic, resulting in a finger-like pattern. Histological differentiation of an oligodendroglioma from an astrocytoma with mucoid degeneration may be difficult. Aside from the degree of cellularity, the rule of thumb can be used that in the astrocytoma the cell nuclei lie at the intersection of the cytoplasmic strands, whereas in the oligodendroglioma they lie inside the vacuoles. Calcification always speaks in favor of oligodendrogliomas, since it only occasionally occurs in astroblastomas.

METASTASIS AND RECURRENCE

Astrocytomas do not metastasize; recurrences always follow incomplete removal, particularly in the diffuse forms. Small circumscribed astrocytomas can be radically removed with lasting cure. Small astroblastomas also seem to have quite a good prognosis. The "malignant astrocytoma" carries a bad prognosis.

5. THE MALIGNANT GLIOBLASTOMAS

(*Synonyms: Glioblastoma, spongioblastoma multiforme, polymorphic glioma, gliosarcoma, "Buntes Gliom;" a large part of the glioma telangiectaticum and the glioma apoplecticum group belongs to the glioblastoma, a smaller part to the oligodendroglioma.*)

HISTORICAL NOTE AND DEFINITION

The malignant glioblastomas were recognized by Virchow (1863, 1865) as gliomatous tumors and can be found in each of the earlier classifications of brain tumors under the name of "variegated", "hemorrhagic" glioma, glioma apoplecticum and telangiectaticum, or under the general term of "gliosarcoma." Around the turn of the century a widespread controversy arose over the nature of this neuroepithelial tumor type. Beginning with the name of the tumor itself, the argument went on to the question of the sarcomatous component of this tumor, which up to then had been considered gliomatous. This controversy, despite some attempts to revive it, can be considered settled, since it has been possible to separate a true sarcoma from tumors previously considered glioblastomas (*see* Sarcoma monstrocellulare, p. 206). The modern histogenetic approach began with Strauss and Globus (1918), who deserve credit for the description of this group, and with Bailey and Cushing (1926). Glioblastomas appear in the works of Roussy and Oberling (1932) as "polymorphic gliomas," in Hortega's (1932) along with the "isomorphic" gliomas. Grades 3 and 4 of Kernohan's (1949) astrocytomas correspond to the glioblastomas. Three histological subtypes of the malignant glioblastoma are well-known— globuliform, fusiform, and multiform. It has been definitely confirmed, however, that despite marked cytological differences the biological behavior of this immature glial tumor is quite uniform, as evidenced by the common histological features of fatty degeneration, necrosis, hemorrhages and pronounced reaction and involvement of the connective tissue.

Busch and Christensen's (1947) proposed subdivision into angionecrotic, multicellular, and magnocellular subtypes seems to us of little advantage since the criteria on which it is based vary. Moreover, the magnocellular type seems to deviate from the usual picture of glioblastoma in regard to macroscopic appearance, histology, and biological behavior; thus it destroys the uniformity of the group. The "magnocellular glioblastoma" corresponds largely to our large-celled (or to some of our malignant) astrocytomas. The subdivision of Davis, Martin *et al.* into angioproliferative and angiothrombotic glioblastoma, furthermore, is not based on any really essential characteristic in our experience.

Further references: Bergstrand (1933); Hasenjäger (1938, 1939); Netsky, August and Fowler; Perria and Sacchi; Schiefer and Udvarhelyi; Udvarhelyi, Walter, and Schiefer.

INCIDENCE AND SITE

The incidence of glioblastomas in various age groups is rather clear. They occur only rarely in the young, becoming more frequent after the age of 30, and having a definite incidence peak around the ages of 48–52

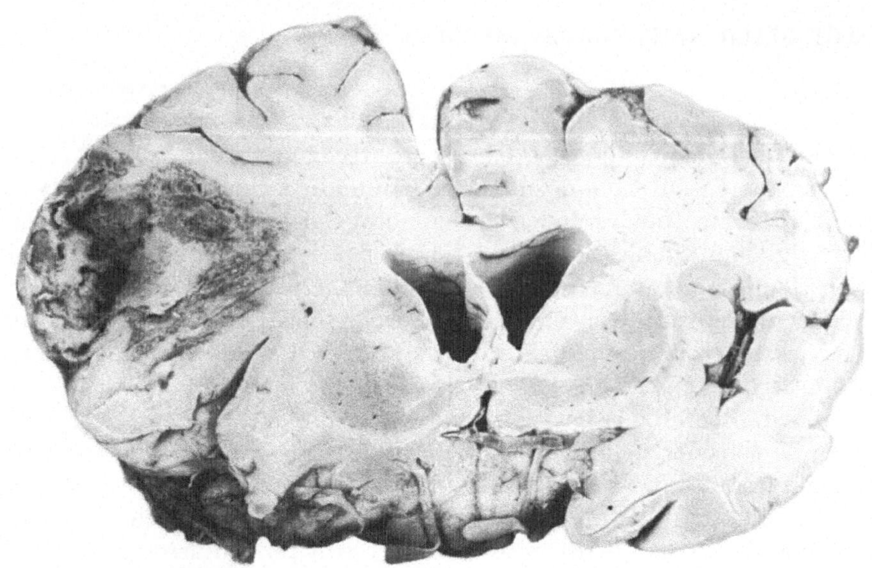

Fig. 43. Frontolateral glioblastoma. The tumor is wedge-shaped (similar to an nfarct) and is necrotic in the center. There is intense brain swelling. (Case 132)

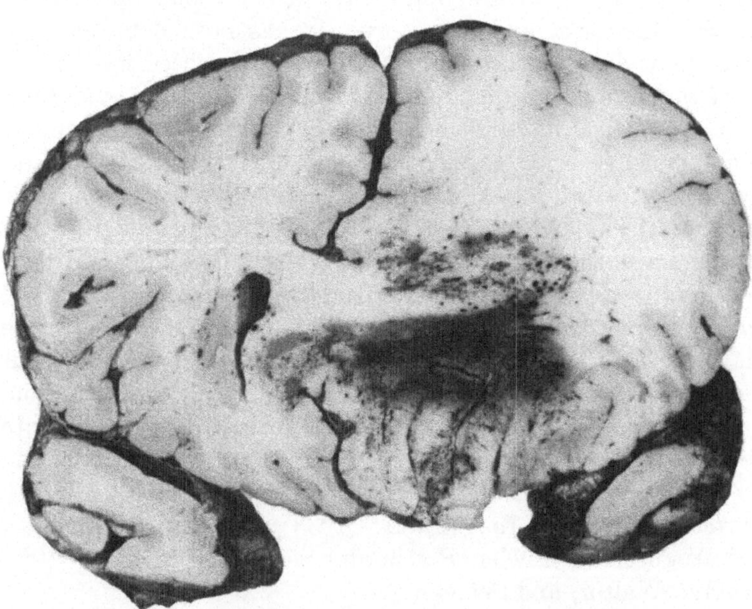

Fig. 44. Frontobasal glioblastoma infiltrating the gyrus rectus and the adjacent gyri and spreading through the frontal white matter. Intense brain swelling. There is a certain similarity to the "hemorrhagic infarct," due to numerous engorged vessels. The splitting of the white matter overlying the orbital convolutions is an artefact. (Case 365)

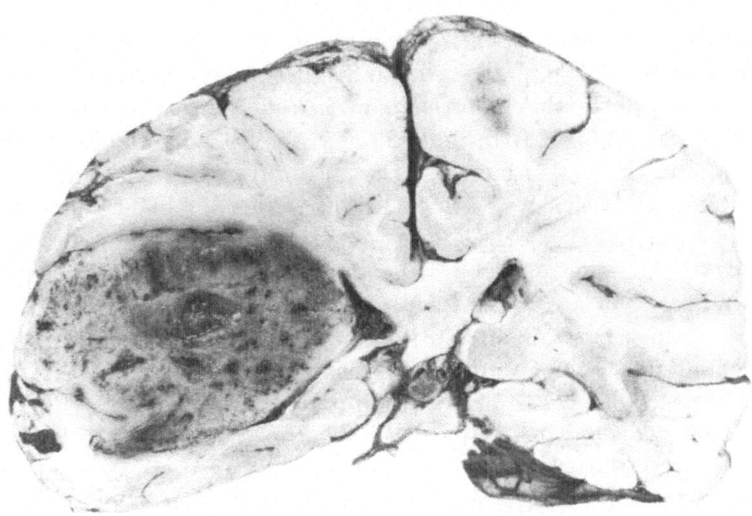

Fig. 45. Temporolateral glioblastoma which extends from the cortex over to the trigonum. Displacement of the midbrain and pineal gland. Inside the tumor are small hemorrhages and cysts. The tumor is sharply delineated from the surrounding tissue. (Case 159)

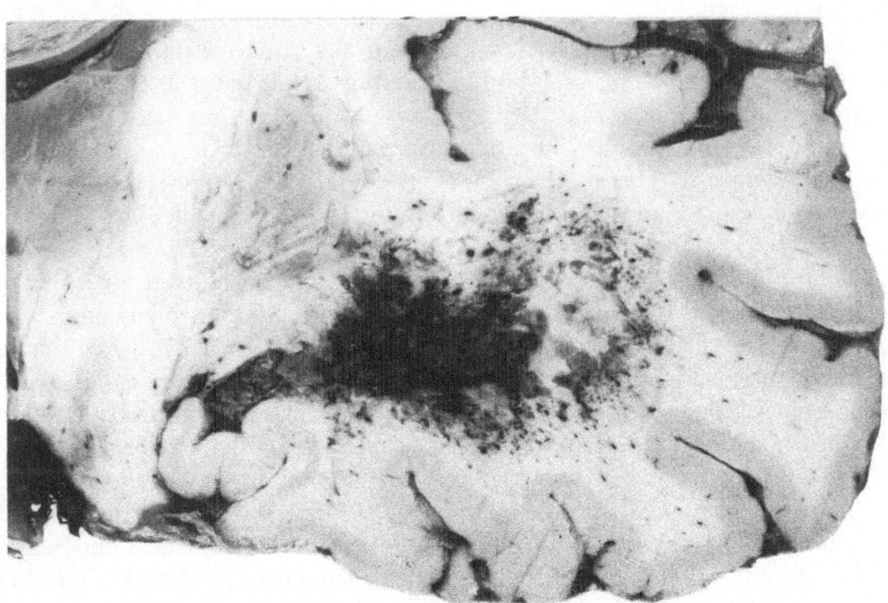

Fig. 46. Close-up of a glioblastoma with central necrosis and a zone of marginal engorged vessels which can be demonstrated well on arteriogram. (Case 158)

(*see* Fig. 8). Our youngest patient was seven, the oldest 78. The glioblastomas constituted 13.1% of all intracranial tumors in our material. In Bailey and Cushing's series they represented 10.3%, Foerster and Gagel's, 15%, and in that of Davis, Martin *et al.*, 29.5%. We find the highest incidence—37% of all intracranial tumors—in the material of Elsberg and co-workers, and in Bennett's series, with 22.9%. In our series of 4,000 tumors, 354 were men, 176 women.

For the glioblastomas, too, it is now possible to point to various sites of preference: they are found in frontolateral location (the size of a hen's egg), in the third frontal convolution (*see* Fig. 17, No. 27 and Fig. 43), and in the subcortical white matter; in frontodorsal location in the first and second convolutions reaching to the tip of the anterior horn (Fig. 17, No. 26); and in frontobasal location in the gyrus rectus and in the adjacent basolateral convolutions, from where they occasionally spread through the corpus callosum to the opposite side (Fig. 17, Nos. 25, 28; Fig. 44). More caudally, we find them in parietolateral location, extending subcortically from the foot of the third frontal convolution (Fig. 17, No. 30) through the middle and inferior part of the pre- and postcentral gyri into the inferior part of the parietal lobe; and in the parietodorsal region, likewise subcortical, originating in the foot of the first and second frontal convolutions (Fig. 17, No. 29), but this time extending through the superior third of the pre- and postcentral gyri into the superior parietal lobe. In the temporal lobe we recognize 1) the temporolateral and 2) the temporomedial glioblastoma. The temporolateral glioblastoma extends from the temporal tip, through the first and second convolutions, and through all of the white matter of the lobe (Fig. 17, No. 31; Fig. 45). While the medial convolutions in this instance remain tumor free, they are particularly affected in the temporomedial glioblastoma, (Fig. 17, No. 32). The main bulk of the tumor lies in the neighboring white matter, with extensions spreading to the pole and the occipital lobe. Glioblastomas of the occipital lobe lie either occipitolateral or occipitobasal and can grow across to the opposite side, through the posterior portion of the corpus callosum; these types, however, have not been too clearly characterized. Certain glioblastomas loop from the frontal into the temporal lobe (Fig. 17, No. 33). They may spread in butterfly pattern from the corpus callosum into the depths of the white matter, bilaterally, as "anterior or posterial callosal glioblastomas" (Fig. 17, Nos. 34, 35). Or they may infiltrate the white matter on one side only as a glioblastoma of the anterior (Fig. 17, No. 37) or posterior (Fig. 17, No. 38) callosal radiation. Or, finally, they can grow along the fornix (Fig. 17, No. 36), particularly in its frontal, parietal, or temporal portions. Glioblastomas are also found in the thalamus (Fig. 17, No. 39), but rarely in the region of the quadrigeminal plate (Fig. 17, No.

40), and only exceptionally in the pons and the spinal cord; they have never been verified in the cerebellum.[5] Generally speaking, glioblastomas spread subcortically; on frontal section they appear wedge-shaped, like an infarct (Fig. 43). But they can also—especially in the temporal and occipital regions—assume a cylindrical form and extend along the long axis of the lobe. The almost "photographic" likeness which two tumors may have was explained by their origin from certain "trouble spots" beside the ventricles (Ostertag, 1936, 1941).

APPEARANCE TO THE NAKED EYE

The variegated color which all glioblastomas, despite their cytological variations, have in common is explained by the necroses (gray), fatty degenerations (yellow, ochre-yellow), and hemorrhages in various stages (brown to red), (Figs 43, 45). These variously-hued regions with their geographical-like borders (Fig. 43) alternate in the depths of the tumor with undegenerated marginal zones which appear more white, yellowish, and glassy. Occasionally, glioblastomas resemble a "necrotizing inflammation" of the brain (Fig. 44). The tumor can not frequently be identified from the surface of the brain, since it grows in the white matter and the convolutions are only widened and flattened—as with other gliomas—and the necroses revealed only when the brain is cut. Dilated blood vessels (Fig. 46), with lumens sometimes as large as a knitting needle, surround many of the tumors or their peripheral zones; only a few of the vessels are thrombosed. They represent the surrounding lacunar vessels and form a specifically recognizable pattern on the arteriogram. Taken as a group, the glioblastomas are often unusually well-circumscribed for gliomas.

HISTOLOGICAL APPEARANCE

The recognized subtypes include the small round cell, spindle cell, and giant cell pleomorphic types (Figs 47, 48), depending on which cell-type predominates.[6] On the whole, the glioblastomas tend to grow along the fiber tracts or the vascular pathways, with an occasional approximation to the streaming architectural pattern of spongioblastomas. Regressive changes result in secondary architectural patterns, such as perivascular cell cuffs (Figs. 25b, 48b), and a pseudopalisading around necrosis (Fig. 23d). Reactive processes lead to "tertiary" histological patterns, such as blood vessel proliferation with subsequent dense networks of blood

---

[5] It is an interesting fact that the two malignant neuroepithelial tumors have mutually exclusive sites: the medulloblastoma occurs only in the cerebellum, the glioblastoma only in the remaining portions. These two tumors are almost mutually exclusive with regard to age incidence as well.

[6] These types correspond to the subdivision referred to above: 1) globuliform, microcellular (Gagel) or protoplasmatic (Bergstrand); 2) fusiform; 3) multiform.

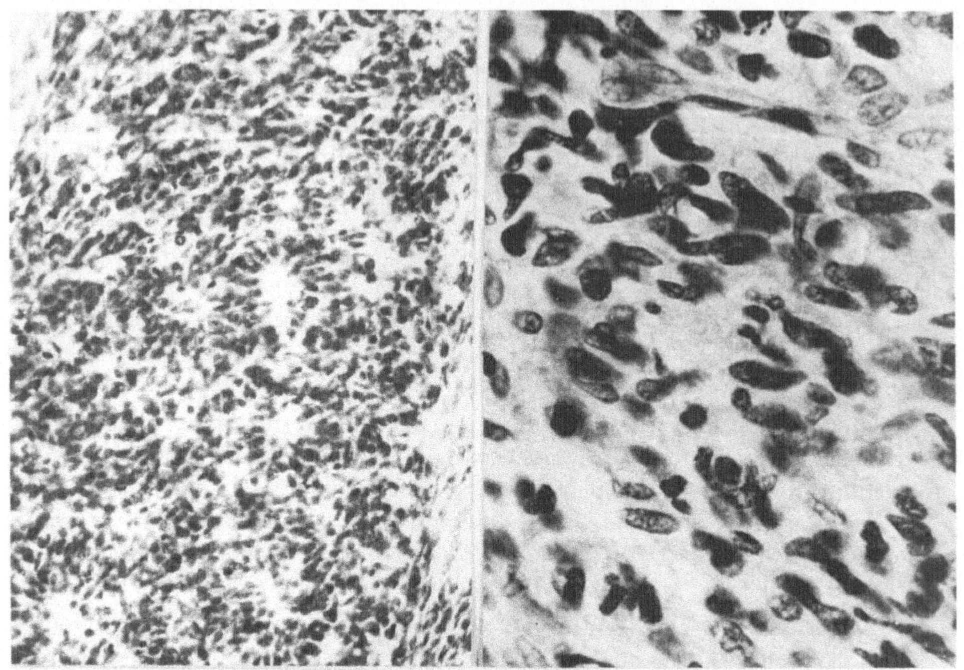

Fig. 47. a) *left:* Small-cell glioblastoma containing predominantly isomorphic round cells and only a few chromatin-rich giant cells. Numerous mitoses. (x120, Nissl stain); b) *right:* Spindle-cell glioblastoma with occasional giant cells and numerous mitoses. (x480, Nissl stain)

vessels (Fig. 26c). Glioblastomas seem to grow from the depths upward toward the cortex; they occasionally permeate and engulf the lepto-meninges. The surrounding brain sometimes shows a progressive astro-cytic gliosis.

The tumor cells of the three mentioned subtypes produce scarcely any glial fibers. The (fusiform) spindle cell types are most common; they contain only scattered giant cells which, naturally, occur most often in the multiform type. The rarest are the round-cell glioblastomas, and they may occasionally be confused with oligodendrogliomas. The speed of growth in all three types is considerable, with a corresponding number of mitotic figures. The connective tissue in glioblastomas is very prominent (*see* p. 93 ff.). Large lacunar vessels, of predominantly venous type, lie in the mantle zone of the tumor or in the immediately adjacent brain. In the marginal zones there are numerous vascular coils and loops (Fig. 26b) which, as part of the reactive process, occur with great frequency and regularity along the margin of necrosis (Fig. 26a). We can distinguish a number of different forms of vascular reaction: 1) capillary networks; 2) barriers of vessels around the margin of necrosis; 3) proliferation of the intima and adventitia of the indigenous blood vessels; 4) large, recon-

160

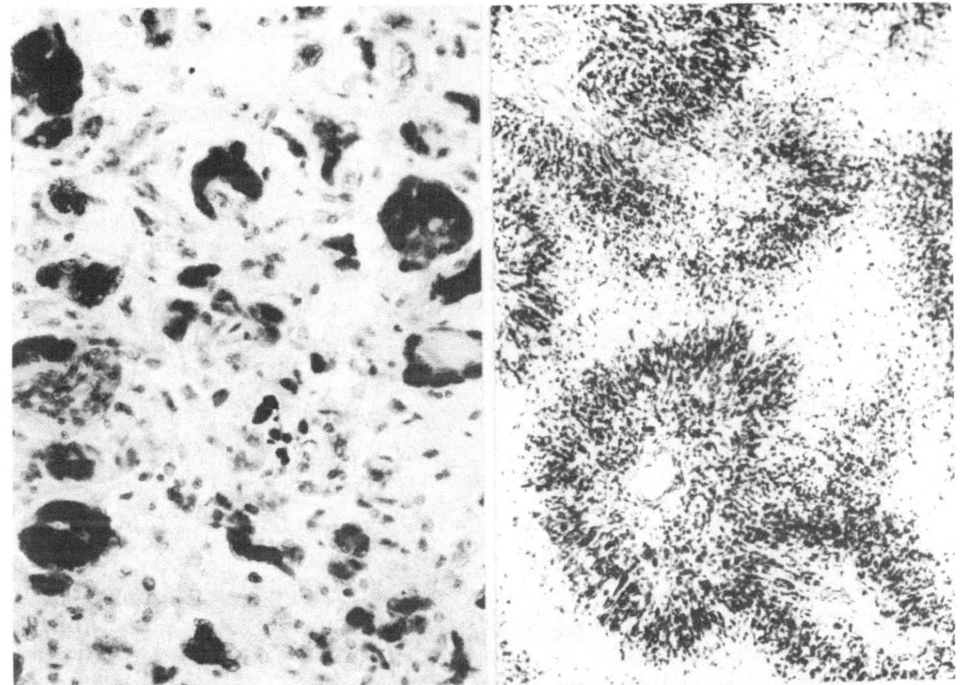

Fig. 48. a) *left:* Giant-cell glioblastoma with numerous hyperchromatic multinucleated cells, atypical mitoses, and vascular proliferation. (x150, Nissl stain); b) *right:* Numerous necroses in a predominantly spindle-cell glioblastoma. Cuffs of cells around blood vessels due to favorable nutrition in these regions. (x78, Nissl stain)

stituted blood vessels with endovascular proliferation (Fig. 26c); 5) remnants of larger vessels with outgrowth of fibroblasts from their walls, and 6) ectatic middle-sized to large blood vessels, indigenous or newly-formed, which form fistulous dilatations and lacunar sinusoids. The blood vessels within the tumor have a great tendency to thrombotic occlusion. Whole regions of the tumor thus undergo regressive fatty degeneration. Particularly striking are the layers of compound granular corpuscles at the margins of necrotic areas (Fig. 48b). The connective tissue forms part of the blood vessels and also participates in the reparative organization of the necrotic regions by the formation of collagenous or reticulin-fiber scars. Cyst formation is rare, and calcification an exception. The excessive proliferation of the blood vessel walls and the high degree of ectasia of the giant lacunar vessels seem to be responsible for the fragility of the blood vessel walls, and the consequent occurrence of small and large hemorrhages. Glioblastomas spread purely by infiltration, and the permeated tissues together with the tumor undergo necrosis quickly. Even after total extirpation, glioblastomas customarily recur within one year at the latest, and end fatally. Metastases take place by way of the cerebrospinal fluid (small ependymal nodules or implants along the ventricles, which may reach the size of a cherry, but are never diffuse as in medulloblastomas), but they seem to be able to spread by other pathways as well. How the rare cases of multifocal glioblastoma occur is not quite known (for instance, tumors in the second and third frontal convolutions and occipital lobe without any connecting bridges, as in four of our own cases). The glioblastomas have the dreaded tendency to produce brain swelling with a high degree of expansion of the adjacent white matter. Even with small tumors the size of a plum, this process can progress to the point of diffuse swelling of the whole hemisphere, something which is seen to a similar degree only with metastases and monstrocellular sarcomas. We have never seen distant metastases.

GROWTH AND CLINICAL PICTURE

The clinical picture can be explained by the tumor's great rapidity of growth (accounting for the short clinical history), and the frequently tremendous expansion of the tumor (causing hemiplegia). Hemorrhages and thromboses of large vessels are related to the tendency to apoplectiform episodes. The markedly elevated intracranial pressure is accounted for by the associated cerebral swelling which often spreads to involve the entire hemisphere.

DIFFERENTIAL DIAGNOSIS

Identification of this tumor on sectioning the fixed brain is easy: the variegated color and the numerous necrotic regions settle the problem clearly. More difficult is the histological differentiation from astrocytoma and oligodendroglioma when studying a very small region, or the marginal zone, or when only a biopsy is available. The oligodendroglioma is nearly always more cellular than the glioblastoma. The way to distinguish these three tumors from one another has already been presented under astrocytomas (p. 153). At operation the surgeon will often recognize the true nature of the tumor only when he encounters necrosis in its depths, or when he recognizes the characteristic fistulous blood vessels containing arterial blood—provided that he had not already appreciated the malignant nature of the neoplasm on the pre-operative angiogram (possible in 50–70% of cases).

Occasionally, it is difficult to distinguish glioblastoma from monstrocellular sarcoma (*see* p. 206). Grossly, the latter does not usually appear so variegated, and, in contrast to the glioblastoma, cyst formation is prominent, necroses are rare, and the tissue is fibrous and "asbestos-like." Histologically, the disproportionately huge monster cells, the presence of spindle and monster cell regions one next to the other, and the isolated presence of generally hyperchromatic giant cells adjacent to capillaries in the *normal* brain, all favor a sarcoma. Large vessels, such as can be demonstrated arteriographically, are more frequent in glioblastoma; vascular budding of the capillaries in the marginal zone, but outside the tumor, point to the monstrocellular sarcomas. In many cases differentiation is possible only after use of the reticulin stain; in the sarcoma this shows abundant production of fibers between the spindle-shaped cells, whereas in the glioblastoma—in those regions which have not yet undergone regressive changes—the reticulin fibers are confined to the blood vessels. In all doubtful cases, silver staining has to be used. Biologically, however, there is little difference between the two kinds; they are of almost equal malignancy.

CHAPTER X

NEUROEPITHELIAL TUMORS: THE PARAGLIOMAS

6. THE EPENDYMOMAS

(Synonyms: Adenoglioma, glioependymoma, ependymoepithelioma, ependymoglioma, ependymocytoma, "Pfeilerzellgliom," blastoma ependymale, "neuroepithelioma;" occasionally they are also described as angiosarcomas.)

HISTORICAL NOTE AND DEFINITION

The first description was by Virchow (1863, 1865). Muthmann and Sauerbeck related the ependymoma to the ependyma as the tissue of origin, and this was proved by Mallory (1902) with his demonstration of blepharoplasts; as a distinct group it was set apart by Bailey and Cushing (1926). Roussy and Oberling (1932) distinguished ependymomas, ependymoblastomas, ependymocytomas and ependymogliomas; Kernohan and Fletcher-Kernohan recognized the epithelial, myxopapillary and cellular types. Many true ependymomas have been described in the general pathological literature, some as neuroepitheliomas (for example, by Storch; Besold; Roman; Marburg (1927); Gold; Rinke; Ribbert (1918); Cimbal; v. Hasselbach; Rosenthal; Bittorf; Saxer; Antoni (1936), and others.) Detailed descriptions can be found in Kernohan and Fletcher-Kernohan (1935); Fincher and Coon; Roussy and Oberling (1932); Foerster and Gagel (1934, 1936); Gagel (1938); Tönnis and Zülch (1937), and Zülch (1940, 1955, 1956).

Further references: Benedek and Juba; Doernbach; Giampalmo; Hardman and Jefferson; Hildebrandt; Hirsch and Elliot; Lüthy and Irsigler; Pimenta *et al* (1950); Naeslund; Rauch; Ringertz and Reymond; Seifarth; Svien, Mabon, Kernohan and McK. Craig; Tönnis and Borck (1953); *see* also Zülch and Kleinsasser. Ztbl. f. Path., 1957 (in press).

INCIDENCE AND SITE

The ependymomas of the cerebral hemispheres occur almost exclusively in childhood and adolescence; the other groups show a predilection for the second to fourth decades. Our youngest patient was seven months

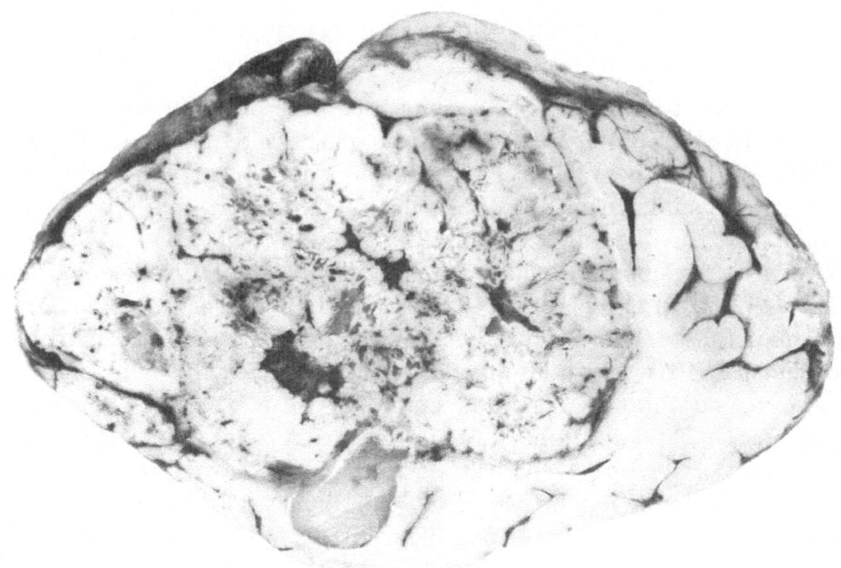

Fig. 49.   Fist-sized ependymoma which reaches the surface of the brain in the occipital region. Note the lobulated appearance of the tumor on the cross-section. The tumor growth is by expansion. A few cysts the size of a peanut are seen in the center of the tumor. (Case 1568)

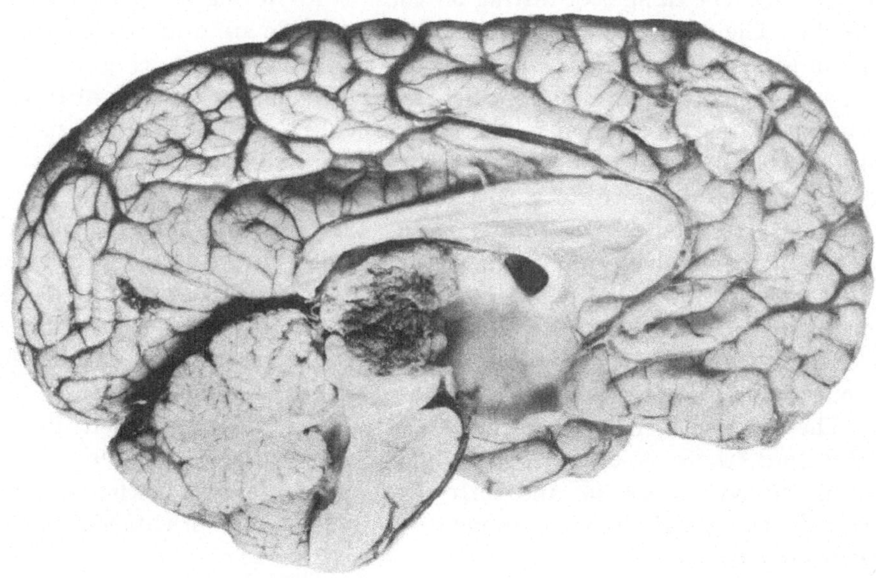

Fig. 50.   Lobulated ependymoma in the caudal portion of the third ventricle. The localization is similar to that of a pinealoma. There is a non-communicating hydrocephalus. The floor of the third ventricle is distended and paper-thin. The quadrigeminal plate is displaced upwards. (Case 932)

of age, the oldest 81 years. The peak of incidence lies between the ages of
eight and 15 (Fig. 9). The ependymomas of the cerebral hemispheres are
the most common hemispheral gliomas of childhood. The ependymomas
of the spinal canal, according to Kernohan, form 60% of the gliomas in
the spinal cord. All in all, 4.6% of all intracranial tumors in our series of
4,000 cases were ependymomas; the comparable figure in Cushing's material was 1.3%, in Olivecrona's (Ringertz and Reymond) 6.3%, and 9.1%
of all gliomas at the Mayo Clinic (Svien *et al.*). Of our patients with
ependymomas, 94 were males and 90 females.

The ependymomas occur predominantly in the vicinity of the
ependyma. The sites in order of frequency are as follows: fourth ventricle,
lateral ventricles, third ventricle, aqueduct. The ependymomas of the
cerebral hemispheres reach the size of a small fist and may lie in any lobe,
with a predilection for the temporo-parieto-occipital junction (Fig. 49).
They lie up against the lateral ventricle (particularly at the trigone) and
from there can grow out and push against the overlying cortex (particularly
the supramarginal and angular gyri); they may occasionally even reach the
cortex (Fig. 17, No. 41). The surface of the ependymoma is lobulated and
tufted, resembling the surface of a placenta or a cauliflower (Fig. 17, No.
44; Fig. 50). The danger of tearing off these tufts during operation is considerable. The ependymomas in the fourth ventricle are usually the size of
a plum and are attached firmly to the floor of the ventricle (Fig. 17, No.
44); a process often extends into the cisterna magna or the lateral recess,
occasionally reaching down to the midcervical cord (down to C 5 in our
case No. 1012). Less frequently, ependymomas lie in the lateral ventricle
at the foramen of Monro (Fig. 17, No. 42) or in the third ventricle rostral
and dorsal to the quadrigeminal plate (Fig. 50), and finally—though
rarely—in the cerebello-pontine angle or actually in the aqueduct. In the
spinal cord they appear either in the shape of a pencil, extending over
several segments (Fig. 17, No. 45) in the region of the posterior columns,
or as large white gelatinous tumors in the region of the cauda and on the
filum terminale where they may reach a length of 9–11 cm.

The cerebral forms usually have a large cyst rostrally placed; in the
spinal cord, there is often a cavity both above and below the tumor,
resembling syringomyelia, and corresponding to the cyst in the cerebral
form; the elongated shape conforms to the longitudinal orientation of the
spinal cord tracts.

APPEARANCE TO THE NAKED EYE

The ependymomas are reddish, nodular and lobulated, often resemble
a placenta or cauliflower, and adjust themselves in form and size to their
surroundings; they grow into the surrounding tissue purely by expansion.

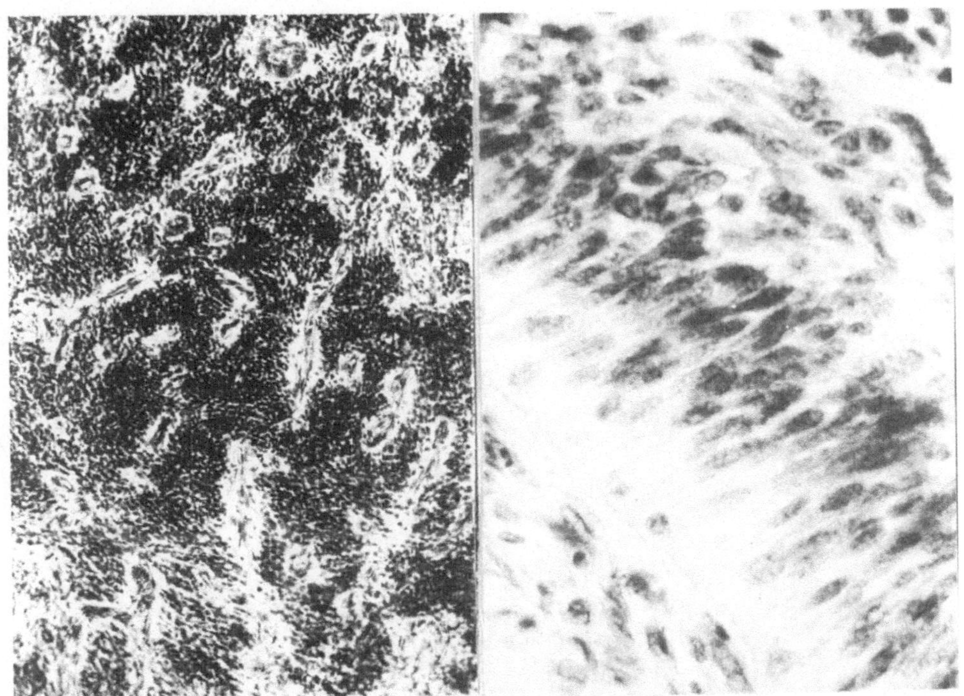

Fig. 51. Ependymoma. a) *left:* Low power view: cellular tumor with uniformly distributed blood vessels. Nucleus-free zones are seen around the blood vessels. (x64, Nissl stain); b) *right:* Columnar arrangement of cells along the wall of a blood vessel. Endothelial proliferation is seen in the left lower corner. (x480, H. & E. stain)

HISTOLOGICAL APPEARANCE

The ependymomas are, uniformly, very cellular, isomorphic tumors with densely packed cells. They tend to show two architectures: one rather mosaic-like, the other an epithelial arrangement along the blood vessels (Fig. 51). They derive their characteristic pattern from the uniform distribution and particular arrangement of blood vessels within the masses of tumor cells, whereby nucleus-free halos form a cuff-like space around the vessel (Fig. 51a). (When only a nuclear stain is used, the section takes on a spotted leopard-skin pattern.) The more or less clearly visible and coarse cell processes, which attach themselves to the vessel walls, extend through the nucleus-free zones around the blood vessels. These processes, forming the so-called crown-like pattern, can often be demonstrated only with special stains (Figs. 52a, 25a). Occasionally, single rosettes (Fig. 52b) may be noticed or—particularly in the spinal ependymomas—one or several ependymal tubules (Fig. 24a). This is of absolutely no significance in the biological evaluation of these tumors and should under no circumstances lead to the obsolete diagnosis of "neuroepithelioma." The cells are poor in cytoplasm; the nuclei have abundant chromatin and are round

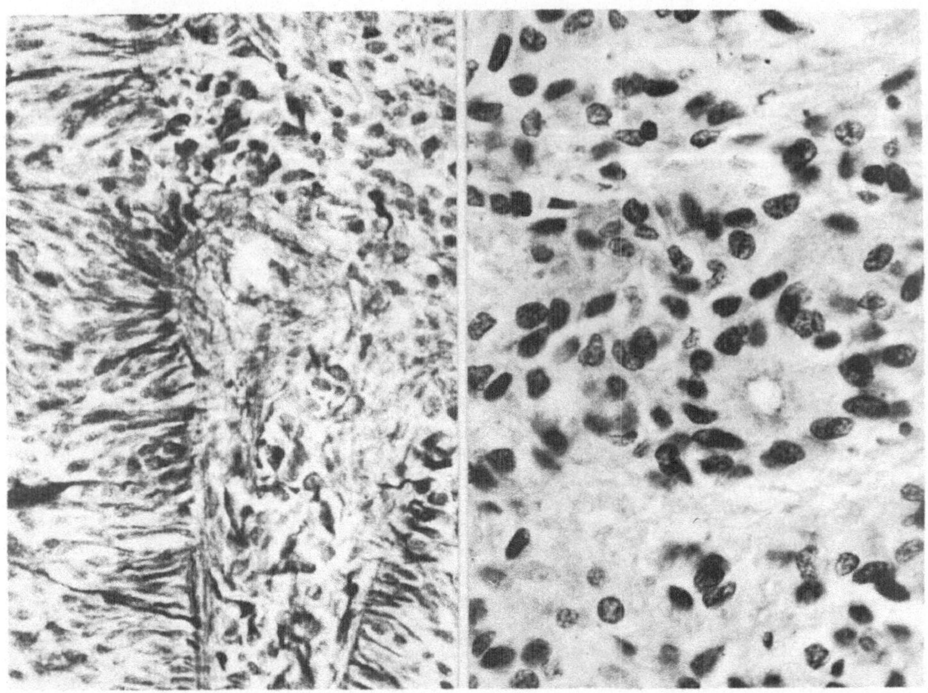

Fig. 52. Ependymoma. a) *left:* Vascular foot-plates demonstrated with gold sublimate. (x200); b) *right:* "True rosettes" in an ependymoma of the fourth ventricle. (x350, H. & E. stain)

or oval. Mitoses occur almost only in the cerebral forms. With special stains, blepharoplasts can be demonstrated (visible only under oil immersion). The intima of the blood vessels tends to proliferate with closure of the lumen, which results in the tendency to undergo regressive changes, including cyst formation. Occasionally there is necrosis as well, though no real fatty degeneration. Ependymomas of the filum terminale, which are clearly broken up into papillae, have a tendency toward mucoid-hyaline degeneration of the vessel walls (myxopapillary forms), and toward cell destruction between the papillae. The end stage, therefore, often reveals only swollen finger-like processes, covered with a single cell layer (Foerster and Gagel, 1936). True glial fibers never occur, except in association with the vascular feet (Fig. 52a). Ependymomas owe their firm consistency to their abundance of branching blood vessels. Generally, the ependymomas grow by expansion but in the marginal zone growth occasionally occurs by means of advancing papillae. Metastases occur spontaneously only occasionally (case No. 1548) but are not uncommon after operation on the hemispheral forms (the whole cerebrospinal fluid system may be involved with nodules and plaques; Zülch, 1940). In the hemispheral forms, recurrences even after "total removal" are frequent; not so in other ependymomas.

168

Ependymomas can be distinguished from medulloblastomas of the fourth ventricle grossly by the harder consistency and microscopically, by the absence of mitoses and the presence of nucleus-free cuffs and crown-like patterns around the vessels, as well as by the presence of blepharoplasts. Occasionally, the cells, through regressive processes, can swell so that the tissue assumes the appearance of an oligodendroglioma. In our opinion, and contrary to Kernohan (1935), this represents a secondary alteration of the tissue and not a primary kinship between the two tumors.

The cerebral forms occurring during childhood often remain clinically silent for long periods in spite of cyst formation. Ependymomas of the fourth ventricle may have a long history and, after decompression, run a benign course over many years. Total removal is dangerous because of the intermeshing of the tumor and the cranial nerve nuclei in the fourth ventricular floor.

Ventricular tumors in tuberous sclerosis

The ependymomas are distantly related to the ventricular tumors that occur in tuberous sclerosis (*see* p. 44); the latter are especially apt to occur in the lateral ventricles around the foramen of Monro.

These tumors, growing on the floor of the anterior horn and being attached to it, to the septum pellucidum, and to the region of the foramen of Monro, range in size from a cherry to a tangerine, are medium hard, often calcified, nodular and produce a block at the foramen of Monro. In this way they often displace the septum pellucidum to the opposite side.

Histologically, these tumors have the same structure as the ependymal granulations of tuberous sclerosis, a structure that is almost type-specific. The tumor is of medium cellularity; the cells are arranged in streams and whorls, with the tissue either more reticular or fascicular. Numerous blood vessels break up the tumor, with the cells arranged radially around them. This arrangement results in a crown-like pattern similar to that of the ependymomas. The cells are small or large with an eccentric nucleus, which in either case is vesicular and has a large nucleolus. These growths form abundant glial fibers and tend to calcify. They correspond to the subependymal astrocytomas described by Roussy and Oberling and are amenable to surgical therapy (Stender and Zülch). Of course, the question to what extent the other changes of the disease make an operation worthwhile still remains.

The "subependymomas"

Tumors described under this term by Scheinker (1945) do not, in our opinion, deserve a separate category. As we have known for a long time and as was described first by Giampalmo, the ependymomas can lose their architecture and much of their cellularity due to pressure atrophy, e.g., such as occurs in the tumor lobules extending into the cisterna magna. These cases reveal a hyalin-appearing region which is relatively acellular but fiber-rich, containing infrequent blood vessels and isolated groups of cells while other portions of the tumor have remained unchanged. Those portions that have undergone secondary pressure atrophy resemble the small ependymal granulations which are occasionally seen as incidental findings (but which should not be confused with the ependymitis granularis seen in chronic infectious processes).

The ependymal cysts

(*Synonyms: Colloid cysts, plexus cysts, cysts of the foramen of Monro, paraphysial cysts.*)

The name ependymal cysts includes a variety of cysts whose common feature is their origin from the ependymal lining of the ventricles. Ependymal cysts occur in three forms: 1) diverticuli of the ventricles, particularly of the tips of the ventricles. These are without pathological significance. 2) Ependymal cysts with a tendency to grow, in which case they act as space-occupying lesions. They represent malformations with one or more chambers and occasionally reach considerable proportions. They lie in the region of the quadrigeminal plate or in the cerebello-pontine angle and are occasionally multicystic in this latter location. They are lined with a single layer of ependymal cells without cilia. 3) The common so-called colloid cysts or "tumors." Cysts the size of a pea have been encountered as incidental findings[1] (Fig. 53); others, reaching the size of a cherry, have acted as space-occupying lesions; they all lie between the foramina of Monro and beneath the roof of the third ventricle (Fig. 17, No. 46). The site of origin is probably a pinched-off remnant of the embryonic paraphysis.[2] They lie under the fornix and are lined with a single layer of ependyma, often ciliated.

Since the cysts protrude into the third ventricle from above, pushing the ependymal lining of the ventricular roof before them, their undersurface is covered with a double layer of ependyma. They are filled with a colloid-like fluid which subsequently coagulates. By blocking the foramen of Monro they lead to hydrocephalus of both lateral ventricles. They are readily amenable to operation.

Further references: Hambücher; Haymaker and Yenerman; McLean (1936); Foerster and Gagel (1934).

[1] *See* Fig. 11, Zbl. Neurochir. **10**, 26–38, 1950.
[2] *See* KAPPERS, A., J. Comp. Neur. **102**, 425–510, 1955.

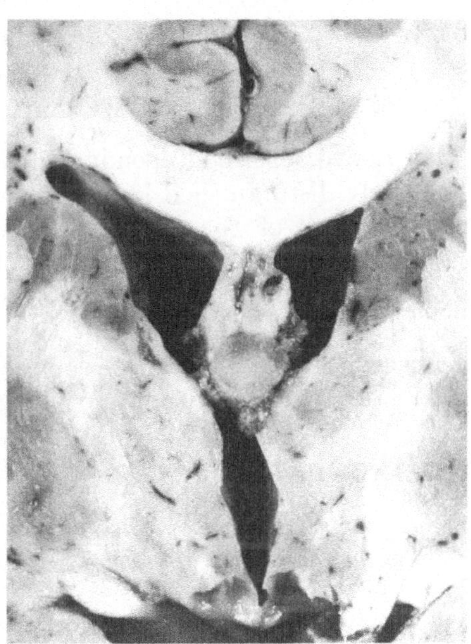

Fig. 53. Ependymal cyst the size of a pea between the foramina of Monro (accidental finding). (Case 1033)

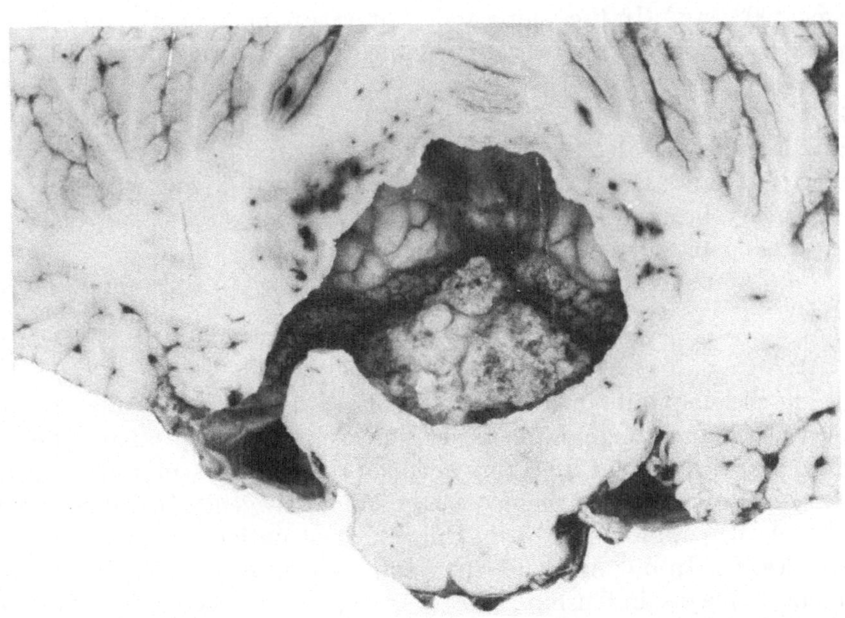

Fig. 54. Small plexus papilloma in the posterior portion of the fourth ventricle. Attachment to the choroid plexus of the roof of the ventricle is well seen. (Case 228, 1939)

Cysts of the septum pellucidum

The above-described ependymal cysts at the foramen of Monro have
to be clearly distinguished from the so-called cysts of the septum pellucidum, and cysts of the cavum Vergae (the so-called "fifth ventricle"),
which represent a cystic enlargement of the very narrow slit between the
two leaves of the septum pellucidum; they rarely act as space-occupying
lesions. They often communicate with the ventricular system and on encephalography have a diagnostic appearance—a uniform widening of the
septum either with or without air filling (Kautzky and Zülch).

7. PLEXUS PAPILLOMAS

(*Synonyms: Epithelioma, carcinoma, or adenoma of the choroid plexus,
choroid epithelioma, choroid papilloma.*)

HISTORICAL NOTE AND DEFINITION

Singl. cases of this tumor have often been described in the pathological
literature particularly from the point of view of differentiation from
ependymal tumors (Studnicka; Agduhr; Vonwiller; Schmidt; Askanazy;
Saxer, 1902; etc.). In the neurosurgical literature only a few comprehensive
studies have appeared until now; nonetheless, they furnish us with a nearly
exhaustive description of the subject (Davis and Cushing; van Wagenen,
1930; and more recently Ringertz and Reymond). I am convinced that
many cases, especially those in the older literature, are not plexus papillomas (Le Blanc; Bielschowsky and Unger; Bouwdijk, and others; *see* also
the primary brain carcinomas, p. 222). Kernohan (1952) and others list
the plexus papillomas with ependymomas.

Further references: Norlén (1950); Perthes; Walker and Horrax;
Zander.

INCIDENCE AND SITE

The plexus papillomas occur particularly in the first decade of life; in
fact, this tumor probably appears earlier in life than any other. There are
indeed four cases in the literature in which the earliest symptoms appeared
in the first year of life; of these, one case of van Wagenen (1930) apparently
had a plexus papilloma at birth. Our youngest patient was two years old,
our oldest 60. In our material, these tumors comprised 0.5% of the brain
tumors of all ages, in Cushing's 0.6%. In our series (4,000 cases) there were
ten males and ten females with plexus papillomas.

Plexus papillomas are understandably confined in location to those
portions of the ventricles which contain choroid plexus, but they have
certain preferential locations. In order of frequency they are: 1) in the

fourth ventricle (the size of a plum) (Fig. 54), where they expand the lumen; 2) in the lateral ventricles (reaching the size of a fist), particularly in the left trigone, where they completely obliterate the lumen and expand all the way out to the cortex; large cysts can occur next to the tumor; 3) in the third ventricle, where they reach the size of a chestnut; and 4) in the cerebello-pontine angle where they are cherry-sized.

APPEARANCE TO THE NAKED EYE

The plexus papillomas are well demarcated from the surrounding tissue, but tufts of tumor may be forced into the cerebral substance by pressure. Plexus papillomas are gray-pinkish, have a fine or coarsely tufted surface, and even though they have a certain general firmness, are tender, friable, and tear easily. On occasion they are highly calcified (Bertha and Sorgo).

HISTOLOGICAL APPEARANCE

Histologically, the plexus papillomas duplicate the normal structure of the choroid plexus, and the cells which cover the tufts of stroma are usually columnar epithelium, similar to that of the choroid plexus of embryos or infants (Fig. 55a). Consequently these tumors have a papillary structure (Fig. 24d) with a single layer of epithelium which tends to be more columnar than flat; the cells often contain small cytoplasmic granules in the Nissl stain. They have no cilia and no blepharoblasts. The connective tissue stroma shows mucoid and hyalin changes, is widened, and occasionally contains calcified foci in the form of laminated spheres or psammoma bodies. On X-ray these can sometimes be visualized. There is no tendency toward degeneration.

DIFFERENTIAL DIAGNOSIS

Plexus papillomas may be distinguished grossly from the coarsely lobulated ependymomas by their delicately tufted, friable structure. When their cells are markedly compressed, they are often confused, histologically, with papillary ependymomas. This mistake may be avoided by taking into consideration the vascular architecture and the absence of blepharoplasts. Distinguishing this tumor from simple cystic hypertrophy—particularly around the glomus—is not difficult.

METASTASIS AND RECURRENCE

Removal of plexus papillomas without recurrence is difficult since the tumor itself is so friable; small fragments, easily torn off, can be liberated and may lead to the artificial seeding of tumor "transplants." The plexus papillomas are very apt to metastasize spontaneously by transplantation.

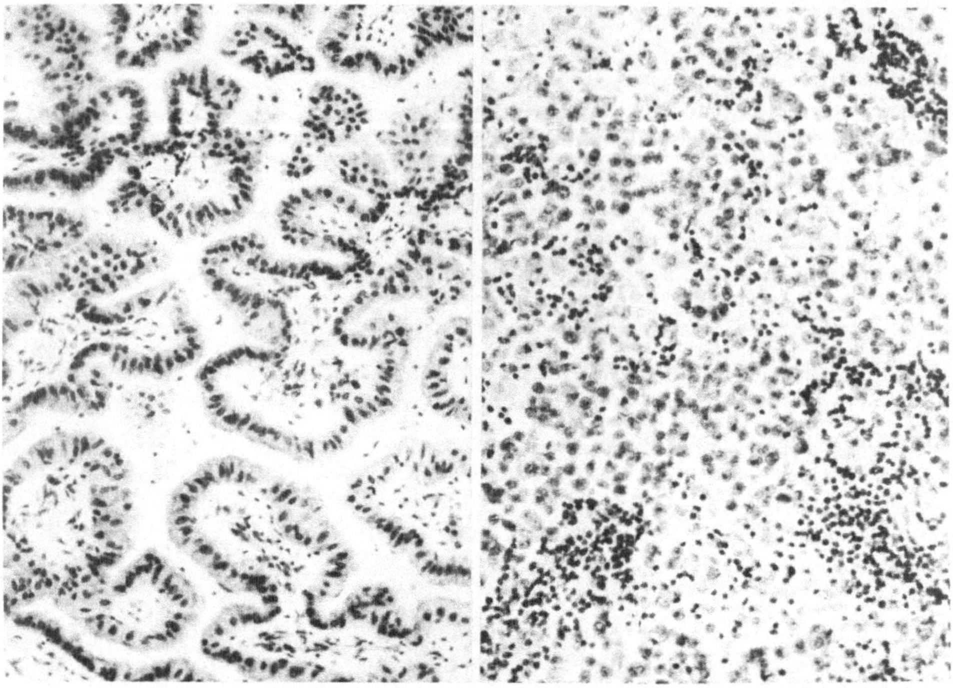

Fig. 55.   a) *left:* Typical architecture of a plexus papilloma: papillae containing blood vessels are covered with one layer of epithelial cells which are cylindrical in some places. The connective tissue of the stroma is expanded and swollen. (x240, Nissl stain); b) *right:* Typical architecture of a pinealoma: large, epithelial-like cells lie in between clusters of small, chromatin-rich lymphocyte-like cells. (x150, Nissl stain)

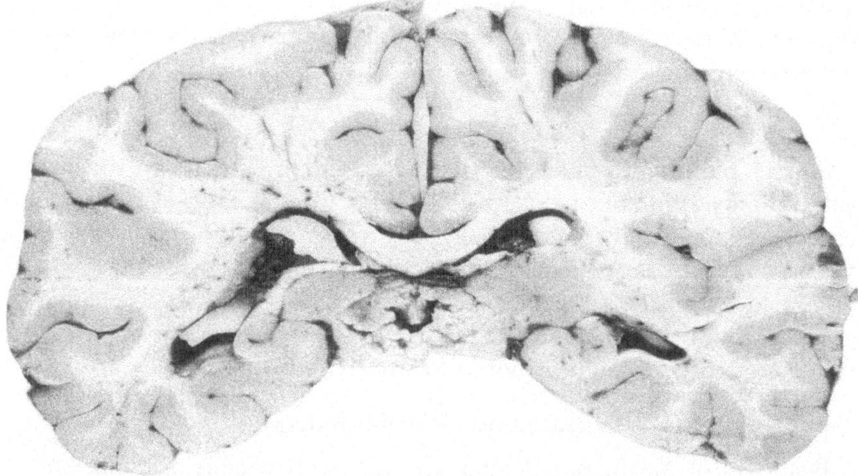

Fig. 56.   Heavily calcified pinealoma. In the marginal zone the tumor grows by infiltration. In the center there is calcification and degeneration due to inadequate nutrition. (Case 1096)

There exist, therefore, a number of cases of multiple plexus papillomas with definite evidence of spread via the cerebrospinal fluid (Ostertag, 1941; Zülch, 1938, 1956). Disregarding these implantation metastases, this tumor generally grows slowly and only by expansion. The few cases described as having been malignant from their very inception might well have been metastases from some primary malignancy elsewhere in the body (*see* Primary Brain Carcinomas, p. 222). We have seen definite malignant changes recently in two cases:

1) a 23-year-old man, with malignant change of the epithelium of the tumor but preservation of the basic pattern;[3]

2) a ten-month-old child with complete carcinomatous alteration of the pattern. (We are grateful to Dr. van Hoytema for an opportunity to examine this case.)[4]

By and large the plexus papillomas cannot be recognized clinically before operation unless they happen to be supplied by one of the choroidal arteries, as was demonstrated arteriographically in one of our own cases.

8. THE PINEALOMAS

(*Synonyms: Adenoma, adenocarcinoma, psammoma or psammosarcoma of the pineal body, pineocytoma, pineoblastoma.*)

HISTORICAL NOTE AND DEFINITION

We owe our knowledge of the pinealomas to the work of Virchow (1863, 1865); Marburg;[5] Krabbe (1944); Berblinger (1925, 1930, 1944), and Globus and Silbert as well as Mahaim. Bailey and Horrax (1920, 1925), too, have concerned themselves extensively with the pathology of pineal tumors. I would like to avoid the expression "spongioblastoma of the pineal," since it may lead to confusion with the true spongioblastoma which also occurs in the midbrain. I am unable to find a genetic relationship between these tumors and the seminoma (germinoma) (*see* Russell, 1944); I only see a morphological similarity. Moreover, I do not believe that pinealomas should be called teratomas, even though a sort of mixed tumor occasionally occurs. I have described the undifferentiated tumors of the pineal under the medulloblastomas. Reference may also be made to the contributions of Askanazy; Baggenstoss and Love; Bailey and Jeliffe; Foerster (1928); Friedman; Haldeman; Horrax; Horrax and Wyatt; Kalm and Magun; Mahaim; Müller and Wohlfart (1947); Pappenheimer; Ringertz and Flyger; Russell (1944, 1954); van Wagenen (1937), and Werner (1939).

[3] *See* CARDAUNS, Zbl. f. Neurochir., 1957.
[4] *See* VAN HOYTEMA and W. WINCKEL, Zbl. f. Neurochir, 1957, in press.
[5] Arb. neurol. Inst. Wien **17**, 217, 1909; Erg. inn. Med. **10**, 146, 1913.

INCIDENCE AND SITE

The bulk of the pinealomas make their clinical appearance in the second and third decade, but some also occur in the first and fourth decade, and beyond. Our youngest patient was one-and-a-half-years old, our oldest 74. It is difficult to obtain an accurate idea about their incidence. In our own collection of 4,000 cases they comprised 0.4%, in Cushing's, 0.7%.

Pinealomas lie, rather understandably, in the region of the quadrigeminal plate. Seeding of the embryonic rests to any great distance probably does not occur[6]. They range in size from a hazelnut to a chestnut (Fig. 56 and Fig. 17, No. 47) and grow mainly by expansion, except for infiltration in the marginal zone. Pinealomas may be quite distinctly circumscribed. They displace the quadrigeminal plate downward, may later push the posterior third of the corpus callosum upward, the thalami to the sides, and penetrate the caudal portion of the third ventricle. Finally, they press the superior vermis downward and force themselves beneath the tentorium. Patients with pineal tumors are predominantly males (3:1 in our series). In our own review of 53 cases from the literature, only nine cases were females.

APPEARANCE TO THE NAKED EYE

The color of the pinealoma is grayish-pink, the consistency tough and hard, or friable if calcified (Fig. 56). Single small cysts occur in the tumor substance. Occasionally, the pineal is still recognizable, rather well demarcated from the tumor, and displaced caudally.

HISTOLOGICAL APPEARANCE

Histologically we have to distinguish three types: 1) the so-called pineoblastomas (medulloblastomas of the pineal, *see* Medulloblastomas, p. 132); 2) the anisomorphic, and 3) the isomorphic pinealomas. The anisomorphic type duplicates the normal structure of the pineal and is therefore the easiest to diagnose. Large, polygonal or round "epithelioid" cells, rich in cytoplasm, are arranged in acini (Fig. 55b); they form pale nests that are separated from each other by a network of round, chromatin-rich, "lymphoid" cells. The blood vessels lie within this network. At the expanding border, pinealomas are mainly composed of small cells. Mitoses do occur. Pinealomas, just like the normal pineal, often show calcification (visible on X-ray). Small areas of necrosis may be present, but other

---

[6] We look upon the so-called "ectopic" pinealomas of the infundibulum as metastases from small tumors of the quadrigeminal plate. However, we have observed two parietal tumors of pineal-like structure in the absence of any primary tumor of the pineal.

regressive processes are absent. There are pinealomas with ependymal tubules, or remnants of squamous or stratified epithelium—indeed, there even exist true double tumors (combination with teratomas). The second, isomorphic form of pinealoma is composed of uniform cells of a single sort which are slightly smaller than the "large" cells of the anisomorphic pinealoma; this constitutes the "pineal spongioblastoma" of the American authors. There is no gathering of cells into nests, and the cells tend to be arranged in rows along the blood vessels. This tumor somewhat resembles the ependymoma, though nucleus-free spaces around the vessels are absent and the cytoplasm of the cells is slightly more abundant. There are no mitoses. Just how far malignant de-differentiation may take place in pinealomas is not clear. Our own case (No. 118/35) of a 74-year-old man was highly pleomorphic with multinucleated giant cells, grew by infiltration, and spread diffusely throughout the subarachnoid space. (*See* Zülch, 1956).

Since the number of pinealomas operated upon is still small, we lack experience with which to evaluate their biological behavior. Neither do we know whether the two forms of pinealoma behave differently in this respect. Our one case of the isomorphic type did not show any infiltrating growth. Operation, even "total extirpation," seldom insures freedom from recurrence. Besides, total removal is difficult due to the pinealomas' close relationship to nervous centers and important blood vessels, and their growth by infiltration in the marginal zone. Nonetheless, several years of postoperative improvement can be hoped for. One more unfavorable point is the tendency of pinealomas to metastasize spontaneously by transplantation into the subarachnoid space, the infundibulum (the "ectopic pinealomas"), for example (case No. 1096), or (occasionally) diffusely over the whole of the leptomeninges (Werner, 1939). An endocrine function of the pinealomas has not been definitely established, and earlier claims to this effect have been rejected. Endocrine changes (pubertas praecox, macrogenitosomia) have been observed more frequently in teratomas of the pineal and are more likely related to the effects upon periventricular centers of the infundibulum, caused by the hydrocephalus. Moreover, diabetes insipidus is often found in cases with implantation metastases to the infundibulum. This latter symptom, along with simultaneous signs of a lesion of the quadrigeminal plate, can be used to make a specific diagnosis of pinealoma (Horrax 1947, 1949, 1950; Kalm and Magun). However, since the diabetes insipidus resulting from the metastases to the infundibulum often forms the main symptom, the metastases are occasionally treated as primary tumors and operated on as "tumors of the chiasm" ("ectopic pinealomas"—our own case E 893). Metastases to other portions of the body (lungs) have also been described for pineal tumors. From the point of view of differential diagnosis, the possibility of metastases of seminomas to the brain should be considered, since they are similar to the anisomorphic pinealomas.

9. THE NEURINOMAS

(Synonyms: Perineurial fibroblastoma, neurofibroma, Schwannoma, lemmoma, lemmoblastoma, chitoneuroma, gliofibroma, neurolemmoma, peripheral glioma.)

HISTORICAL NOTE AND DEFINITION

Neurinomas had already been described at the beginning of the 19th century, but Virchow was the first to recognize them for what they were. The considerable contributions of von Recklinghausen, Verocay (1908); Antoni (1920); Mallory (1902), and Penfield (1932) have not yet definitely clarified the nature of neurinomas. There are still two opposite schools of thought: opinion remains divided over the mesodermal vs. the ectodermal origin of these tumors, and the argument hinges on the interpretation of the silver-impregnated fibers. The thought that this tumor is a "glioma" does not warrant serious consideration today. Tissue cultures seem to have proved that neurinomas originate from Schwann cells (Stout, 1949). The "central neurinomas" of the older literature most likely were spongioblastomas with a special tendency towards rhythmic cell patterns.

Further references: Dermann; Gagel (1935); Gardner and Frazier; Gardner and Turner (1938); Graf (1952); Henschen (1910, 1955); Korbsch (1930, 1939); Krayenbühl; Krayenbühl and Lüthy; Masson (1935); Olivecrona (1927, 1941); von Orzechowski; Ratzenhofer; Rhoads and van Wagenen; H. J. Scherer (1934); Tegerter and Smith; Zschau.

INCIDENCE AND SITE

The solitary neurinomas occur particularly in the middle decades of life (with the peak around 35–40 years, Fig. 10) and only exceptionally in childhood. Our youngest patient was 11 years old, the oldest 67. In the latter decades of life neurinomas are encountered as incidental findings in the region of the cauda, and are asymptomatic. Of our patients, 97 were males and 200 females. The neurinomas comprised 7.5% of all the brain tumors in our series (4000 cases), and 14% of neuroepithelial tumors; in Cushing's series 8.7% were neurinomas.

The neurinomas occur most frequently on the eighth nerve, where they probably arise from the vestibular portion. They form tumors in the cerebellopontine angle of hazel- or chestnut-size (Fig. 57); they indent the pons and medulla, push them aside, (Fig. 17, No. 48)—and force the

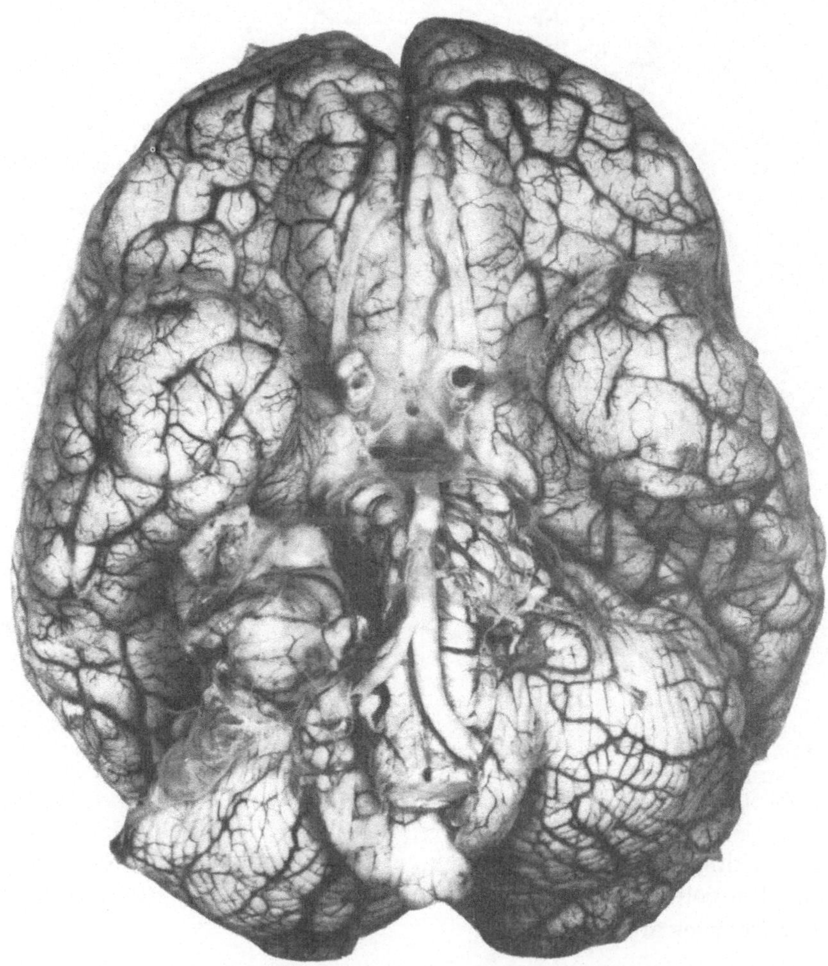

Fig. 57. Chestnut-sized acoustic neurinoma on the right, with a marked bilateral cerebellar pressure cone. Posteriorly from the tumor one sees a large arachnoid cyst which can be clearly recognized since the brain was photographed under water. (Case Las)

cerebellum both up and downward (forming a superior and inferior cerebellar pressure cone). The caudal end of the tumor is often the site of one or more arachnoidal cysts (Fig. 57). As a result of pressure or disturbances in circulation, small areas of softening often develop in the pons. Bilateral cerebellopontine angle neurinomas are looked upon as a *forme fruste* of von Recklinghausen's neurofibromatosis. Neurinomas in the spinal canal may be distributed over one or more segments, are attached to the posterior roots, and may be finger-shaped or resemble a lima bean. Dumbbell forms may arise when the tumor grows through the intervertebral foramen. Neurinomas rarely occur on other cranial nerves (III and V). In the course

179

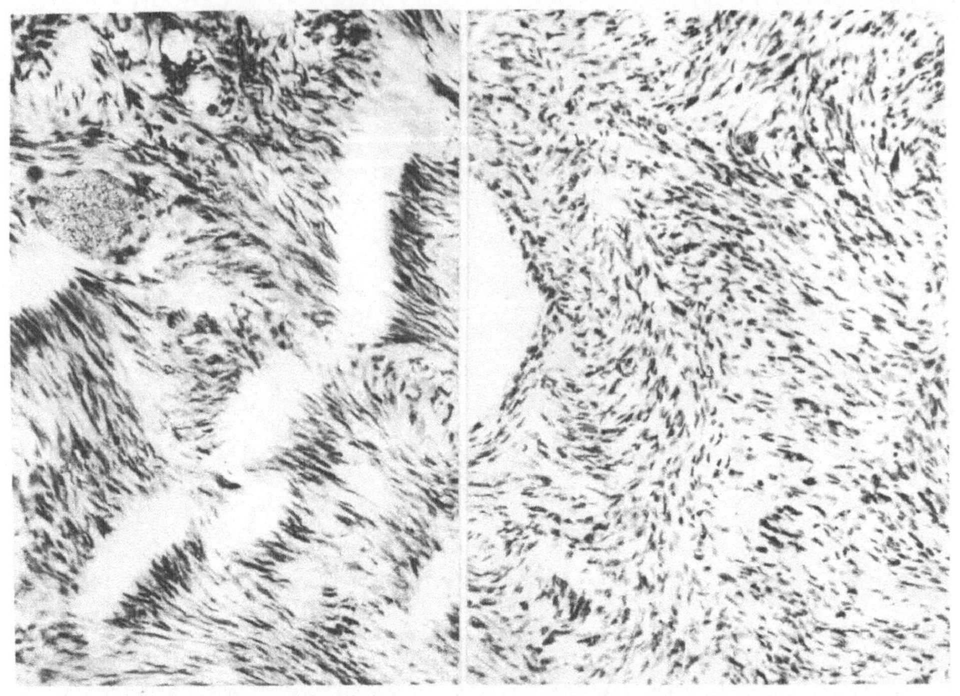

Fig. 58. a) *left:* Marked palisading in a spinal neurinoma. (cf. Fig. 23c) (x150, Nissl stain); b) *right:* Typical "fascicular" architecture of a neurinoma. The cells are arranged in long streams and show a certain tendency towards formation of whorls. (x90, Nissl stain)

of von Recklinghausen's disease they can be noticed on every cranial and peripheral myelinated, or unmyelinated, nerve. Solitary neurinomas of peripheral nerves are rare.

APPEARANCE TO THE NAKED EYE

The neurinomas are smooth, well-encapsulated tumors, often with a finely nodular appearance. The vessels course in the arachnoid capsule that covers the tumor. Color ranges from pinkish gray-yellow to deep yellow, or translucent gray. Consistency varies, depending on the amount of regressive change that has taken place; it is rubbery in the marginal zone but friable in its center, so that the tumor may easily be curetted out. At operation it is not always possible to distinguish the cerebello-pontine (Fig. 17, No. 48), or posterior root, neurinomas from meningiomas in these locations, although the meningiomas have a dural attachment.

HISTOLOGICAL APPEARANCE

Histologically the neurinomas consist of cells of moderate density which appear to be arranged in a syncytium and show patterns in streams, loops, and palisades (Figs. 23a–c). The spinal forms are particularly apt to

180

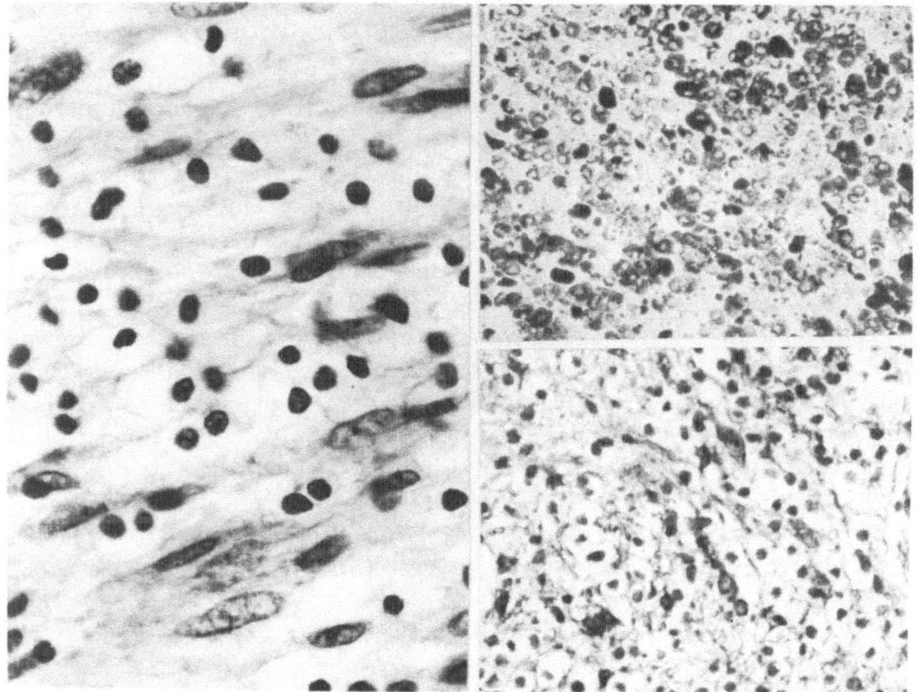

Fig. 59. a) *left:* "Reticular" tissue-type of a neurinoma. Some cells show distinct fatty degeneration (vacuolated cell body), other cells have foamy cytoplasm. (x650, Nissl stain); b) *top right:* Fatty degeneration and rounding-up of the tumor cells in a neurinoma. Nuclei are transformed into small, clear vacuoles. (x150, Scharlach-red stain); c) *bottom right:* A region of neurinoma showing fatty degeneration. This picture forms the "negative" to (b). The tissue has a honeycomb appearance similar to that of an oligodendroglioma (cf. Fig. 37a) (x150, H. & E. stain)

show the classical palisading of nuclei (Figs. 23c, 58a). Otherwise the nuclei, which have a rod or cigarette shape and contain a medium amount of chromatin, lie in long and wavy streams, loops and whorls (Fig. 58b). There are two particularly prominent architectural types: the dense *fibrillary* structure of tissue type "A" (Fig. 58a), and the loosely *reticular*, less cellular structure, of tissue type "B" (Fig. 59a), the latter being the result of regressive changes (hyalinization and fatty degeneration).

Using the silver method, it is possible to demonstrate fine fibrils which probably are not of connective tissue nature, however.[7] True reticulin fibers are found in the marginal zone and apparently originate from the

[7] Because of the uncertainty over the interpretation of these argentophilic fibers, there is still a controversy over the mesodermal or ectodermal origin of neurinomas. The content of connective tissue in peripheral neurinomas (neurofibromas) of von Recklinghausen's disease is much greater than that of the intracranial and spinal neurinomas, since the perineural connective tissue has undergone pronounced reactive proliferation. But, in the same way, a scirrous carcinoma does not become a sarcoma simply because the stroma shows excessive proliferation.

arachnoidal connective tissue. The blood vessels there are more numerous, and their walls have a tendency toward hyalinization. Occasionally they accumulate there to the extent that they resemble a cavernoma. The growth of neurinomas is slow; mitoses are never seen. The tendency to fatty degeneration is extraordinarily marked (something which may lead to a rounding out of the cells and the formation of a honeycomb-like pattern similar to the oligodendroglioma—Fig. 59c). The fat is birefrigent.

Intracranial neurinomas are somewhat different from those in the spinal canal: the former contain an abundance of the reticular type B tissue, with true palisades being less numerous; fatty degeneration and hyalin change are very pronounced. Mucoid degeneration with cyst formation is rare. The spinal neurinomas, however, more often show the strict type A tissue, frequently with true palisades, and fatty degeneration is less prominent than mucoid degeneration and cyst formation; various sized hemorrhages occur from the cavernous blood vessels into these cysts.

DIFFERENTIAL DIAGNOSIS

The neurinomas of the cerebello-pontine angle and in the spinal canal can be macroscopically differentiated from meningiomas. Histologically, differentiation from the fibroblastic meningiomas is occasionally difficult. The mixture of fibrillary and reticular tissue types speaks for a neurinoma but the demonstration of true reticulin fibers (see above) against it. The possibility of confusion with oligodendrogliomas and chordomas, particularly in paraffin-embedded material stained with H. & E. has been pointed out. Differentiation of this tumor from tumors of the glomus jugulare is not difficult.

Prognosis: Metastases have not been observed, and malignant degeneration occurs only in the peripheral neurinomas of von Recklinghausen's disease. Recurrence always occurs after incomplete removal, and reoperation is usually rewarding. Total removal results in a permanent cure. Sudden paraplegia may develop in cases of spinal neurinomas, following massive hemorrhages into the cysts (Krayenbühl and Lüthy).

CHAPTER XI

NEUROEPITHELIAL TUMORS: THE GANGLIOCYTOMAS

10. THE GANGLIOCYTOMAS

(*Synonyms: True neuroma, ganglioglioma, ganglioneuroma, glioneuroblastoma, neuroastrocytoma, ganglioma, Purkinjeoma, etc.*)

HISTORICAL NOTE AND DEFINITION

The gangliocytomas were first described by Virchow (1863, 1865) for the sympathetics, and subsequent cases of Loretz, Parker, and Manasse followed. Most of the cases were published only after the advent of the Nissl stain for ganglion cells. Here our knowledge has been enriched particularly by Bielschowsky and Henneberg; Herxheimer; Pick and Bielschowsky; Schmincke (1909, 1910, 1914); Courville (1930); Christensen (1937), and above all by Foerster and Gagel (1932, 1933). There is considerable lack of clarity on the classification and interpretation of this group. Attempts at subdivision have resulted in the setting up of such subgroups as: neuroblastomas (from immature stages of development), gangliocytomas (ganglion cells and their precursors), ganglioneuromas (gangliocytomas with formation of myelinated fibers—gangliocytoma myelinicum, or axis cylinders alone—amyelinicum), ganglioglioneuromas (gangliocytomas with formation of glia and axis cylinders or myelin sheaths), etc. For neurosurgical purposes, a simpler, all-inclusive concept of gangliocytomas is entirely sufficient, since there is no evidence that the above-mentioned features of autonomous glial participation, or axis cylinder, or myelin formation (if they really occur at all) have any biological significance, i.e., influence the manner of growth or the degree of malignancy. If completeness in a pathological sense is desired, it is sufficient —according to the above data—to add to the name of gangliocytoma the corresponding characteristics. We consider it more important, however, to distinguish three different types depending upon location: 1) in the cerebral hemispheres, brain stem and spinal cord; 2) in the cerebellum; and 3) in the sympathetic trunk. In the subdivision of the neuroepithelial tumors, I have placed the gangliocytomas as a fourth group beside the medulloblastomas, gliomas and paragliomas.

Further references: Alpers and Grant; Amstad; Bailey (1932); Bielschowsky (1925); Bielschowsky and Simon; Pick and Bielschowsky; Foerster and Gagel (1932, 1933); Heinlein and Falkenberg; Lhermitte and Duclos; Lichtenstein and Zeitlin; Kernohan, Learmonth and Doyle; Olivecrona (1919); Robertson (1914, 1915); Schär and Christensen; Schöpe (1942); Tönnis and Zülch (1939); Töppich (1936); Wolf and Morton.

INCIDENCE AND SITE

Since the gangliocytomas are rare tumors, it is difficult to determine their age incidence accurately. There is a definite predilection for the first three decades. Tönnis and Zülch (1939) described a series of operable tumors of the temporal lobe. These patients had long histories; the average age of onset of symptoms was 11 years, and the average age at operation was 19. Our youngest patient of the whole group was five years old, the oldest 52 years. The gangliocytomas of the sympathetics are also found predominantly in childhood and adolescence. The gangliocytomas accounted for 0.2% of Cushing's series, and in our series (4,000 cases) made up 0.7% of neuroectodermal tumors, and 0.4% of all cases. Of our patients, eight were males and five females. Gangliocytomas of the sympathetics are supposed to occur more often in women than men.

In order of frequency their preferential sites are as follows: 1) cerebral hemispheres (particularly the medial part of the temporal lobe, where they form large cysts and show a marked tendency to nodular growth into the leptomeninges); 2) tuber cinereum and third ventricle, where they reach the size of a plum or a chestnut; 3) medulla oblongata (which they permeate diffusely); 4) cerebellum (where they form hyperplastic-looking cerebellar folia within a circumscribed "neoplastic" region, particularly in the anterior lobe; 5) sympathetics, where a tough tumor, partly necrotic inside, growing by expansion and varying in size from a chestnut to a child's head, may arise. The order of frequency in the sympathetics is lumbar, thoracic, and cervical. For the tumors of the non-chromaffin ganglia, so-called glomus tumors, *see* Kleinsasser, O.: Zbl. f. Neurochir. 17, 155–168, 1957.

APPEARANCE TO THE NAKED EYE

With the exception of the rare cerebellar forms which look like hyperplastic convolutions, the gangliocytomas do not have any very characteristic appearance. In any event, in cases of tough cystic tumors of the medial basal temporal lobe it would do well to think of gangliocytomas.

HISTOLOGICAL APPEARANCE

Because of the number of different forms (see above), it is difficult to draw a consistent histological picture. Of fundamental importance is the

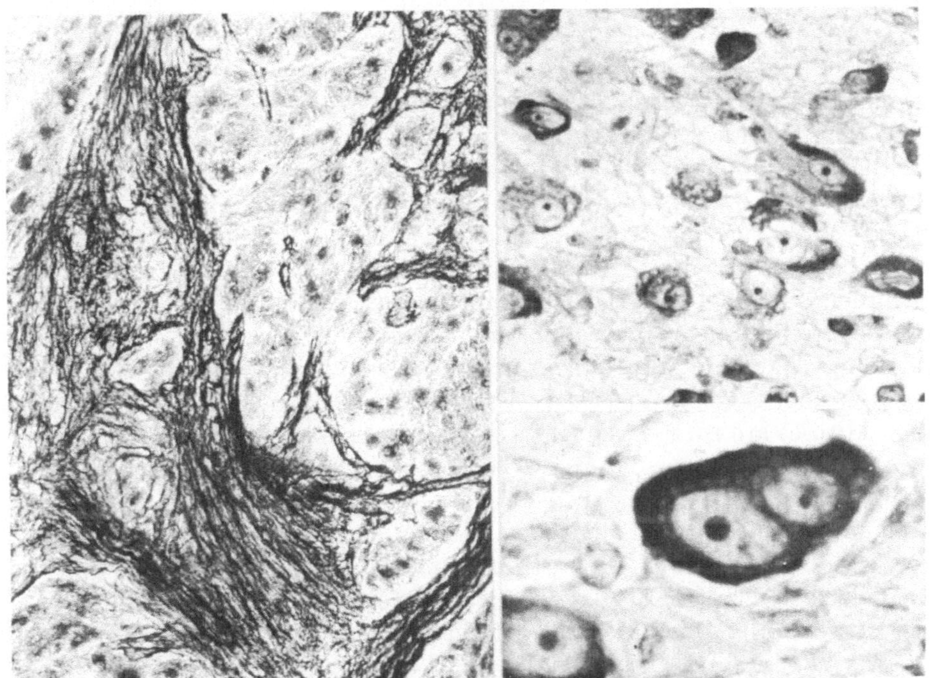

Fig. 60. Gangliocytoma. a) *left:* In most gangliocytomas the tumor tissue is subdivided into islands by abundant connective tissue (x100, tannin-silver method); b) *top right:* The tumor cells containing one or more nuclei lie in nests and show the typical structure of large nerve cells. (x250, Nissl stain); c) *bottom right:* A nerve cell with two nuclei. (x650)

decision whether the cells under consideration are really ganglion cells at all and, if so, whether they are of neoplastic origin. The mere finding of a "ganglion-like" vesicular nucleus with a large nucleolus does not suffice. That can be found in sarcomas (*see* Monstrocellular Sarcoma, p. 206), carcinomas, proliferating connective tissue, and in fresh reactive astrocytes as well. One can only be certain about such a diagnosis when there is Nissl substance in the cytoplasm (Figs. 60b, c).

When that kind of a neoplastic ganglion cell has been demonstrated, a more positive interpretation of the immature precursor forms seems justified. Neurofibrillae can only rarely be demonstrated in neoplastic ganglion cells.

The next step is to be certain about the *neoplastic* nature of the ganglion cells. Care should be exercised not to confuse with the gangliocytoma a gliomatous tumor invading a region of abundant nerve cells—for example, one of the large vegetative nuclei of the hypothalamus. The normal anatomy has to be kept in mind, and the possibility that the cells have preexisted there has to be excluded. Particularly noteworthy in gangliocytomas is the frequent abundance of reticulin fibers, with the cells often lying, in groups and acini, within little compartments of connective tissue (Fig. 60a). This latter situation is usually due to the invasion and nodular growth of these tumors into the neighboring leptomeninges, as is particularly apparent in the temporobasal forms. Finally, "lymphoid" infiltrates around blood vessels, such as are not infrequently seen in oligodendrogliomas, may often be observed in the marginal zone of the tumor. Their true nature (neuroblasts?) has not yet been clarified. We can find in gangliocytomas of the cerebral hemispheres mature nerve cells (Fig. 60b), frequently neuroblast-like immature stages, and occasionally newly-formed myelin sheaths and axis cylinders—all associated with proliferating neoplastic glia. Mitoses are rare, except in very malignant forms, as in our own case (No. 36) of an 18-year-old male. The cerebellar forms have a particularly characteristic appearance: the cerebellar cortex is expanded as a result of abundant proliferation of large ganglion cells, corresponding to the Purkinje cell layer. In the sympathetics, the undifferentiated tumors correspond to medulloblastomas (*see* p. 132). The mature forms, on the other hand, consist of well-formed ganglion cells of the sympathetics, a few less mature representatives, and a thick network of axons and Schwann cells. The hemispheres contain occasional (anaplastic?) malignant gangliocytomas which behave like malignant glioblastomas (our own case No. 36). Here there occur multinucleate ganglion cells with numerous mitoses (Fig. 60c).

METASTASIS AND RECURRENCE

Even for the temporobasal form, which, biologically, is quite benign, a metastasis has once been described. Otherwise, due to the lack of wider experience, this question cannot be answered. Post-operative recurrences are known. The biological behavior of the gangliocytomas cannot yet be evaluated with any certainty. Nonetheless, the generally cystic gangliocytomas of the temporobasal region are benign, operable, and of importance to neurosurgeons. Moreover, the mature tumors of the sympathetics can be easily operated upon and do not recur. Immature gangliocytomas of the sympathetics can metastasize.

DIFFERENTIAL DIAGNOSIS

The question of what the ganglion-cell tumor group should include is important and was taken up above. It should further be stressed that numerous monstrocellular tumors, described previously as "ganglioglioneuromas," "glioblastoma ganglioides," etc., do not belong to this group at all, but are most likely sarcomas (*see* Monstrocellular Sarcomas, p. 206).

CHAPTER XII

MESODERMAL TUMORS

11. THE MENINGIOMAS

(Synonyms: Fungus durae matris; psammoma, fibroma, sarcoma, endothelioma, exothelioma or mesothelioma of the dura mater; meningeal fibroendothelioma, meningeal or arachnoidal fibroblastoma, meningothelioma; arachnothelioma; leptomeningioma, etc.)

HISTORICAL NOTE AND DEFINITION

The meningiomas are in all probability the brain tumors that have been known longest. Because of the occasional production of grotesque cranial deformities, they had already attracted the interest of doctors and laymen alike even before the advent of classical pathological anatomy. (*See* also Cushing and Eisenhardt's monograph, 1938; for example, the case of Kaufmann, Crellius, Heister and Haller.) A series of excellent reports began with that of Louis, followed by Cruveilhier and Rokitansky, and ended with Virchow, who produced the first precise description of the "sarcomas" and "endotheliomas" of the dura, and the "psammomas."

Golgi's concept of the endothelioma started the controversy over the origin of the meningioma from the dural endothelium which subsequently also involved Marburg (1935). The question seems to have been settled now, largely because of the findings of M. B. Schmidt, and Ferner, i.e., the derivation of this tumor from the arachnoidal granulations. However, only the collection of large numbers of these meningeal tumors in certain North American clinics has made possible the final classification of their tissue type, localization, and clinical symptomatology. This information resulted from the investigations of Mallory (1920), Bailey and Cushing (1926) and their co-workers, and was finally set down in a comprehensive monograph by Cushing and Eisenhardt (1938). In the German literature, Essbach's monograph treated the subject thoroughly from the anatomico-pathological point of view. However, even today there are two opposing points of view, since one group would like to relate the meningioma to the arachnoidal endothelium, the other to the fibrous connective tissue (arachnoidal fibroblastoma). On the other hand, attempts to prove the neuroectodermal origin of meningiomas (Oberling, 1922) have failed to gain adherents, although this point has been taken up again recently by Diezel.

Further references: Aoyagi and Kyuno; Arlt; O. T. Bailey (1940), Bailey and Bucy (1931); Benedek and Juba; Bergstrand and Olivecrona (1935); Bland and Russell; Bostroem and Spatz; Buckley and Eisenhardt; Castellano, Guidetti, and Olivecrona; Courville and Abbott; Echols (1941); Frazier and Alpers (1933); Globus (1937); Gutmann and Spatz; Kalbfleisch and Grebe; Laas; Lapresle, Netsky, and Zimmerman; Learmonth (1927); Majerszky-Sántha; Noetzel (1951); Olivecrona (1934, 1935); Peters (1951); Prym; Ribbert (1910); Russell (1950); Tönnis (1938); Tönnis and Schürmann; Wolf and Cowen.

INCIDENCE AND SITE

The meningiomas show a clear predilection for the middle and latter decades of life. They begin to become more frequent with the third decade, a fact that is useful in differential diagnosis (for example, in the prechiasmal region the craniopharyngiomas occur around the second decade, pituitary adenomas around the third decade, and meningiomas thereafter). However, the age incidence of meningiomas is seen to be variable, depending on whether the material to be studied comes from a neurosurgical clinic, a pathological institute, or a mental hospital, where many meningiomas are discovered only as asymptomatic incidental findings. In our collection, made up of material from mixed sources, the peak of incidence lay around the age of 45 years (Fig. 11). The average age of Cushing's patients was 46.6 years for both sexes; the average of the males alone was 52, and that of the females 42.9. Our youngest patient was three years old, the oldest 86. The youngest case of Cushing's seems, however, to have been a five-year-old child with a spinal meningioma. Of our patients, 319 were males and 404 females. In Cushing's material, the meningiomas accounted for 13.4%, in ours (4,000 cases) for 18.1% of all tumors. Essbach summarized the statistics of 6,116 intracranial tumors of which 14.3% were meningiomas. Of 888 spinal tumors, however, 32% were meningiomas—a figure that was only 25.9% at the Mayo clinic.

The increased incidence of meningiomas in certain regions has been recognized for a long time and corresponds to the distribution of the arachnoidal granulations. Arranged in order of frequency we have the following groups (we have followed Cushing's groupings with only slight changes):

1. Meningiomas of the sagittal sinus or parasagittal meningiomas (of all three thirds of the sagittal sinus—Olivecrona, 1934). Reaching the size of a tangerine or an apple, these round tumors lie in the angle formed by the sinus and the dura; they are most common in the middle third of the sinus,

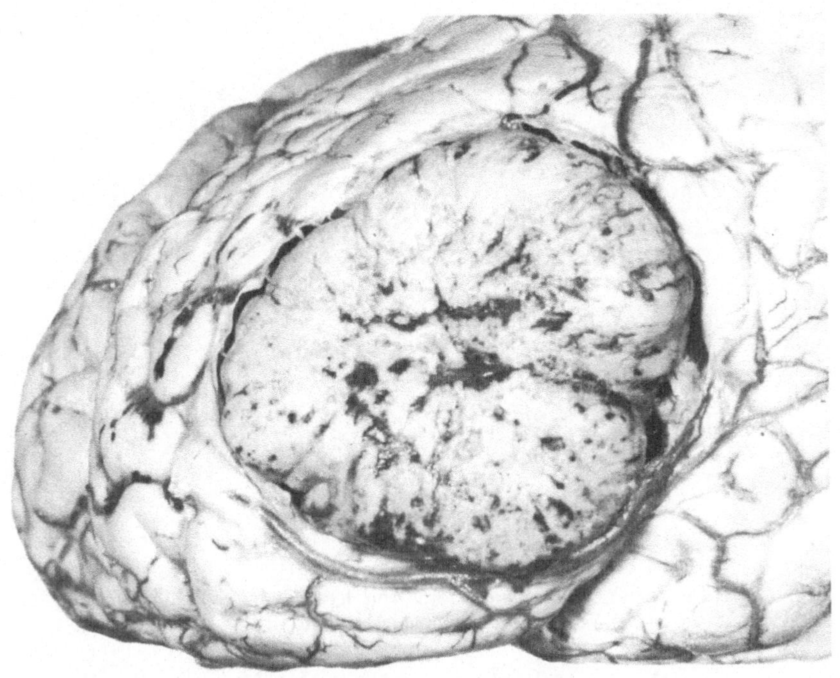

Fig. 61. Meningioma of the left frontolateral region (meningioma of the convexity). (Case 73/37)

Fig. 62. Right parasagittal meningioma of the posterior third of the sagittal sinus. The falx is curved slightly to the opposite side. No displacement of the midbrain. (Case 1743)

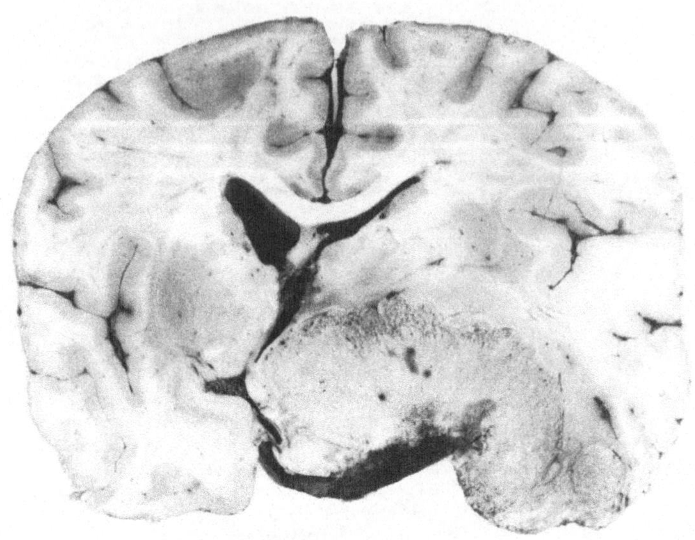

Fig. 63. Meningioma *en plaque* along the lesser wing of the sphenoid on the left. The tumor crosses the midline and extends on caudally along the clivus.

less common in the anterior third, and rare in the posterior third. The overlying bone is often infiltrated or hyperplastically thickened (Fig. 21, Nos. 51, 53; Fig. 18, No. 1; Fig. 62).

2. Meningiomas of the convexity. These differ from the foregoing type by their lack of any relationship to the falx. They are distributed over the whole convexity, with the majority lying anterior to the Rolandic fissure. We find here, too, local or diffuse hyperostoses, with or without actual infiltration of the bone (Fig. 17, No. 54; Fig. 18, No. 5; Fig. 61).

3. Meningiomas of the sphenoid ridge and the Sylvian fissure. They lie along the sphenoid ridge and are round or flat like a plaque or carpet. They vary in extent and may grow into either the anterior or middle fossa. The structures at the base (vessels, cranial nerves) can be surrounded by the tumor's carpet-like outgrowth. More than any other type, these meningiomas tend to produce hyperostosis of the sphenoid wings and the base of the skull. Meningiomas lying more laterally around the Sylvian fissure merge with the group over the convexity. In this type, frequently growing *en plaque*, there are some portions of the tumor which occasionally interdigitate with the brain (Fig. 17, Nos. 55–57; Fig. 63).

4. Meningiomas of the olfactory groove (or of the cribriform plate). These lie on the lateral or medial floor of the anterior fossa, reach the size of a tangerine, are hemispheral in shape, and push the brain upward. They may straddle the falx, and extend caudally to the chiasm (Fig. 17, No. 58; Fig. 18, No. 9).

5. Meningiomas of the tuberculum sellae (suprasellar meningiomas or prechiasmal meningiomas). They are cherry- to tangerine-sized, lie in the

190

midline posterior to those of the olfactory groove, often have a finely nodular surface, and displace the chiasm, the carotids, and adjacent structures upward. There are also small tumors which spread out along the sheath of the optic nerves (Fig. 17, No. 59).

6. Meningiomas of the tentorium (peritorcular meningiomas). These tumors grow either supratentorially, expanding beneath the temporal or occipital lobe, or infratentorially over the superior surface of the cerebellum. They may grow in both directions and assume the shape of a dumbbell. In general, they are most frequent around the torcular Herophili (Fig. 17, No. 60).

7. Meningiomas of the temporal fossa and Meckel's cave. These tumors are round and, lying beneath the temporal lobe, form a transition between the meningiomas of the cerebello-pontine angle, the sphenoid, and of Meckel's cave itself (where they usually lie *en plaque* at the petrous tip and send processes into the surrounding regions).

8. Meningiomas of the falx. These tumors are different from those of the sagittal sinus in that they possess a broad attachment to the falx (usually bilateral) and are covered toward the top by a mantle of brain tissue. Their attachment is therefore at a distance from the sinus. Most of them occur oral to the central fissure (Fig. 17, Nos. 49, 50; Fig. 18, No. 11).

9. Meningiomas of the cerebello-pontine angle. These are cherry- to plum-sized and lie along the medial portion of the petrous pyramid; they may lie at the same site as acoustic neurinomas, but seldom expand into the porus acousticus, more often growing toward the foramen magnum (Fig. 17, No. 62).

10. Meningiomas of the lateral ventricle. They occur as egg-shaped tumors that reach the size of a fist, and lie mainly in the trigonal region where they are firmly attached to the choroid plexus. Meningiomas of the velum interpositum project into the third ventricle (Fig. 17, No. 63).

11. Meningiomas of the clivus, or craniospinal meningiomas. These proceed from the lateral or medial clivus toward the temporal lobe, anterior surface of the cerebellum, or the pontine region, and may send a tongue of tumor down into the foramen magnum or the spinal canal (Fig. 17, No. 64).

12. Spinal meningiomas (or meningiomas of the cord). These are bean- or acorn-sized, occasionally finger-shaped, and extend over several segments. They are most common in the thoracic region, but most extensive in the cervical or caudal regions. They have a firm attachment to the dura, usually dorsolaterally, but occasionally elsewhere. At times they cannot be distinguished macroscopically from neurinomas (here the site of attachment may be of some help). (Fig. 17, No. 61; Fig. 64.)

On rare occasions meningiomas are multiple, their size ranging from that of a lentil to an apple, and are encountered in any of the above-

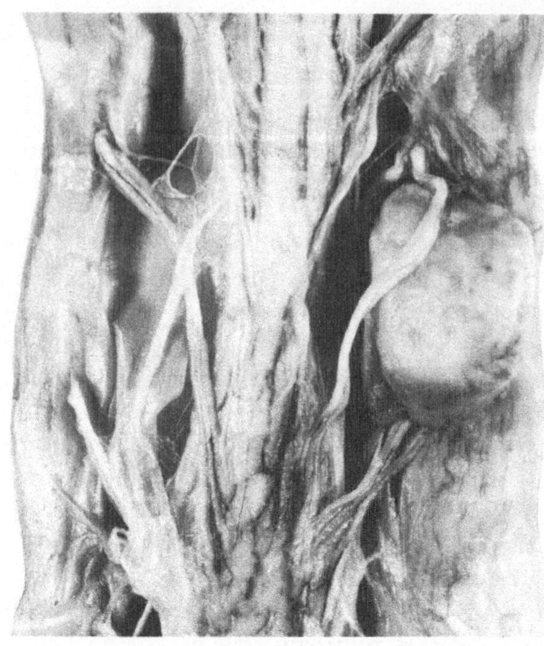

Fig. 64. Bean-sized spinal meningioma located dorsolaterally. (Case 807)

mentioned sites; there may be as many as 100 of them. They are often associated with acoustic nerve tumors, or other neurinomas and neurofibromas in von Recklinghausen's neurofibromatosis (*see* pp. 43 ff.; 76). Some authors apply the term *diffuse meningeal meningiomatosis* to the primary, usually sarcomatous, tumors in the subarachnoid space, and refer to the metastatic spread of gliomas throughout the cerebrospinal fluid pathways as *meningeal gliomatosis* (*see* pp. 116 ff.).

APPEARANCE TO THE NAKED EYE

The fresh operative specimen is dark red with lighter translucent parts; the cut section is coarsely fibrous, and cysts are found only rarely. The angioblastic type may be recognized by the coarse vascular meshwork on the cut surface. Meningiomas range in size from a pinhead to a man's fist, depending on location and type of growth (Figs. 61–63). Their form may be spherical, hemispherical or conical, or they may grow out *en plaque* or carpet-like (Fig. 63). Rarely are both types of growth combined, a conical tumor growing out of a flat one. The hyperostosis which they not infrequently induce leaves a corresponding impression, an umbilication, in the tumor. When meningiomas sit astride a bony ridge like the sphenoid wing, falx or petrous ridge, a corresponding saddle-shaped impression results (Fig. 63). If the growth takes place in two directions, as it does in tumors of the tentorium, a dumbbell form develops (Fig. 17, No. 60). The weight of meningiomas ranges from a few grams to 835 gms, and in one case has even reached 1300 gms, including the infiltrated bone; the average weight is 50–300 gms. Meningiomas are smoothly encapsulated, or coarsely, or finely nodular. The consistency varies, depending on the size, amount of degeneration (hyalinization, cyst formation), formation of fibers and calcification, and is described as rubbery or hard. At the site of dural attachment, where the connective tissue of the meninges radiates into the tumor, meningiomas are often harder than in other regions. The brain substance adjacent to the meningioma can either be pushed aside and compressed or can be both softened and edematous (edema necrosis —Jacob); it may even have undergone cystic degeneration.

HISTOLOGICAL APPEARANCE

Meningiomas behave differently, depending on the structure with which they are in contact. They generally only displace the brain and spinal cord but on rare occasions interdigitate by means of finger-like processes. The dura and the sinus are infiltrated rather consistently, which explains the tumor's firm adherence to these surfaces. The overlying bone, too, is not infrequently invaded and portions of the tumor extend uninterruptedly along the Haversian canals. This usually results in hyperplastic bony overgrowth, accounting for the protuberances and projections on the skull. Occasionally, large parts of the base of the skull become hypertrophic because of overlying tumor growth *en plaque*. However, there are also many instances of bony hyperplasia without actual tumor infiltration. The disproportion in size between the paper-thin tumor, consisting only of a few rows of cells, and the emormously thickened bone is sometimes grotesque.

Histologically, Bailey and Bucy (1931) first distinguished nine subgroups and subsequently Cushing and Eisenhardt (1938) recognized 22. In Globus' (1937) complicated subdivision the basis for classification frequently changes.

Aside from the fact that such a subdivision can scarcely find a practical application and would be advantageous only if each subgroup behaved biologically in a consistent manner—something which Cushing himself denied—we have often been unable to distinguish the subgroups even in Cushing's and Eisenhardt's own pictures. It is sufficient to distinguish three main tissue types of this macroscopically uniform tumor. Taking into consideration historical and pathological viewpoints, we have termed them as follows:

1. Endotheliomatous meningiomas
2. Fibromatous meningiomas
3. Angiomatous meningiomas

To these must be added a fourth group of meningiomas, showing malignant or sarcomatous de-differentiation.

1. The endotheliomatous meningiomas comprise all examples which form densely cellular tissue consisting of large "endothelial" cells, some-

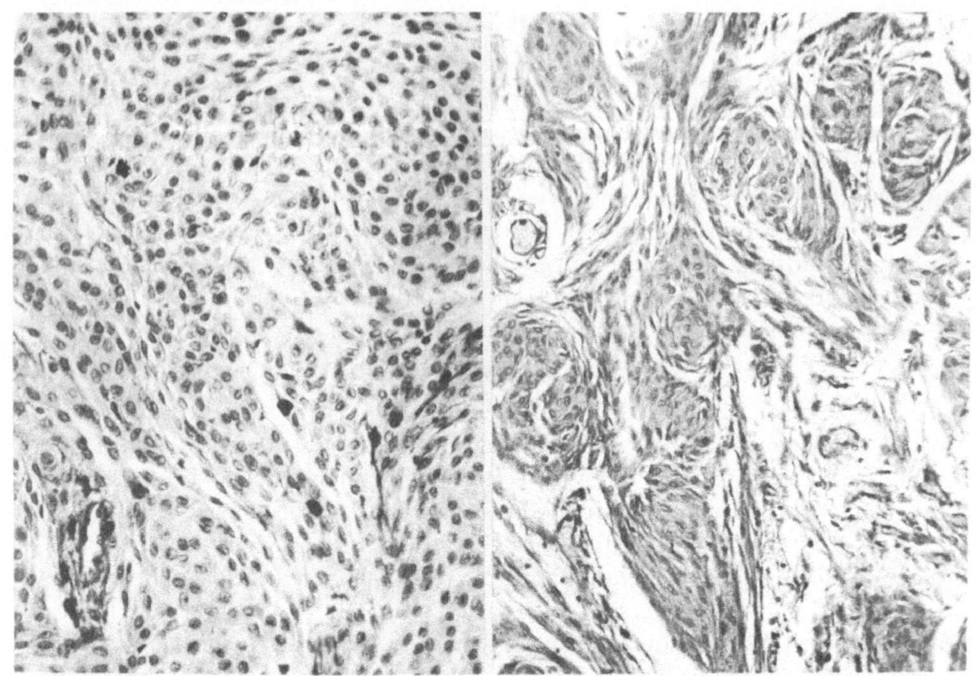

Fig. 65. a) *left:* A typical "endotheliomatous" meningioma. Islands and finger-like processes of cells forming a syncytium are seen. (x180, H. & E. stain); b) *right:* The division into islands is more pronounced as the interstitial tissue is better developed. Only a few capillaries are seen. (x150, H. & E. stain)

times without, but more frequently with, an interstitial tissue which divides the cell masses into islands, nests, and other cell groups (Figs. 65–67). An identifying characteristic of this form is its similarity to the nests of normal arachnoidal endothelium (Fig. 65a). The cells usually form a syncytium, are large, and their distribution is uniform, diffuse, or in long streams. The interstitial tissue is sparse, limited to a few vessels and fibers, and separates the individual cell groups from each other (Figs. 65b, 67). Silver methods allow one to identify this form particularly well (Fig. 67b), as the reticulin fibers are confined to the stroma. The cell nests not infrequently show a subdivision with concentric cellular arrangement (onion-skin) into rings (Fig. 66), whorls (Figs. 25c, 66a), or other patterns in which psammoma bodies develop (*see* below). Some meningiomas consist exclusively of such onion skin patterns with central hyalinization and calcification ("psammomas," Fig. 66a).

2. The fibromatous meningiomas comprise most of the "fibroblastic" forms and are very similar to a fibroma. The long, spindle-shaped cells lie in streams and whorls (Figs. 23b, 68a), but do not form palisades. Around the capillaries are loop-shaped formations and concentric layers of cells which bear a certain resemblance to the similar formations of the first

194

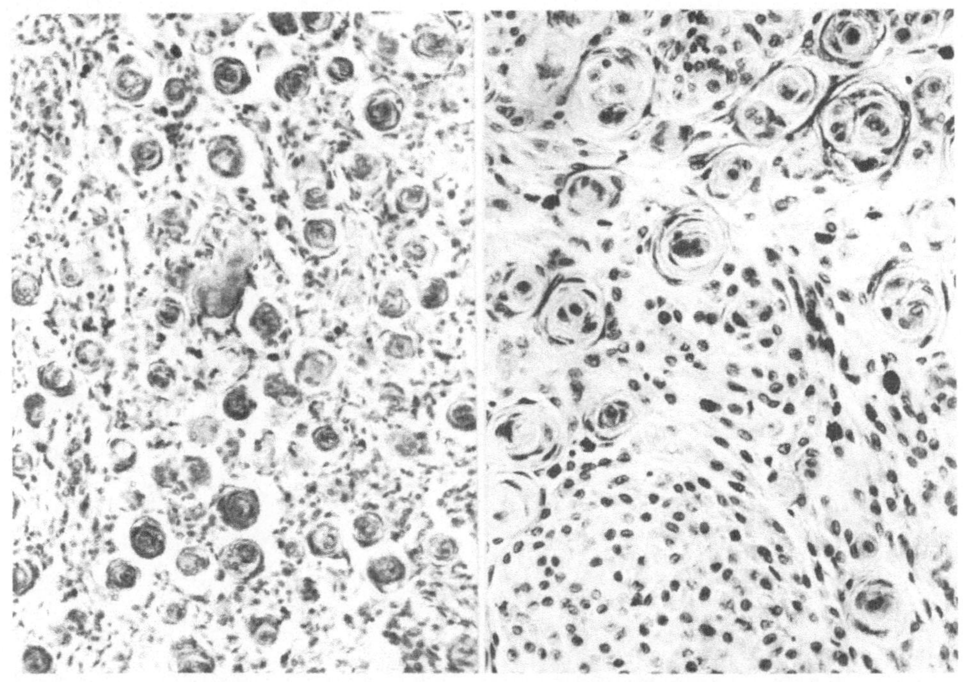

Fig. 66.   a) *left:* Certain meningiomas of endotheliomatous subtype tend to form cell groups arranged in an onionskin pattern. The centers of these cell groups undergo hyaline degeneration with subsequent calcification and formation of psammoma bodies. (x120, cresyl violet); b) *right:* Endotheliomatous meningioma with simultaneous presence of large islands of cells and small groups of cells arranged in onionskin pattern. (x360, Nissl stain)

group, where the central capillary, however, is missing. Metal impregnation reveals a dense network of true reticulin fibers between the cells (Fig. 68b), thus providing the best point for differentiation from neurinomas. Calcifications are spear- or club-shaped.

3. The angiomatous meningiomas represent the rarest form of meningiomas. This is in no way a particularly "vascular" meningioma but rather a type with a special architecture. The tissue consists of capillaries arranged in a network, interspersed with large lining cells. The endothelium of the vessels is of a single layer. There is a certain kinship with the angioblastomas, and occasionally histological differentiation between the two is not possible. However, the meningiomas are always well-encapsulated and grow by expansion. Here, too, the angiomatous structure is best revealed by silver staining. A few examples of this type, despite their benign biological behavior, present the histological picture of a pleomorphic tumor with atypical cells, hyperchromasias, etc. These are, however, secondary regressive processes and are in no way indications of malignancy. This last varient represents a transition to the endotheliomatous type (type IV, 2 of Cushing).

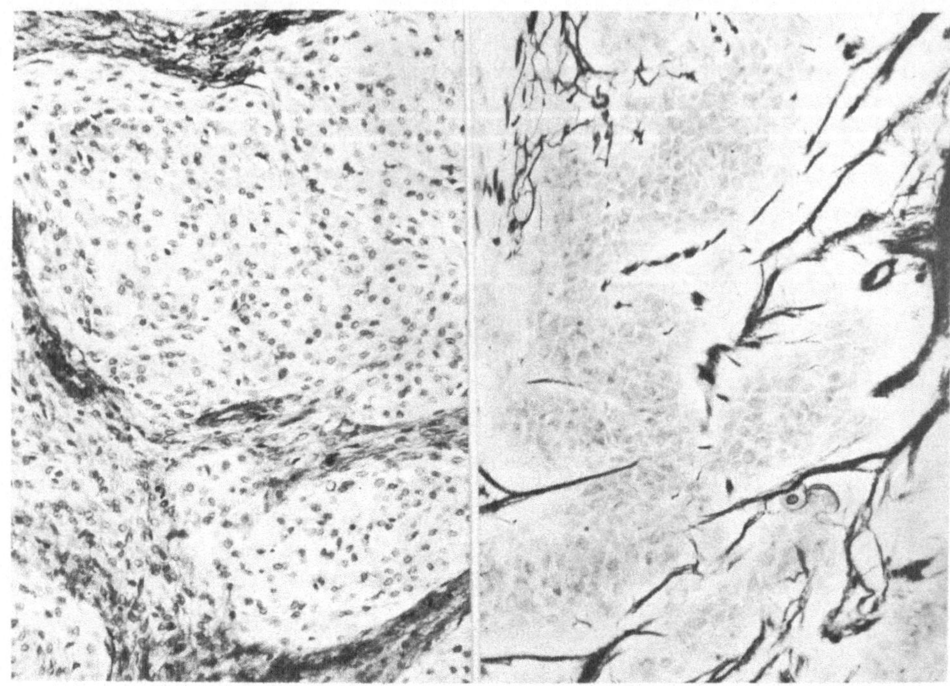

Fig. 67. a) *left:* Endotheliomatous meningioma with large cell-islands and abundant interstitial tissue (x136, Nissl stain); b) *right:* Similar tumor with silver impregnation of the connective tissue. (x136, Perdrau impregnation)

4. Meningiomas with sarcomatous degeneration are rare. Though they possess a sort of capsule, they are poorly demarcated from the brain tissue. These tumors are more cellular, have numerous blood vessels and a disorganized architecture, and grow rapidly (mitotic figures). They form a transition to the fibrosarcomas (*q.v.*), and, after some decades may metastasize to other organs.

Beside these main types, there occurs in rare instances the formation of fatty, cartilagenous, or bony tissue in the tumor. These cases can be characterized by the addition of the word "lipo-chondro-osteoblastic." Regressive processes are not uncommon in meningiomas. Most prominent is the tendency toward hyalinization of the interstitial tissue and blood vessels. In the fibromatous type, particularly, we find broad hyalinized swathes of tissue to a point where the architecture is lost. Calcifications in the form of psammoma bodies occur mainly in the endotheliomatous type, and in spear-shaped or plaque-like deposits in the fibromatous type. These regressive changes can, in rare cases, lead to the complete calcification of the whole tumor, so that the tumor can be demonstrated roentgenologically. There may also be calcification of the blood vessels. Fatty degeneration, though, is less apparent but can occur diffusely in scattered cells in the fibromatous type, or in the center of the cell islands in the

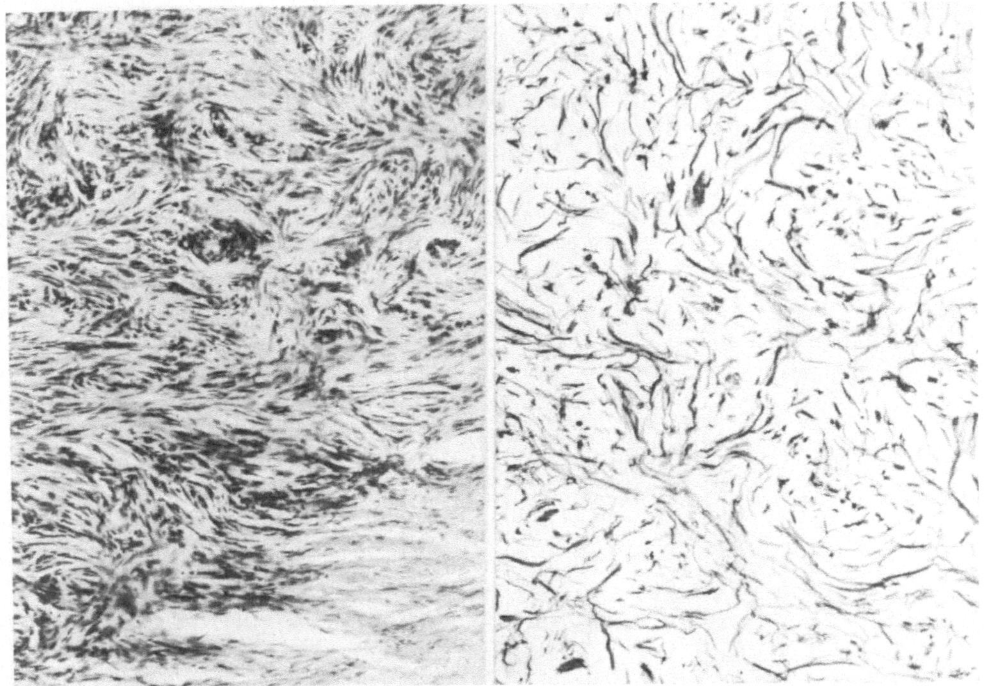

Fig. 68. a) *left:* Fibromatous meningioma. Spindle-shaped cells are arranged in streams and whorls. In the right lower corner one sees capsule tissue containing fewer fibers. (x120, H. & E. stain); b) *right:* Similar tumor with silver impregnation of the connective tissue. Numerous connective tissue fibers are seen. (x120, Perdrau's stain)

endotheliomatous type. A few meningiomas tend to undergo diffuse mucoid degeneration (Fig. 69b), with resulting small or large cysts (the size of a cherry-stone). Hemorrhages into the tumor are rare.

METASTASIS AND RECURRENCE

Meningiomas practically never metastasize. In a few cases, spread via the C.S.F. (Kalm, 1950), or via the blood stream to other organs (Cushing and Eisenhardt; Zülch, Pompeu and Pinto) has been described. A permanent cure by operation is possible only if the surrounding structures into which the tumor grows—sinus, dura, bone—are completely removed, too. It is often preferable to excise apparently healthy tissue as well, as the infiltration of hyperplastic bone is difficult to judge. Cushing himself had numerous recurrences, as is apparent from the fact that 522 operations were performed on 282 patients with meningiomas.

DIFFERENTIAL DIAGNOSIS

At the beginning of the operation, a surgeon may mistake an oligodendroglioma attached to the dura, or more rarely also a metastatic tumor, tuberculoma, or gumma attached to the dura, for a meningioma. However,

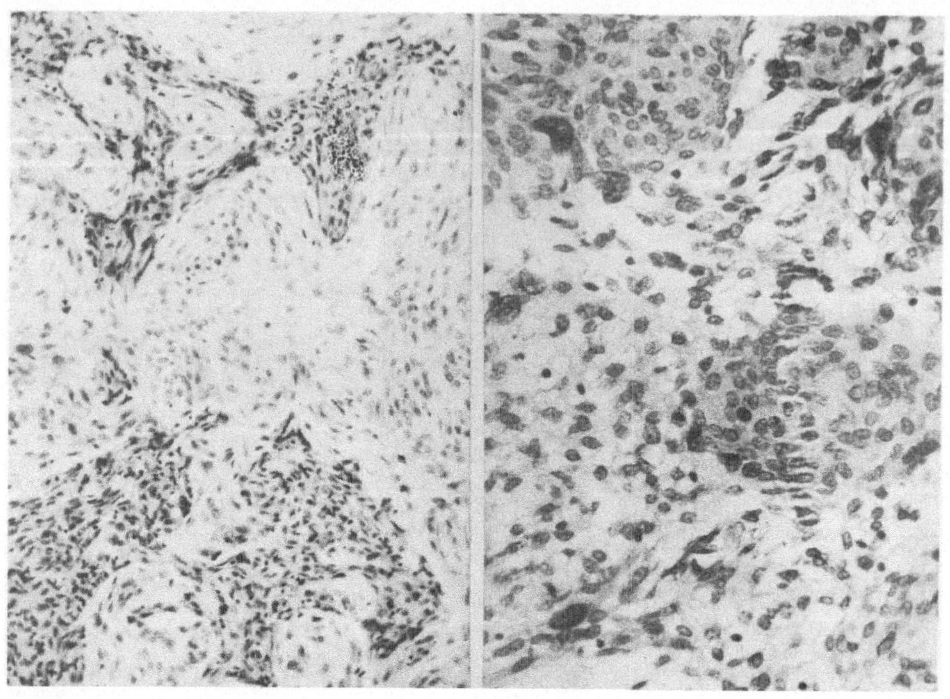

Fig. 69. a) *left:* Endotheliomatous meningioma in which the "parenchyma" and "stroma" are present in equal proportion. The stroma is very cellular. (x136, H. & E. stain); b) *right:* Mucoid and hydropic degeneration of an endotheliomatous meningioma. (x250, Nissl stain)

the nature of the tumor usually becomes apparent during the operation. In the cerebello-pontine angle or in the spinal canal, meningiomas are often difficult to differentiate from neurinomas, unless they are calcified on X-ray (which is rarely demonstrable in the spinal forms). Histologically, too, this differentiation is difficult, particularly with the fibromatous form of meningioma. The spindle-shaped nuclei of the neurinoma, its true palisading, the co-existence of tissue types "A" and "B," and the pronounced tendency to undergo fatty degeneration all favor a neurinoma, while any calcification favors a diagnosis of meningioma. Only the meningiomas form concentric whorls and show a dense intercellular network of true reticulin fibers; the neurinomas possess delicate "specific" argentophilic fibers. These tumors sometimes must also be distinguished from those of the glomus jugulare because of a certain similarity between these latter tumors and the endotheliomatous variety of meningiomas.

TUMOR GROWTH AND CLINICAL COURSE

Meningiomas, because of their slow expansile growth, can remain clinically silent for a long time although they may have reached enormous size, especially in the frontal lobe. Restoration of function after removal is therefore usually good. The history of the disease often extends over many years before symptoms of increased intracranial pressure set in. A history with an apoplectiform onset is unusual. The expansile growth leads to specific patterns of vessel displacement on the arteriogram, where vessels from the external circulation, or a diffuse network of capillaries within the tumor, are often filled. Because of the slow displacement of the adjacent brain, obstruction of the cerebrospinal fluid pathways is less frequent than with tumors that arise from the brain proper; the ventricles in cases of meningiomas tend to be rather small. The significance of bony changes on X-ray—vascularization, erosion, and hyperostosis—in diagnosing the specific tumor type need only be mentioned. Calcification of the whole tumor to the point where it is roentgenologically visible is specific for meningiomas. The abundance of blood vessels in certain meningiomas is so great that in the venous phase of the arteriogram the tumor appears "stained." The prognosis of meningiomas is the best of all brain tumors. Total removal leads to permanent cure. With recurrence, reoperation is usually successful. Malignant de-differentiation of a once benign tumor scarcely ever occurs (*see* however the case of Dorothy Russell, operated upon by Cushing, which showed malignant de-differentiation at the 17th operation, and died from pulmonary metastases (Cushing and Eisenhardt). Likewise, in a case of Zülch's, Pompeu and Pinto, death occurred from distant metastases after 22 years.

12. THE ANGIOBLASTOMAS

(Synonyms: Lindau's cysts or disease, angiomatosis of the central nervous system, cerebellar angiomas, epithelial angiomas, angioreticulomas, cerebellar hemangioendotheliomas.)

HISTORICAL NOTE AND DEFINITION

During a study of cerebellar cysts in 1926, A. Lindau found that a number of them contained hemangiomatous mural nodules and that they were often associated with small angiomas of the retina (the so-called retinal angiomatosis of von Hippel). He named this syndrome angiomatosis of the central nervous system. In the meantime, the name "von Hippel-Lindau's disease" became generally accepted. Berblinger (1928) had previously noticed a relationship between spinal angioblastomas and cysts of the pancreas. Roussy and Oberling (1930), on the other hand, had emphasized the relationship of the angioblastoma to the reticulo-endothelial system (angioreticuloma). However, their recognition of a special type, the "epithelial angioma," does not seem justified. Bailey, too, opposed the establishment of a special group of "angiogliomas." Again the angiogliomas of Bergstrand (Bergstrand, Olivecrona, and Tönnis) were nothing more than vascular spongioblastomas (the so-called cerebellar astrocytoma). Jung's term "cerebellar angioma" fails to take histological structure properly into account (*see* Angiomas and Aneurysms). Von der Hoeve classified von Hippel-Lindau's disease together with the phacomatoses (*see* Hamartoblastomatosis). It can also be related to other hamartoblastomatoses (Pennybacker).

For detailed studies we are particularly indebted to Cramer and Kinsey; Corradini and Browder; Davison *et al.*; Lotmar (1935); Putschar (1935); Olivecrona (1952); Cushing and Bailey (1928); Kautzky and Vierdt; Koella; Kufs (1932); Jung; Möller; Perlmutter, Horrax, and Poppen; Schuback; Silver and Hennigar; Tannenberg; Urban (1936); Vincent, Puech and David (1930); and Zeitlin (1942).

INCIDENCE AND SITE

There is a definite peak of age incidence of angioblastomas between 35 and 45, with the curve beginning to rise more steeply at 20, and trailing off between 50–60 (Fig. 12). Our youngest patient was 16 years old, the oldest 69. 41 patients were males and 19 females. Angioblastomas comprised 1.2% of intracranial tumors in Cushing's series, in our material (4,000 cases) 1.5%, and of 560 tumors (Gagel, 1938), 10 were angioblastomas.

The site of angioblastomas is usually restricted to the metencephalon and the spinal cord. Only isolated cases have been described in the cerebral hemispheres (Rochat; Kautzky and Vierdt).

The angioblastomas lie either 1) in the cerebellar hemispheres and vermis or 2) in the roof of the fourth ventricle (area postrema). In the cerebellar hemispheres we usually find them near the cortex, and less often solid than cystic (Fig. 70). The cysts are often many times larger than the solid portions. Occasionally, we can discover the cherry-pit sized, blue-red mural nodule (Fig. 71) but only after a prolonged search. The cysts are usually unilocular, only rarely multilocular, and almost never are large clusters of cysts encountered. The angioblastomas of the second group lie between the tonsils and the exit of the fourth ventricle at the calamus scriptorius in such a way that the underlying cysts firmly interdigitate with the floor of the fourth ventricle; (Fig. 17, No. 66), they may, therefore, at first be considered as large tumors of the medulla. In rare cases, a tongue of tumor reaches down to the level of the upper cervical segments. Multiple angioblastomas can occur, as in our case (No. 3347) of a 31-year-old man who had five tumors in the cerebellum and spinal cord. Multiple tumors are probably responsible for the sudden appearance of so-called recurrences (Pennybacker). In the full-blown syndrome, cysts in the kidney and pancreas are often found.

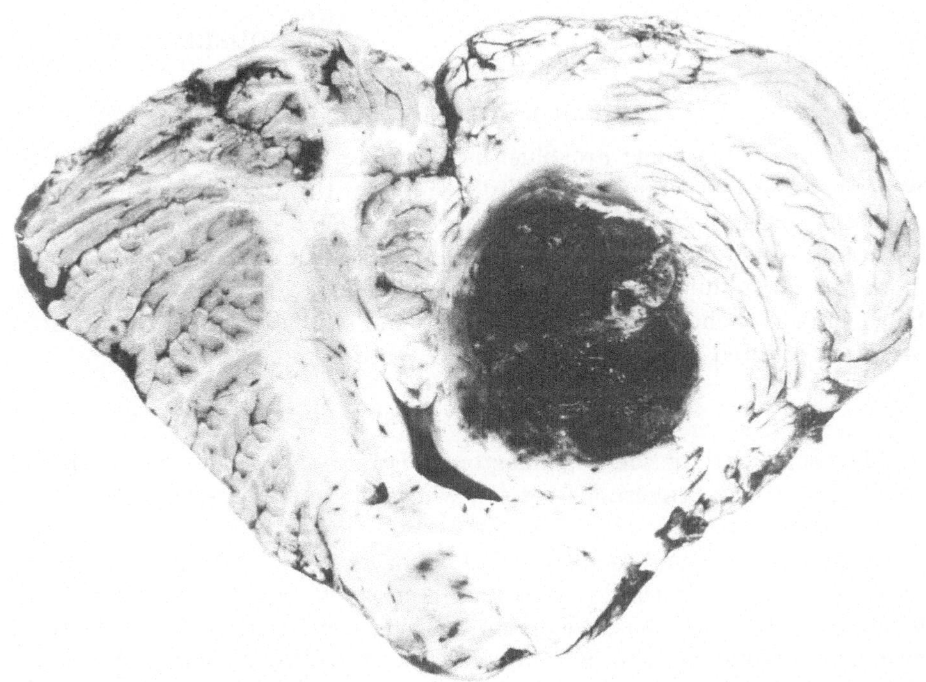

Fig. 70.   Angioblastoma of the size of a chestnut without cysts and with numerous massive hemorrhages. (Case 444)

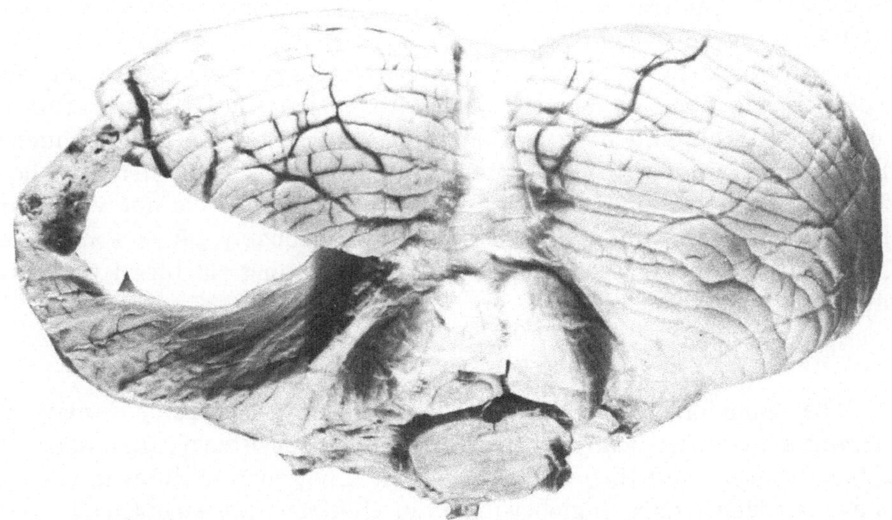

Fig. 71.   Huge cyst formed by a small angioblastoma seen in the upper left-hand corner of the picture. Marked herniation of both tonsils. (Case M 3528)

APPEARANCE TO THE NAKED EYE

The angioblastomas are blueish-red ("like a cherry") to brown-red, well-circumscribed tumors (Fig. 70), usually with large cysts which may be brown on the inside due to hemorrhages. The cyst fluid coagulates spontaneously upon cooling, and is yellowish or brown. The consistency of the mural nodule is soft and elastic. The size of the solid tumors can be as large as a chestnut, of cysts like a child's fist (Fig. 71); the tumors are often covered with tortuous cortical vessels.

HISTOLOGICAL APPEARANCE

The solid part of the angioblastomas is formed by dense networks of capillaries or large cavernous vessels, whose walls are covered with lining cells (interstitial cells), (Fig. 72a). In certain types, these interstitial cells predominate and form broad epithelial bands, or nests, which are separated by capillaries. While the interstitial cells are usually small, elongated, or triangular elements, these "epitheloid" cells can be large. They have a pronounced tendency to accumulate fat (pseudoxanthoma cells with birefringent lipid) which develops by infiltration rather than by degeneration. The capillary network consists of endothelium and a meshwork of abundant reticulin fibers. Numerous mast cells often are found between the blood vessels. Growth seems generally slow, and mitoses do not occur. In the growth zone, the tumor advances into the adjacent nervous tissue (Fig. 72a) by infiltration of the capillary loops. The angioblastomas also grow into the leptomeninges and infiltrate them. Lastly, they can even invade the dura, muscles, and skin—at least after operation (Pennybacker). Noteworthy among regressive changes are in particular hyalinization of connective tissue and degeneration into small cysts (concerning mucoid degeneration and mast cells, *see* Regressive Processes, p. 100 ff.). Just how the giant cysts, so characteristic of this tumor, develop is not yet clear. Transudation into small degenerative cysts probably plays some role. Calcification is never seen. Macrophages, containing old blood pigment, often lie in the vessel walls.

DIFFERENTIAL DIAGNOSIS

The spongioblastomas (so-called cerebellar astrocytomas) may be recognized macroscopically by their firm, tough consistency, their sparcity of blood vessels, and their midline position. They tend to differ in respect to age incidence, since angioblastomas in childhood are exceptional. Cyst formation is about the same in both. On inspection, metastatic hypernephromas may show a certain similarity to angioblastomas (brown-red color, etc.). Histologically, too, the "epithelial" forms of the angioblastoma bear

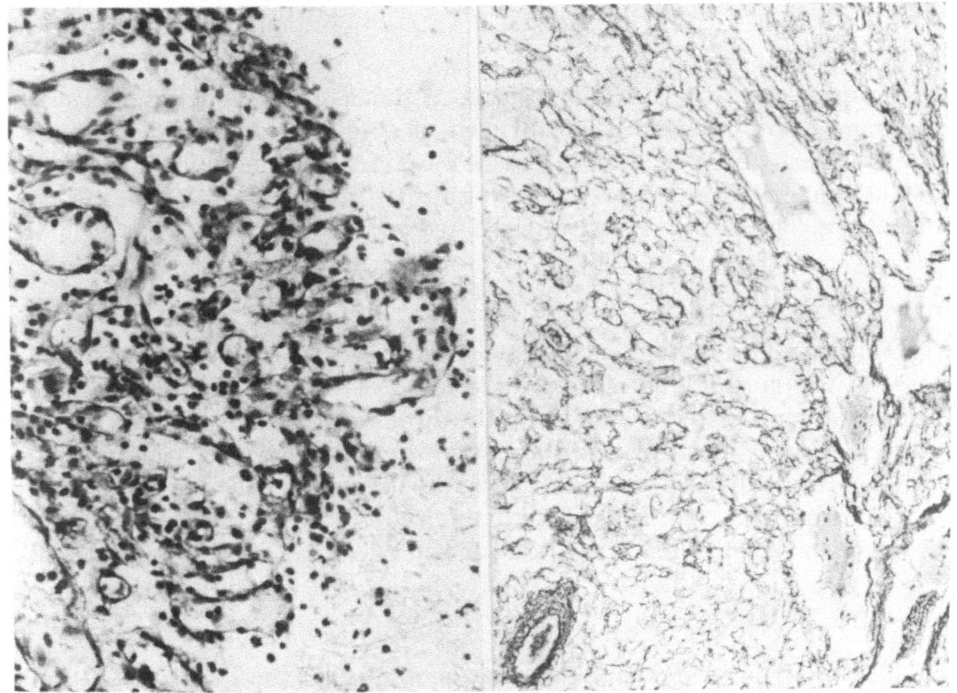

Fig. 72. a) *left:* Capillary network in the marginal zone of an angioblastoma. In between the loops of capillaries one sees interstitial cells showing fatty degeneration. (x136, Nissl stain); b) *right:* Capillary network in an angioblastoma as seen on the reticulin stain. A few small cysts are seen on the right side. (x84, Perdrau impregnation)

a certain resemblance to some hypernephromas, as was pointed out by Lindau (*see* also Hueck: *Morphologische Pathologie*, 1941, p. 722, Fig. 714). One of our own cases resembled this picture so much that a diagnosis of metastatic hypernephroma was first made, with an experienced pathologist concurring. The diagnosis had to be revised after the patient survived many years without any signs of a renal tumor. Angioblastomas—after surgical exposure—can sometimes be easily identified by the overlying veins in the leptomeninges.

Correlation between the pathology and the clinical picture: the clinical symptoms are accounted for by the tumor's location in the cerebellum and, in particular, by its tendency to form large cysts. These cysts fill up progressively (by transudation), produce signs of marked displacement of the intracranial contents—especially of the cerebellar tonsils—with obstruction and recurrent attacks of hydrocephalus. Clinically, a few of the angioblastomas are associated with polycythemia; if this is present, it may give an indication of the tumor type before operation. Prognostically, the angioblastomas should be listed among the benign intracranial tumors, even though they grow within the nervous parenchyma. Total removal results in permanent cure but recurrence should be expected if the cyst has merely been opened. Clinically it is often difficult to decide whether one is dealing with a recurrence or a new tumor, since multiple tumors are not uncommon. Malignant degeneration does not occur, and there is no metastasis. The tumor is moderately X-ray sensitive.

13. THE FIBROMAS

Once the fibromatous meningiomas have been eliminated, only a few cases of true intracranial fibromas are left. Nevertheless, there are some tumors without any connection with the dura—a proportion of them intra-cerebral—which fully deserve the name fibroma. They tend to undergo various degenerative processes, such as hyalinization, calcification (as in one of our own cases), or mucoid degeneration. (*See* also the contributions of Baker and Adams (1937), and Meyer and Scheller.)

14. THE SARCOMAS

The group of intracranial sarcomas is quite small after the elimination of meningiomas, medulloblastomas, oligodendrogliomas, and glioblastomas; this should be kept in mind when reading the older literature.

Presently we include in this group only the malignant tumors derived from connective tissue—from the vessels and meninges.

In accordance with the above definition, a separate group of sarcomas has been established, subdivided into four different types:

a) Diffuse sarcomatosis of the leptomeninges (meningeal sarcoma)

b) Diffuse sarcomatosis of the blood vessels (the so-called adventitial sarcoma)

c) Circumscribed sarcoma of the arachnoid (of the cerebellum)

d) Circumscribed sarcoma of the blood vessels (the so-called monstro-cellular sarcoma)

The following tumors qualify as transition forms from the meningiomas to the sarcomas:

e) Fibrosarcomas, both inside and outside the dura, that grow into the brain by infiltration and show signs of accelerated cell growth even though externally they may be similar to a meningioma (*q.v.*). There is a question when to call them "malignant meningiomas," and when "sarcomas." I would like to propose capsule formation as the fundamental distinguishing characteristic. Malignant meningiomas have a capsule and grow only by expansion; sarcomas of the dura grow into the brain by infiltration. The sarcomas generally have more mitoses than the malignant meningiomas. However, a good deal of caution is indicated when making the diagnosis of sarcoma. The time is past when such a diagnosis could be made simply because one was at a loss for something else. The term, however, remains appropriate for the following four types (*see* Zülch, 1953):

Further references: Abbott and Kernohan; Bailey (1929); Black and Kernohan; Connor and Cushing; Döring (1940); Gömöri; Hsü; Környey (1933); Marquardt; Neubürger and Greene; Nonne; Rössle (1939); Schaltenbrand and Bailey; Schmincke (1924); Wilke (1950, 1952); Winkler.

a) Diffuse sarcomatosis of the leptomeninges (meningeal sarcomas)

This is a well-known group, into which several medulloblastomas have previously been placed erroneously. It is a tumor of the young or middle-aged, where, macroscopically, the leptomeninges are clouded, as in meningitis, and the thickened cisterns are plugged with whitish masses. Single small nodules may occur but large circumscribed tumors are not found. In the leptomeninges, whose reticulin framework is increased and thickened, microscopic examination discloses a diffuse accumulation of lymphoid and chromatin-rich, or elongated and polygonal cells with scanty cytoplasm. Growth is rapid (mitotic figures). The infiltrates mold themselves into the leptomeninges and the subarachnoid spaces, and penetrate into the brain along the blood vessels and directly. Locally they often cannot be distinguished from the infiltration of the meninges by medulloblastomas. (*See* Fahr (1936); Fried (1930); Gömöri; Connor and Cushing.)

b) Diffuse sarcomatosis of the blood vessels (the so-called adventitial sarcomas)[1]

We can distinguish this form from the preceding one by the way it restricts itself to infiltration around the intracerebral vessels, while the leptomeninges are not involved at all, or infiltrated secondarily, and only in exceptional instances. The picture of this tumor, which occurs mainly in adults, is characterized by the growth of tumor cells along the vessel wall, by moderate pleomorphism, a high rate of cell division and simultaneous widespread nuclear degeneration (Fig. 75a). The areas of diffuse perivascular spread may merge with individual tumor-like accumulations of neoplastic cells. A gradual transition leads to the "special granulomas" (Wilke, 1955) mentioned below. On superficial examination of the sparsely cellular regions of this tumor, there is danger of confusing it with the lymphoid cell infiltrates of encephalitis.

[1] Conclusive proof in the important case of Környey is unfortunately not available since a complete autopsy was not performed.

c) **The circumscribed sarcomas of the arachnoid**
(of the cerebellum)

These tumors were described for the first time by Foerster and Gagel (1939) and have been confirmed in the literature many times since. They are sharply circumscribed nodular tumors, often spreading over the surface of the cerebellum like a mushroom, and occur in the middle decades. Histologically, they are characterized by the co-existence of islands of lightlystained, large cells and streams of dark, lymphoid cells. A dense network of reticulin fibers permeates the tumor in places where the leptomeninges could not have been engulfed. We have no cases of our own. This tumor group needs further detailed study.(*See* Marquardt; Neubürger and Greene.)

d) **The circumscribed sarcomas of the blood vessels**
(the so-called monstrocellular sarcomas)

These curious tumors have only recently been distinguished from the group of nerve cell tumors or glioblastomas, to which they seem to be most closely related in growth and external appearance. These were the tumors described as ganglioneuromas or spongioblastoma gangliodes by Schmincke (1914), and later by Wätjen; Paul; Alpers (1931); Foot and Cohen; H. J. Scherer (1933, 1935); and Foerster and Gagel (1939). Their sarcomatous nature had previously been suspected—Foot and Cohen had related them to the reticulo-endothelial system. We called attention to it in 1940 and offered proof in 1947 and 1953. A comparison with certain giant cell tumors (e.g., sarcomas of the spinal column) comes to mind at once, as well as the parallelism to a benign cousin, the giant-cell epulis, which, according to earlier views, was supposed to have originated from vascular buds. In all probability, the circumscribed sarcomas originate from a specially differentiated perithelium. They are not infrequently encountered in large collections of tumors with the mistaken diagnosis of "glioblastoma." It is not yet possible, therefore, to determine their incidence. We suspect that one monstrocellular sarcoma occurs for every 20 glioblastomas. The tumors have been described in patients of all age groups (our youngest patient was five, our oldest 64). They are found in all portions of the brain, with a certain predilection for the brain stem. What is usually first noted on inspection is the tumor's sharp delimitation—occasionally resembling a metastasis—and its fleshy, fine-tufted, fibrous, and asbestos-like surface (Fig. 73). Large cysts are quite common (but are rare in glioblastomas). The variegated color of the glioblastoma is usually not seen, the sarcoma being a uniform gray-pink. Necrosis, fatty degeneration, and hemorrhagic foci, therefore, are not much in evidence. The consistency is firmer than that of the brain itself, and may often be termed tough, due to the abundance of reticulin fibers.

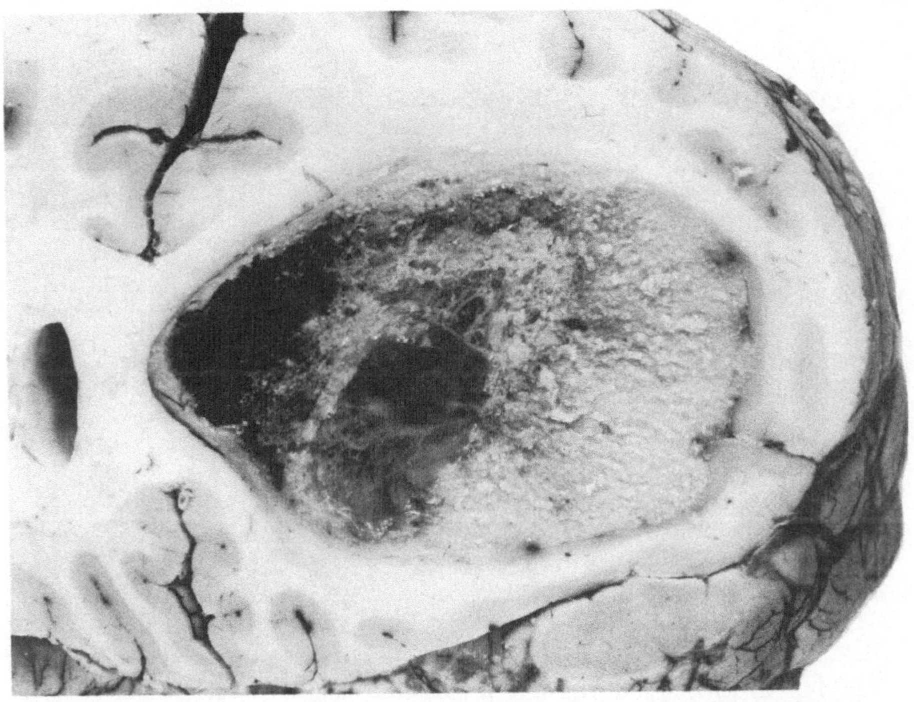

Fig. 73.   Huge monstrocellular sarcoma with large cysts. The tumor is sharply demarcated from the brain and shows a characteristic fibrous cut surface. (Case 946)

These sarcomas are characterized by a great variety in their histological picture, but two architectural patterns predominate: 1) in the periphery are regions containing spindle-cells, densely arranged in streams (Fig. 74a) and 2) in the center, areas of giant tumor cells of the most bizarre and fantastic form, (Figs. 74b, c) "which, because of their form and size, can not be compared to anything else in the human body." Both types can occur together. The monster cells are atypical in every conceivable way: they can assume almost any shape and are up to 400 μ. in size; there are single giant nuclei (Fig. 74b), multinucleated masses, inclusion bodies—as many as 50–80 in a single cell—bird's eye patterns (a central core surrounded by a halo), vacuoles (Fig. 74c), a honeycomb pattern of the cytoplasm, lobulation of the nuclei, hyperchromatic nuclei, neurone-like nuclei and also ghost cells without nuclei. Mitotic figures may also be grotesquely abnormal. In their earlier stages the spindle cells resemble fibroblasts. Occasionally, lymphoid infiltrates in the marginal zone are found. Between these various types of cell, a dense network of reticulin fibers is formed—even in the center of the tumor. In the growth zone the tumor not infrequently spreads by means of vascular buds. Large, hyperchromatic tumor cells detach themselves from the adventitia of these vessels, and are found lying singly in brain tissue which has

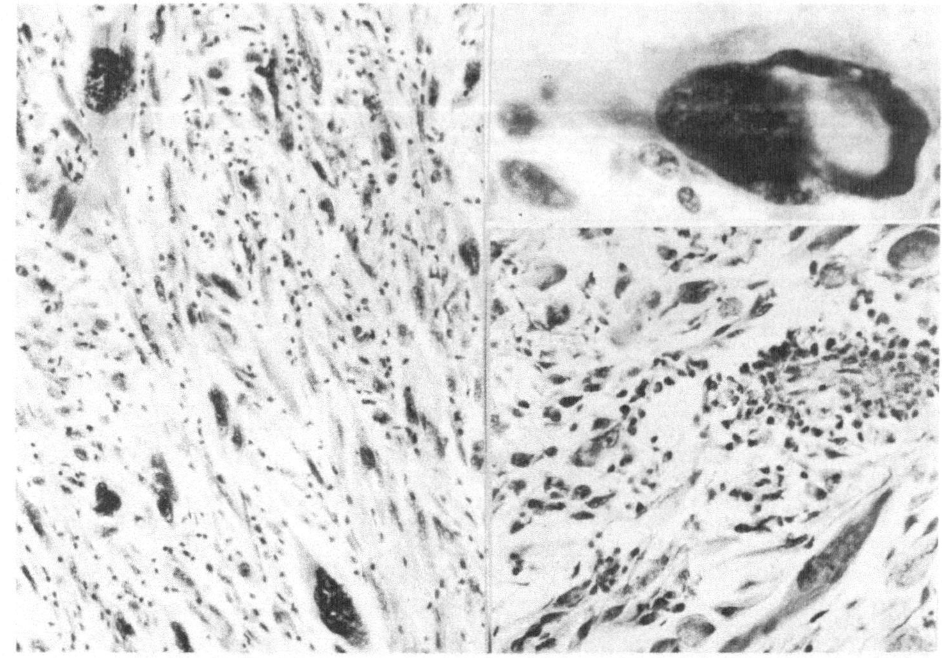

Fig. 74. a) *left:* Typical region of a monstrocellular sarcoma. Cells of all sizes can be seen: giant, monstrous cells with hyperchromatic nuclei, middle-sized spindle cells and small, lymphoid cells. (x86, Nissl stain); b) *top right:* Vesicular (neurone-like) nucleus of a giant cell. (x650, Nissl stain); c) *bottom right:* Giant spindle cell and a blood vessel surrounded by small cells in a monstrocellular sarcoma. (x120, Nissl stain)

scarcely yet been infiltrated. On the other hand, the tumor cells may lie in dense rings, with abundant reticulin fiber formation (Fig. 75b), around the blood vessels. Regressive processes are seen in the form of fatty degeneration of the tumor cells, or of formation of small necrotic foci and cysts. We have never seen calcification. Vascular overgrowth, which is so prominent in glioblastomas, plays a much less important role. The monstrocellular sarcomas seem to manifest a tendency toward diffuse spread into the leptomeninges, something which is quite uncharacteristic of the glioblastoma. As far as we can tell, we are dealing there with very malignant, rapidly growing tumors. They characteristically infiltrate the dura and can grow beyond it—something which never occurs in glioblastomas. For the differential diagnosis between this tumor and the glioblastoma, *see* p. 162.[2]

e) Fibrosarcomas

There is a gradual transition from primary fibrosarcomas of the dura to sarcomatous meningiomas (*see* p. 196). For purposes of distinction I would like to propose that we call the tumors which are still encapsulated

[2] A case recently sent us (E 870) had lung metastases; another cardiac metastases.

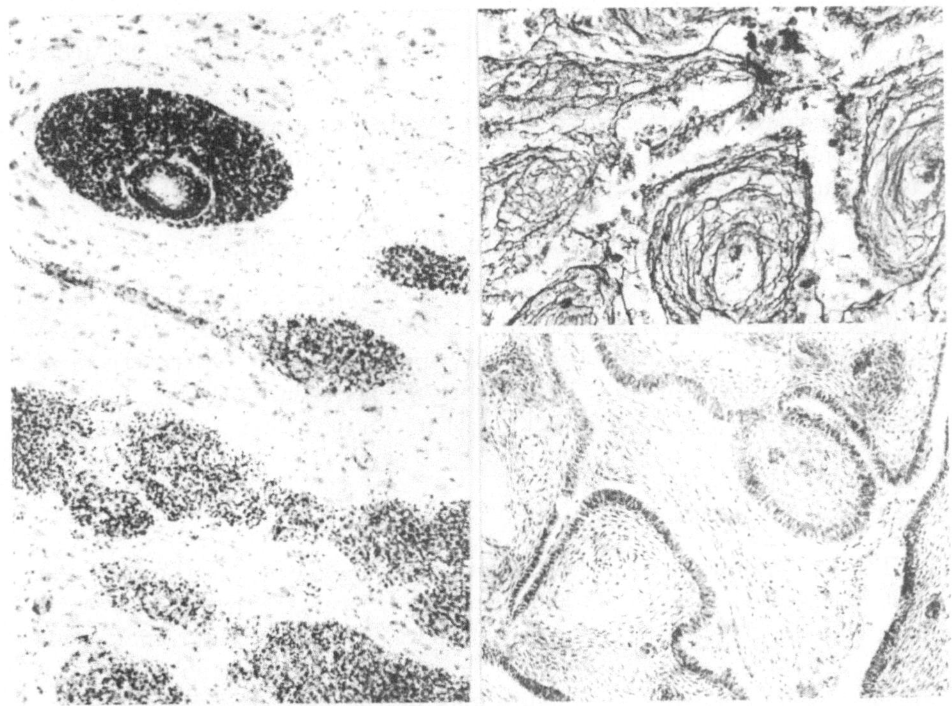

Fig. 75.   a) *left:* Diffuse perivascular sarcomatosis (the so-called perithelial or periadventitial sarcoma). The tumor is composed of small cells spreading along the blood vessels. The centers of tumor growth which are thus formed can merge together. (x80, Nissl stain); b) *top right:* Concentric rings of reticulin fibers around the blood vessels in a monstrocellular sarcoma. (x100, Perdrau method); c) *bottom right:* The marginal zone of a craniopharyngioma. One sees fingerlike extensions of the tumor into the brain tissue, which shows reactive gliosis. (x120, Nissl stain)

but have a rapid growth *malignant (sarcomatous) meningiomas,* and the infiltrating tumors of the dura which grow without a clear border *primary fibrosarcomas.*

Primary diffuse melanomatosis

The primary melanoblastoma of the brain was many years ago related to the chromatophores of the leptomeninges, believed to be their tissue of origin. The pigment of the tumors has to satisfy the staining criteria of the pathologists. The primary nature of these tumors must be assured by excluding the presence of a primary in other organs. The melanomas occur particularly in youth and middle age and are, generally, rare. Macroscopically, the leptomeninges look thickened and smoky-gray or dark brown; occasionally lentil-sized nodules are present. Sometimes only a histological study can reveal the true source of the grayish discoloration of the leptomeninges. The histological picture is very uniform. The melanin-containing cells are either multipolar, or more rounded and elongated.

Some of the cells are amelanotic. These tumors penetrate into the nervous tissue along the blood vessels. Melanomas spread diffusely throughout the cerebrospinal fluid but do not metastasize to other organs (*see* Lence).

Retothelsarcomas (reticulum-cell sarcomas)

In the superior nasopharynx and the neighboring portions of the base of the skull, the retothelsarcomas are not rare. They produce late neurological symptoms from involvement of cranial nerves or the structures of the base. Their existence in the brain itself has been described, but not substantiated. Their histology is described in pathology textbooks (*see* Döring, 1940).

15. THE CHONDROMAS

The chondromas arise from the dura of the convexity, of the falx, and most often of the base (close to the foramen lacerum), but they also occur in the choroid plexus of the lateral ventricles. Multiple chondromas occur on the spinal dura, though they take up very little space. Such tumors are rare on the laminal arches. Chondromas of the nervous system are the same as those elsewhere in the body, growing predominantly by expansion; they can produce bone and are often calcified. When next to bone, they erode it.

Further references: Brütt; Danis and v. Eyck; Green and Childrey; Klingler; Learmonth and Verbruggen; Smitt; Volland (1938); Wolf and Echlin.

16. THE LIPOMAS

The first lipomas were observed by neuroanatomists in cases of aplasia of the corpus callosum. An excellent description was provided by Bostroem (1897) in his fundamental work on dermoids. A large number of case reports and review articles have increased our knowledge of these tumors, which are not—by and large—space-occupying neoplasms. We have, in the following discussion, disregarded all those cases that were observed as part of spina bifida, myelomeningoceles and encephaloceles. The rarer, space-occupying lipomas manifest themselves in earlier decades of life than those that are encountered incidentally at autopsy. The latter type does not seem to be too rare actually (six cases were reported within three years from one mental hospital). Lipomas occur in six places: 1) Above the corpus callosum; when a part or all of the corpus callosum is missing, they appear in the size of either a bean, or a plaque a millimeter or slightly more in thickness; 2) at the infundibulum as a pea-sized lesion; 3) on the quadrigeminal plate as a pea-sized lesion; 4) attached to the choroid plexus of the lateral or third ventricle in the form of a bean- to egg-sized tumor; 5) in the other cisterns or over the convexity (rare); 6) along the spinal cord, where they are found a) in the lower thoracic region over a few segments, or b) drawn out over the whole spinal cord or, c) in the region of the cauda equina. They usually lie in the region of the posterior columns.

The lipomas are sharply circumscribed, but are tightly fastened to the adjacent nervous tissue by penetrating strands of connective tissue and blood vessels, making removal difficult. They are similar to lipomas in other parts of the body. In the brain, they can be surrounded by calcified leptomeninx. The lipomas of the spinal cord are especially important neurosurgically.

Further references: Eckart; Ehni and Adson; Krainer; E. Scherer (1935); Vonderahe and Niemer.

17. OSTEOMAS AND OSTEOSARCOMAS

Osteomas of the skull have to be carefully distinguished from reactive bone formations, such as arise over meningiomas, either without neoplastic infiltration or with the Haversian canals permeated with tumor. True osteomas with a very low growth potential occur either in the form of small exostoses on the outer surface of the skull, or intracranially—particularly on the anterior clinoid processes, on the lesser wing of the sphenoid, or around the porus acousticus. The growth rate of osteomas pressing on the orbital roof or ethmoids is more rapid. Certain spongiomatous osteomas show the growth characteristics of autonomous neoplasms. True osteosarcomas of the calvarium must be distinguished from reactive osteomatous hyperplasia of meningiomas (*see* p. 193). Ossifying fibromas of the nasal sinuses occur particularly in the first decades.

Further references: Abbott and Courville; Christensen and Busch; Geschickter (1939); Herzog; *see* also Kleinsasser, O., Arch. Klin. Chir., 285, 274–307, 1957; the same author's Pathologie der Tumoren des Hirnschädels in Hdbuch. d. Neurochirurgie, Vol. IV, 1, Springer, Berlin, 1958; and Kleinsasser and Albrecht, Arch. Klin. Chir., 285, 115–133, 1957.

18. THE CHORDOMAS

The controversy over the origin of chordomas has a long history that starts with the discussions between Virchow and Müller; Ribbert (1914) was the first to relate the tumors correctly to notochordal rests (Müller actually was of the same opinion but yielded to Virchow). In older people they are encountered as incidental findings on the clivus and scarcely act as space-occupying lesions (the so-called benign chordomas). But they may grow autonomously, occasionally with malignant degeneration, at a variety

of sites where notochordal tissue is found during embryological development. The chordomas produce clinical symptoms in the third and fourth
decades, with only the sacro-coccygeal chordomas manifesting themselves
earlier. They are two to three times more common in males than in females.
Their size varies from that of a millet seed, or cherry (noticed only by
accident) to that of a man's fist. Indeed, in the true pelvis they can attain
the size of a child's head by developing antero-posteriorly. They may lie
at the base—subsellar or on the clivus—from where they expand destructively toward the nasopharynx, or grow toward the chiasm, or the foramen
magnum. Chordomas occurring in the vertebral column lie predominantly around the dens of the axis; others grow in the sacral or coccygeal
regions. The clivus and the last-mentioned regions are most frequently
involved. They rarely metastasize. Macroscopically, the chordomas are
whitish, translucent and gelatinous, or of a somewhat brownish-red color;
occasionally, they are broken up into coarse nodules. Histologically, they
correspond to the basic pattern of notochordal tissue, i.e., vesicular cells
with chromatin-rich nuclei. In a way they resemble plant cells. More or
less hyalinized connective tissue or osteoid regions may traverse the tumor.
The center of the growth often contains packed cells, less vesicular and
with smaller nuclei. Malignant forms show mitoses, hypercellularity,
pleomorphism, and less vacuolization. Regressive processes consist principally of mucoid degeneration, while hemorrhages, calcification, and bone
formation can occur. The chordomas seem to be quite X-ray sensitive but
their operative removal is generally not very successful because of the
way they infiltrate the bone.

Further references: Bailey and Bagdasar; Boemke and Joest; Bormann;
Coenen; Hass; Herzog; Jeliffe and Larkin; Poppen and King; Zeitlin and
Levinson.

CHAPTER XIII

EPITHELIAL TUMORS

19. CRANIOPHARYNGIOMAS

(*Synonyms: Tumors or cysts of the hypophysial duct, cysts or tumors of Rathke's pouch, tumors of Rathke's cleft, craniopharyngeal pouch tumors, suprasellar cysts, pituitary stalk tumors, Erdheim's tumors, adamantinomas or ameloblastomas of the pituitary region.*)

HISTORICAL NOTE AND DEFINITION

Some of the older descriptions of "Markschwämme" or medullary carcinomas of the pituitary were most probably descriptions of craniopharyngiomas. However, we owe to Erdheim (1904) the first correct interpretation and adequate description of these tumors. Among subsequent contributions, the following are especially worth mentioning: Strada; Critchley and Ironside; Frazier and Alpers (1931); McLean (1930); and Wittermann.

Further references: Berckmann and Kubie; Love, Shelden and Kernohan; Müller and Wohlfart; Zeitlin (1935).

INCIDENCE AND SITE

The craniopharyngiomas can definitely be considered as tumors of childhood and adolescence but they occur in adults as well. Cushing himself had two patients over 60 years of age. The peak of incidence occurs between the ages of 13 and 23 (Fig. 13). The oldest of our patients was 62, the youngest five years old. In childhood and adolescence craniopharyngiomas of the chiasmal region are the most common tumors. In our material (4,000 cases) they comprised 2.7% of all tumors, in Cushing's 4.6%. In the series of Frazier and Alpers of 244 lesions around the sella, only 14 were craniopharyngiomas (11 of those were histologically verified), and in McLean's series they formed 30% of the "hypophysial tumors." In our series, 65 patients were males and 42 females.

Since the craniopharyngiomas occur exclusively in the region of the sella, their only variation in site is in their relation to the diaphragma sellae and the direction of spread from this point. Thus there are both intrasellar

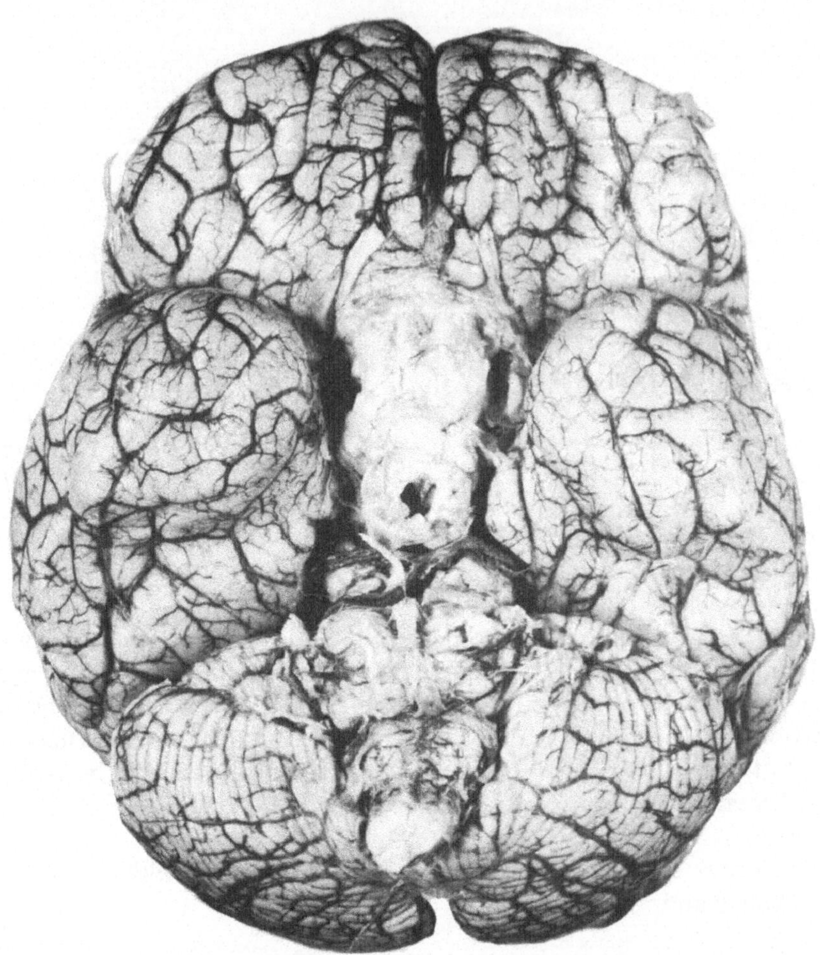

Fig. 76. Large suprasellar craniopharyngioma filling the third ventricle. The fine nodular whitish-gray surface can be distinguished clearly from the brain tissue. The chiasm is displaced upwards and anteriorly. Both olfactory tracts are displaced laterally. Bilateral cerebellar pressure cone. (Case 465)

and suprasellar craniopharyngiomas. Of these, the intrasellar types are at first separated from the brain by the dura and arachnoid. As they grow, however, they push the diaphragma upward—generally breaking through it—growing on in the direction of the third ventricle where they excavate a bed for themselves from below. The suprasellar type (Fig. 76) starts in the arachnoid of the basal cisterns and pushes directly against the third ventricle, whose place the tumor may eventually occupy as it continues to grow (Fig. 17, Nos. 67–69). The ventricular floor thus becomes paper-thin and tears so that the tumor capsule abutts directly against the ventricular wall. The relation of the tumor to the chiasm varies. Some tumors displace it antero-superiorly, stretching it into a thin band; others, from the first,

214

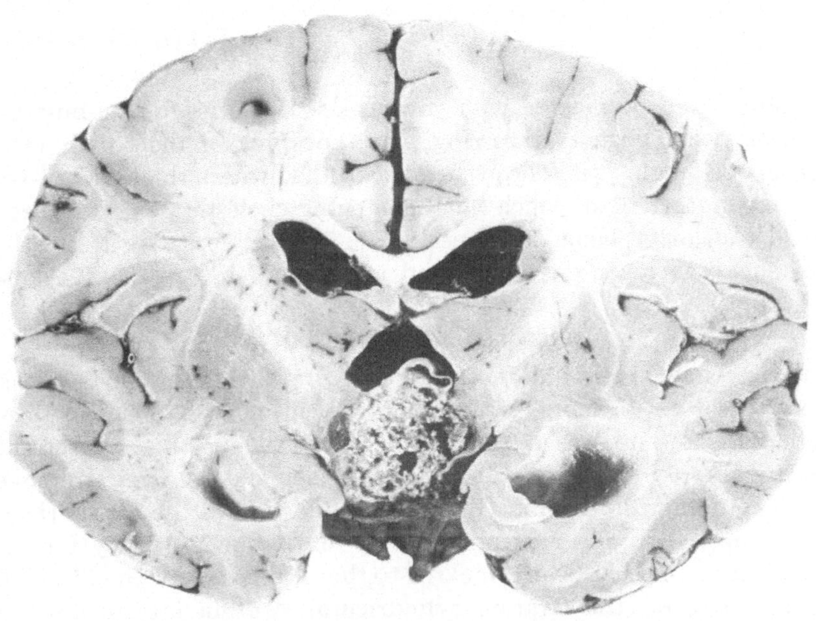

Fig. 77. Suprachiasmatic craniopharyngioma pushing up against the third ventricle. Hydrocephalus of lateral ventricles. (Case 1635)

develop above the chiasm (Fig. 77) and force it downward; still others lie, so to speak, "in the lumen" of the third ventricle and can scarcely be seen on the base of the brain. All of this is very important in the operative removal of these tumors. They also occasionally grow posteriorly, in the direction of the thalamus and pons. They can expand to either side and occupy the region of the frontal or temporal lobes (we saw a tumor at each such site the size of a fist). The pituitary will be displaced downward, flattened out, and damaged by the intrasellar craniopharyngiomas, with the floor of the sella being markedly eroded. On the other hand, the suprasellar craniopharyngiomas often leave the hypophysis and the bony sella undamaged. These various ways of growth can be explained embryologically by the varying primary site of the corresponding "rest" of the hypophysial duct. Occasionally, primary craniopharyngeal cysts are encountered that do not form a solid tumor. They usually lie intrasellar. (This brings up the question of their relation to cysts of the pars intermedia—Müller and Oswald).

APPEARANCE TO THE NAKED EYE

Craniopharyngiomas are well-encapsulated tumors which grow purely by expansion. Their size varies from a pea to a walnut; at times they reach the size of a tennis ball. They have a smooth encapsulated or finely nodular surface, and a gray-pink color (Fig. 76). On cut surface they are spongy and porous, and permeated with various-sized cavities, depending on the degree of cystic degeneration (Fig. 77). The bulk of the tumor often is made up of a single cyst. The cyst cavity is filled with a thick brown-yellow fluid (like motor oil) in which small glistening cholesterol crystals are suspended, the latter being type-specific for this tumor. The tumor has a tough and tenacious consistency and is rather hard in parts because of calcification.

HISTOLOGICAL APPEARANCE

Where they are not degenerated, the craniopharyngiomas consist—like the basal cell tumors—of a system of epithelial bands and bridges, held together and nourished by the connective tissue stroma. The epithelial zones are about 8–20 layers thick; and on their outside they are covered by high columnar epithelium (Fig. 75c), while toward the inside they are less organized and form a progressively more spongy syncytium. This histological picture has been compared to the three strata of the Malpighian layer of the skin: the stratum cylindricum, stratum intermedium, and stratum spinosum. The presence of the latter stratum in the tumor depends, however, on the degree to which regressive changes have taken place. The architecture of the epithelial zones can be either more "adenomatous" or more "papillary," depending on regressive processes and the variation in the amount of stroma (Figs. 75c, 78a). Regressive changes are numerous and consist in liquefaction of the cells, ranging in degree from the first stage, the spiney cell (Fig. 78a), all the way to complete disintegration of the tissue. In addition, there is a type of degeneration in which the cells swell to the point where they lose all stainability without showing any tendency toward cornification and its particular staining properties or the early stages of keratohyalin formation (*see* Epidermoids). True cornified epithelial pearls are not seen. Only a *keratoid* substance is laid down. The deposition of calcium salts in these keratoid regions is a recognized peculiarity of the craniopharyngiomas, allowing them to be visualized on X-ray. The stroma, too, undergoes regressive changes; it swells, becomes edematous and relatively acellular, and finally undergoes cystic degeneration, so that we can observe cyst formation in both the ectodermal and mesodermal portions. The craniopharyngiomas grow very slowly and mitoses do not occur. They do not metastasize; recurrences are the rule, except in the case of total removal—a very difficult technical feat. In the course of tumor growth, a zone of reactive gliosis may arise in the floor of the third ventricle; it sometimes reaches the thickness of ½ cm. and resembles a spongioblastoma both macro- and microscopically. We interpret this as a cicatricial reaction due to the fatty acids that are produced by the regressive processes, particularly to cholesterin, which is also capable of producing a marked inflammatory reaction.

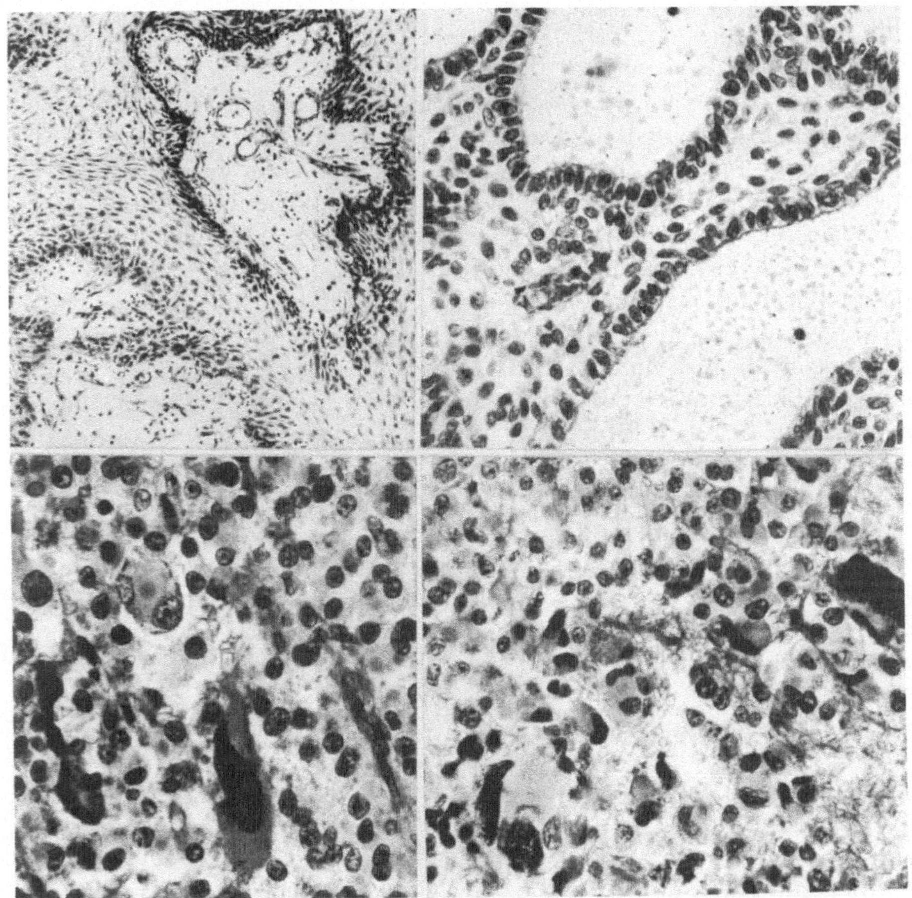

Fig. 78.   a) *top left:* Typical appearance of a craniopharyngioma: epithelial cell bands separate islands of stroma which contain blood vessels. Softening begins in centers of the cell bands. The stroma is swollen and undergoes mucoid degeneration. (x94, Nissl stain); b) *top right:* Cell band in a craniopharyngioma covered by a layer of cylindrical cells. (x250, Nissl stain); c) *bottom left:* Pleomorphic appearance of an eosinophilic adenoma of pituitary. d) *bottom right:* Eosinophilic pituitary adenoma. Epithelial cells and a few giant cells with hyperchromatic nuclei are seen. (x320, H. & E. stain)

DIFFERENTIAL DIAGNOSIS

It is necessary to differentiate between epidermoids and those craniopharyngiomas that have been completely transformed into cysts. In the latter, large cavities are formed, covered with a thin capsule of neoplastic tissue with small mural tumor nodules. Not only is the cyst content of craniopharyngiomas and epidermoids different[1] but the regular deposition of layers of "epidermis," and particularly the true cornification of epidermoids (with keratohyalin granules), facilitates a histological differentiation.

[1] Epidermoids contain concentric layers of swollen, shed-off epithelial pearls; craniopharyngiomas, a brownish, oily fluid.

The secondarily cystic craniopharyngiomas as well as the primary craniopharyngeal cysts have to be distinguished from the ependymal cysts in the
region of the foramen of Monro (*see* p. 00). Only in the earlier literature
was there any confusion between the plexus papillomas or the hypophysial
adenomas of "fetal" type (Fig. 80b) and craniopharyngiomas. The slow
growth of craniopharyngiomas accounts for the long clinical course; their
position in relation to the third ventricle and their frequently firm attachment to the base of the skull present the surgeon with great difficulties.
Drawing off the cyst fluid, or making a permanent opening in the cyst wall,
is adequate to improve the clinical picture for a time; the final aim, though,
must always be the total removal of the tumor or at least the restoration
of the cerebrospinal fluid circulation. The diagnosis of these tumors can
frequently be made on X-ray. It is important to remember that the C.S.F.
serology is occasionally positive in craniopharyngiomas. Unfortunately,
the indifference among clinicians to endocrine disturbances is still so great
that even today a majority of these patients come to the hospital only
because of increased intracranial pressure, by which time the tumor
is already enormous (Müller and Wohlfart).

20. PITUITARY ADENOMAS

(*Synonyms: Pituitary cancer, hypophysial struma.*)

HISTORICAL NOTE AND DEFINITION

It is surprising how little the older clinicians knew about hypophysial
tumors, in spite of the frequently grotesque external disfigurement of those
patients (*see* Nothnagel, 1879). The real study of this group of tumors
began only with Pierre Marie's discovery (1886) of the connection between
acromegaly and the eosinophilic pituitary tumors. A period of definite
progress began with the comprehensive studies of Erdheim, Benda, Kraus
and Berblinger, and of such clinicians as Babinski, Marie, Falta, Simmonds,
and Fröhlich at the beginning of the twentieth century. Once the surgical
approach to this region had been mastered (Hirsch, Horsley and Krause),
Cushing, in 1912, was able to publish a comprehensive monograph on
diseases of the pituitary. Tumors were soon classified, in accordance with
the normal hypophysial cells, into chromophil (those with stainable
cytoplasm) and chromophobe types. The former could be further subdivided into acido- or eosinophil, and baso- or cyanophil types. Of the
three types of adenomas, the basophilic ones—because of their minute
size—are of little surgical importance.

Further references: Antoni (1950); Bailey and Cushing (1928); Bakay
(1950); Dott and Bailey; Frazier (1930, 1936); Henderson; Jefferson

(1954); Kux; McLean (1936); Müller (1954); Müller and Pia; Puech and Stuhl; Röttgen and Peters; Roussy and Oberling (1933); Russell (1950); Salus; Strada; Tönnis (1949); Tönnis, Müller and Brilmayer; Tönnis, Oberdisse, and Weber; Vosskühler.

INCIDENCE AND SITE

Pituitary adenomas practically never occur under the age of 20 and tend to increase in frequency only in subsequent years. The rather blunt peak of the age curve lies around 37–41 years (Fig. 14). The age incidence of the three types is the same. Only the mixed forms seem to occur in somewhat younger patients (Tönnis *et al.*, 1953).

The space-occupying pituitary adenomas[2] comprised 7.0% of intracranial tumors in our collection of 4,000 cases. In Cushing's series, because of the particular interest of the author, they occurred with a disproportionately high frequency of 17.8%. However, the relative proportion of the three subtypes in operated cases is characteristic: of Cushing's 338 cases, 260 were chromophobe, 67 acidophil, and 11 adenocarcinomas.[3] Of our patients with pituitary tumors, 151 were males and 131 females.

Their site is naturally confined to the region of the chiasm. Only in exceptional cases does a pituitary tumor occur in the body of the sphenoid bone.

APPEARANCE TO THE NAKED EYE

By their growth, the pituitary adenomas produce an increase of the sellar contents, so that the sellar walls are forced laterally, toward the sphenoid sinus and in the direction of the third ventricle. Later, the pituitary tumors bulge up next to the pituitary stalk and press on the optic tract or the caudal (less often, the oral) portion of the chiasm, depending on the form and position of these structures. In still later stages, the chiasm is pushed anteriorly (Fig. 17, No. 70) or, more commonly, pushed up and stretched over the tumor. There are exceptional cases, in which the chiasm is compressed without any gross changes in the sella. On the other hand, the acidophilic adenomas generally produce marked clinical (endocrine) changes before they reach the chiasm. Large, space-occupying tumors therefore usually belong to the chromophobe type. After rupturing the diaphragma, the tumor grows toward the floor of the third ventricle and may occupy its lumen (Fig. 17, No. 71). The chiasm can be cut into by the overlying anterior communicating artery, if the former is pushed

---

[2] Microscopically tiny miniature forms of pituitary tumors are found in about 10–20% of the population. Whether these represent the precursors of space-occupying tumors has not yet been established.

[3] This does not correspond to the relative percentage of the different cell types in the normal gland. The chromophobe tumors are therefore relatively more frequent.

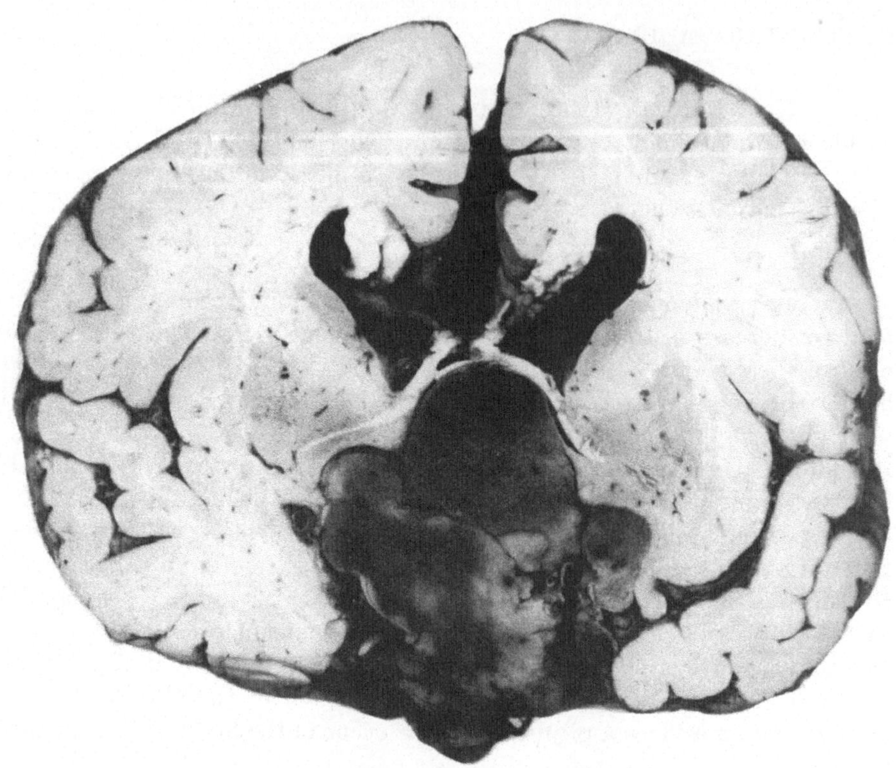

Fig. 79.   Large chromophobe adenoma of the pituitary which grew predominantly in the direction of the third ventricle, and, to a lesser extent, laterally toward the temporal lobes. The carotids are surrounded by the tumor. (Case 1292)

upward enough. The constricting effect of the chiasm can produce an indentation or "waist" in the tumor itself. The larger adenomas can grow around both carotids (Fig. 79), or may grow anteriorly against the frontal and laterally toward the temporal lobes (Fig. 22, No. 70), while extension toward the paranasal sinuses is usually less pronounced. Nonetheless there are cases in which the tumor erodes the spongy bone and spreads out extradurally over the base, leaving the skull together with the exiting nerves and vessels to appear on the under-surface of the skull. The pituitary adenomas appear well-encapsulated, with occasional small nodules protruding from the capsule (Fig. 79). The size of truly space-occupying chromophobe adenomas ranges from that of a plum to a child's fist. During life they are dark to blue-red while the eosinophilic adenomas, because of hemorrhages within the tumor, often have a brownish color. The capsule of the tumor is quite tough, whereas the contents are so soft that they can be removed with a sucker. The adenomas grow into the brain purely by expansion.

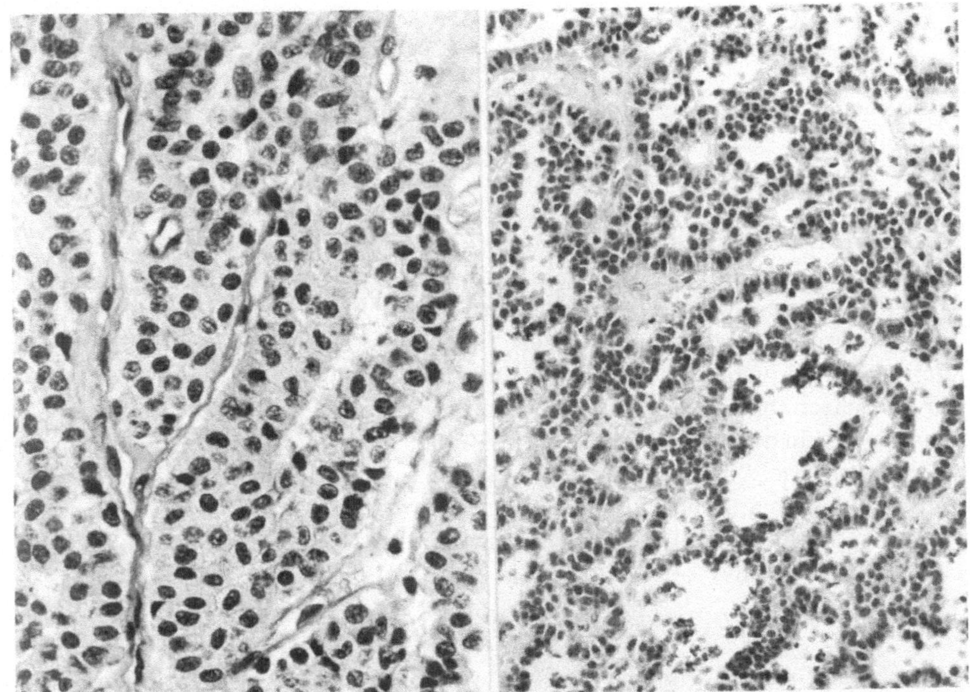

Fig. 80. a) *left:* In a chromophobe adenoma the "cylindrical" cells lie around the capillaries. (x270, H. & E. stain); b) *right:* In a so-called "fetal" subtype of chromophobe pituitary adenoma a "papillary" architecture is predominant. When regressive processes occur, the cells close to the blood vessels survive longer and produce typical architecture—epithelial-like cells covering numerous capillaries. (x120, H. & E. stain)

HISTOLOGICAL APPEARANCE

Histologically, the pituitary tumors have a rather monotonous structure. The pinhead-sized basophilic adenomas are composed of a sharply circumscribed though not encapsulated accumulation of these cells in an otherwise normal hypophysis. The eosinophilic adenomas, definitely larger, are composed of a neoplastic proliferation of the corresponding cells, which, however, assume a characteristic architecture: the eosinophilic adenomas are composed of islands of these cells separated from each other by scanty stroma (Figs. 78c, d). In contrast to the latter, the chromophobe adenomas are distinguished by their "epithelial" cellular arrangement into bands and broad columns which occur predominantly along the numerous capillaries (Fig. 80a). A subtype (the so-called fetal pituitary adenoma of Kraus, 1926) even assumes an almost papillary architecture (Fig. 80b), so that it is easily confused with plexus papillomas and papillary ependymomas (particularly after some dissociation of the tissue due to liquefaction). There are no indications, however, that this form is more malignant than the others, much as the name might suggest it. In addition to these pure types, there are "transitional" forms (Bailey, 1932) between the chromophobe and acidophil types in which the architecture and cell type tend more to one or the other—the "mixed cell" adenomas of Kraus (Tönnis *et al.*, 1953). The cell types of the individual tumors can be recognized on H. & E. staining, but are always verified ultimately with special stains (*see* Technique). There are also multinucleate cells in the eosinophilic adenoma (Figs. 78c, d). The rate of growth is slow and mitoses are rare. Regressive processes, however, are well known. Hydropic swelling going on to liquefaction and cyst formation, for instance, is very common in the chromophobe tumors. In this way, the architecture can become completely lost. Characteristic colloid-filled cysts do occur but calcification is extremely rare. Metastases have been described in only a few cases but are not unequivocal. Recurrence after operation, even after intensive X-ray radiation, is not so rare, and reoperation of recurrent adenomas is usually worthwhile.

The so-called adenocarcinomas

Certain pituitary adenomas, showing cell pleomorphism and rapid growth (mitoses), have been called adenocarcinomas by the American school. They are presumed to infiltrate the dura. This type, however, has not yet been sufficiently described to be judged. In any case, they do not infiltrate the brain. We have seen no cases of this sort. Even the malignant tumors reportedly arising primarily from the hypophysis are not altogether convincing (Budde; Cagnetto; Dandy, 1932, 1938; Fahr, 1918; Köhlmeier, 1944).

The growth rate of hypophysial adenomas is slow and the clinical history therefore long. The endocrine syndromes of the different adenoma types are too well known to warrant description here. Hemorrhages into the tumor can bring about an apoplectiform worsening of symptoms. (List *et al.*, 1952; Brougham *et al.*, 1950; Röttgen and Peters; Müller *et al.*, 1954.)

Primary carcinoma of the brain

Carcinomas of the brain would have to originate from the epithelial structures of the brain or its glandular appendages: hypophysis, epiphysis, choroid plexus epithelium, ependyma, or the immature stages of these tissues. Remembering the theories of embryonic tissue origin, we will have to eliminate even the pineal gland, plexus epithelium and ependyma, since they are really a special form of the nervous parenchyma, which we, together with Hortega, prefer to call paraglia.

The majority of pituitary tumors are benign. There are cases, nonetheless, that erode their way out of the sella by pressure (not by infiltra-

tion); they penetrate far into the bone—as far as the temporal squama—
and then grow back along the structures which pierce the base of the skull
—nerves and blood vessels—forming separate nodules on the under-surface
of the dura. These forms, however, show no signs of malignant invasion of
the overlying brain and therefore do not fulfil the definition of a carcinoma.
(It is curious, on the other hand, that malignant neuroepithelial tumors
never invade mesodermal structures destructively.) Only two "pituitary
tumors" are said to have metastasized via the C.S.F. and those have not
been adequately described. Two cases of craniopharyngioma are supposed
to have metastasized the same way. We have never observed true carcinomatous degeneration, such as was described in an epidermoid (Hug), in
craniopharyngiomas. Among pinealomas, we have studied one tumor which
was histologically similar to carcinoma. It metastasized, however, only
via the cerebrospinal fluid—as is so common—but not to other organs. We
therefore prefer to list it as an anaplastic form of pinealoma. A few cases
of metastasis of pinealomas to the lungs, though, have now been conclusively demonstrated. Finally there remain only the ependyma and choroid
plexus as a source of possible "carcinomas." Both give origin to quite benign
tumors which can metastasize by implantation via the C.S.F., though their
behavior is otherwise consistently benign. When ependymomas undergo
malignant degeneration, they may resemble the medullary carcinoma (*see*
Zülch, 1940), but do not otherwise fulfil the carcinoma requirements. Histologically, plexus papillomas are almost never malignant. However, I
have now observed two cases with definitely malignant degeneration (*see*
p. 175). Cases in the literature described as primary brain carcinomas are
not convincing. Earlier observations (Le Blanc; Bielschowsky and Unger;
v. Lehoczky, 1928) have already been critically refuted by Kufs. After
careful study and comparison with presently known brain tumors, these
carcinomas must be looked upon as metastases from tumors originating
elsewhere in the body, with the primary tumor having remained undis-
covered. This fact is supported by experiences of our own pathological
institutes where autopsies were performed with the greatest of care. We
can therefore conclude this section without having to introduce a group of
primary brain carcinomas.

Further references: v. Braunmühl; Gromelski; Hart; Saxer (1902).

21. CYLINDROMATOUS EPITHELIOMAS

The "cylindromas" (Billroth) or "cylindromatous" epitheliomas occur
intracranially at two sites: 1) beginning as nasopharyngeal tumors, they
force their way from the nasopharynx through the crista galli, displacing
the fronto-orbital part of the frontal lobes upwards; 2) more commonly,

they grow from posterior toward the Gasserian ganglion, forcing themselves into it (Walter, 1955; Zülch, 1956). There they resemble the neurinomas macroscopically. Histologically, they are cellular epithelial tumors which probably originate from the embryonic buccal cavity (nasopharynx, Eustachian tube). They form large epithelial islands and processes which liquefy in their centers, forming the "cylinder." These regressive changes can progress to the point where a colloid-filled lattice-work similar to colloid goitre is formed, and the possibility of actual secretion has to be considered. The cylindromas not only tend to recur (total removal is rarely possible), but some of them undergo malignant degeneration and metastasize to other organs (*see* also Learmonth and Kernohan).

The so-called "nasopharyngeal" tumors

This group is apt to include some benign and some malignant tumors of the nose and pharynx, especially the "cylindromas" (*see* above), and such malignant tumors as the squamous cell carcinomas, lymphosarcomas, reticulum-cell sarcomas, the so-called nasopharyngeal fibromas, and others.

CHAPTER XIV

CONGENITAL AND EMBRYONIC TUMORS

22 and 23. EPIDERMOIDS AND DERMOIDS

(*Synonyms: Pearly tumors, tumeurs perlées, cholesteatomas with and without hair, sebaceous cysts.*)

HISTORICAL NOTE AND DEFINITION

Because of the unusual, fatty content of epidermoids and dermoids, descriptions of them can be found in the early literature. Cruveilhier, as early as 1829, reported on "pearly tumors", and Joh. Müller in 1838 gave a very detailed account about "Perlmutterglänzende Fettgeschwülste" (fatty tumors shining like mother-of-pearl). For the fundamental work dealing with the embryological explanation of their origin, though, we are indebted to the elder Bostroem. Extensive studies, particularly by Critchley and Ferguson; Mahoney; and Wettler, followed. Today the epidermoids and dermoids are sharply separated from other squamous epithelium containing tumors, e.g., craniopharyngiomas, and the inflammatory cholesteatomas of the middle ear. We therefore avoid the use of the name cholesteatoma for this neoplastic condition.

Further references: Bailey (1933); Bauditz; Birkmayer and Hasenjäger; Hug; Findeisen and Tönnis; Krieg (1936); v. Lehoczky; Love and Kernohan; Olivecrona (1932, 1949); Rand and Reeves; Scheinker (1948); Stender (1937).

INCIDENCE AND SITE

The age curve of the dermoids and epidermoids shows a definite peak around the age of 40 (Mahoney[1]); in our material, it lies between 25 and 40 (at the time of operation or autopsy), while in the curve representing the age of onset of the condition it lies far to the left, having its peak around the age of 15. These are therefore very slow-growing tumors (Fig. 15). In

---

[1] A curve derived from purely neurosurgical cases is going to be displaced much farther to the left, toward the younger age groups, since Mahoney included many cases from the literature which were incidental findings at autopsy.

Cushing's material the epidermoids and dermoids comprised 0.7%. In our own series of 4,000 cases the epidermoids formed 1.5% and dermoids 0.1%. Findeisen and Tönnis found 48 cases of epidermoids among 5185 intracranial tumors, i.e., 0.9%. Dermoids are numerically less frequent. Of our patients, 41 were males and 25 females. Verbiest (1938) had six males in eight spinal cases.

Since the epidermoids and dermoids develop in all probability from embryonic rests, their predilection for certain sites is understandable.

Epidermoids occur by preference at the following sites:

Cerebello-pontine angle or parapontine

Chiasmal region or parapituitary

Longitudinal fissure and anterior corpus callosum

Around the quadrigeminal plate and posterior corpus callosum

Sylvian fissure

Lateral ventricles

Third ventricle

Fourth ventricle, and midline cerebellum

Diploë of the skull

Spinal cord

Multiple epidermoids apparently do not occur.

The *dermoids*, on the other hand, are particularly apt to lie around the pituitary, the pons, or along embryonic closure lines. They are most common along the line of closure between the maxillae and orbits (the embryonic naso-optic furrow) and may actually grow into one orbit; they are also encountered along the cerebellar midline and in the sacral region. Neurosurgically the most important dermoids are those of the neck, which penetrate all the way to the dorsal raphé of the cerebellum, those on the face (orbito-ethmoidal dermoids), and those in the region of the cauda equina. It is important to recognize that epidermoids can melt the adjacent parenchyma by setting up inflammatory processes, so that an epidermoid cyst of the fourth ventricle, for example, may have a broad connection with the cerebello-pontine angle through the lateral recess (Birkmayer and Hasenjäger), or an orbito-ethmoidal dermoid can break into the anterior horn of the lateral ventricle. The size varies from that of a pinhead to an orange. The surface of *epidermoids* is covered by a delicate capsule and appears whitish and shiny, like mother-of-pearl. It may be smooth, lobulated, or knobby with daughter nodules (Fig. 81). The blood vessels run in the capsule. On suitable sectioning, the contents consist of shining masses of friable, leafy material arranged in layers like onion-skin. The inside is occasionally softened. The *dermoids* have a firm pod or shell, and are generally filled with a greasy, soapy mass containing numerous short hairs. The contents are formed by the continual proliferation of new

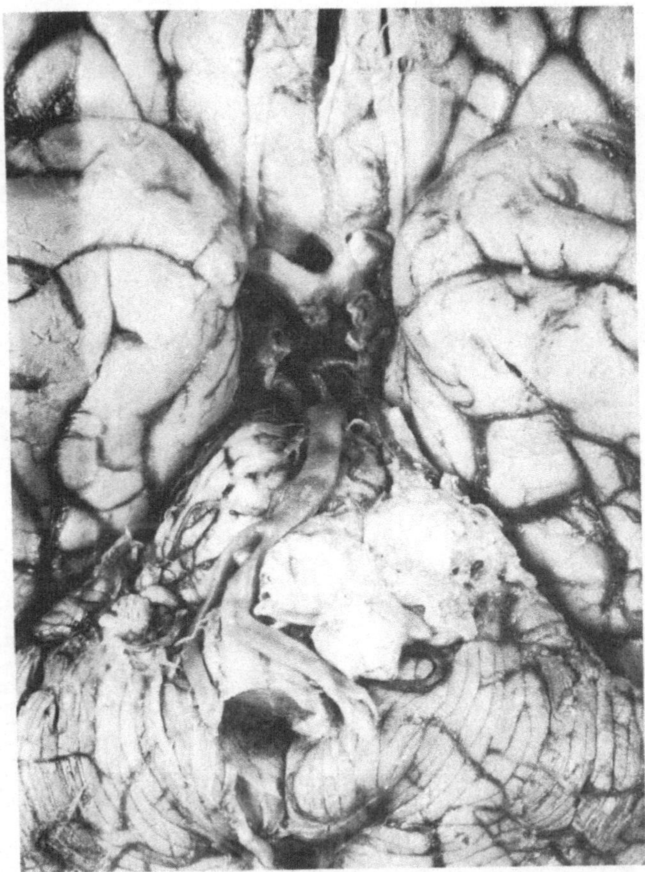

Fig. 81. Parapontine epidermoid (epidermoid of the cerebello-pontine angle). The basilar and vertebral arteries are displaced. Cerebellar pressure cone. (Case HB 6666)

cells of the germinal layer, degeneration of these cells (deposition of kerato-hyalin granules), and finally cornification, along with the simultaneous secretion of sebaceous material and sweat from the corresponding glands, and the formation of hair.

HISTOLOGICAL APPEARANCE

The epidermoids are characterized by great monotomy of their histological picture. In their small external capsule we see the three normal layers of the epidermis: the stratum germinativum, granulosum, and corneum, with a total of between two and five, or occasionally as many as ten, cell layers (Fig. 82a). Certain epidermoids are noteworthy because of the papillary architecture of this capsular layer. The dermoids differ from the epidermoids in that they contain the accessory structures of skin: the dermis, with hair follicles, hairs, sebaceous glands (Fig. 82b), and (sometimes) sweat glands. Of great importance is the inflammatory effect of the

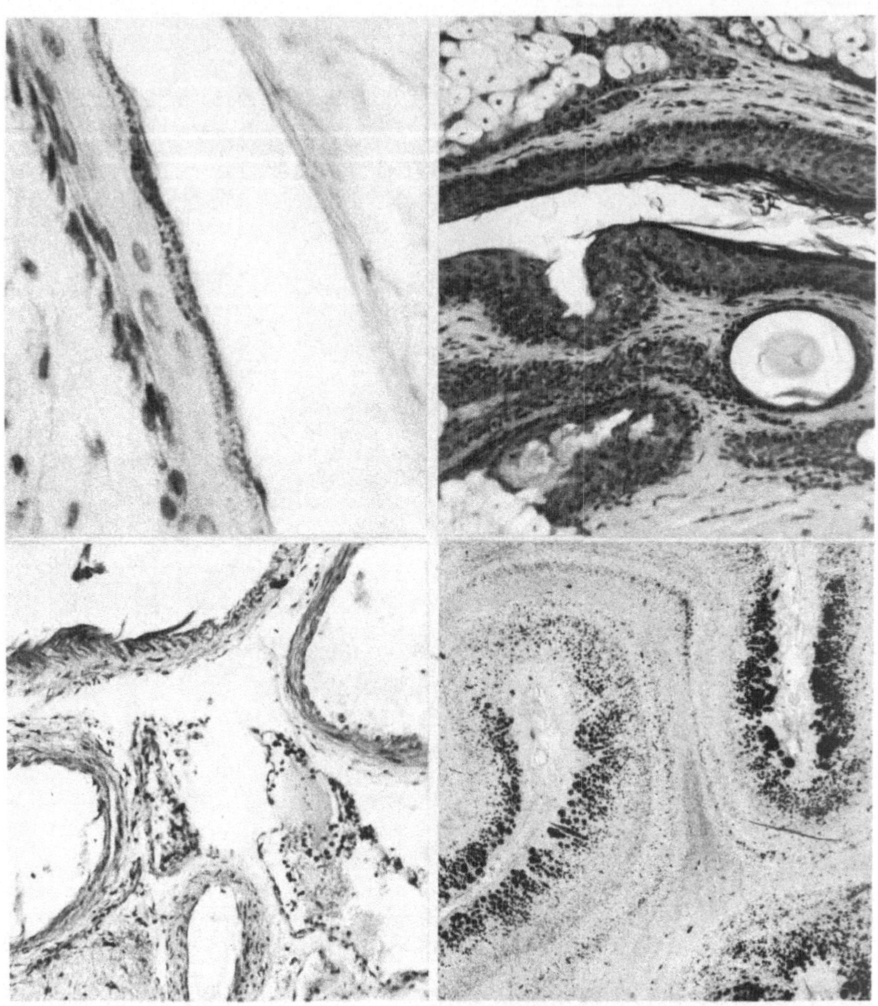

Fig. 82. a) *top left:* Capsule zone of an epidermoid. From left to right: stroma of connective tissue, stratum germinativum,. the stratum granulosum with kerato-hyaline granules, and the stratum corneum composed of desquamated keratinized cells. (x320, H. & E. stain); b) *top right:* Capsule of a dermoid. In addition to the layers of epidermis described under (a) one sees subcutaneous connective tissue and sebaceous glands. (x86, H. & E. stain); c) *bottom left:* Various types of blood vessels in an arteriovenous angioma. (x72, H. & E. stain); d) *bottom right:* Low power view of angiomatosis of leptomeninges (Sturge-Weber's disease). One recognizes the capillaries and veins of the leptomeninges and the intense calcification of underlying convolutions of the brain. (x22, Nissl stain)

capsule contents upon the surrounding parenchymatous tissue; this is especially true of the epidermoids, less so of the dermoids. One can see signs of a neighboring meningo-encephalitis or even a melting of the tissue (*see* above). Clinically this gives rise to symptoms of dysfunction and irritation, and morphologically it results in a fusing of the epidermoids

228

with the neighboring tissue and a chronic sterile meningitis. Calcification of epidermoids usually does not occur, but it has been described in dermoids. If the contents of epidermoids or dermoids ruptures into the cerebrospinal fluid, or if contamination occurs at operation, a very intense aseptic inflammatory reaction of the meninges arises, with resulting arachnoiditis and ependymitis, and even aqueduct stenosis.

METASTASIS AND RECURRENCE

Metastasis is not known. Recurrence always takes place after incomplete removal of the capsule. In one case of Hug's, carcinomatous degeneration was discovered in an epidermoid which had seemed otherwise unremarkable.

DIFFERENTIAL DIAGNOSIS

It is necessary to distinguish these tumors from other squamous epithelium-containing tumors which produce cholesterin-bearing masses (craniopharyngiomas), and this may be difficult if the neoplastic capsule itself is very thin. Attention should be paid to the epidermoids' three-layered structure, and particularly to their true cornification with keratohyalin granules. Their clinical behavior is determined by their slow growth (long clinical history), by the signs of long-standing meningeal irritation in cases of seepage of cholesterin and fatty acids, by sudden exascerbations and even death upon rupture of the capsule, and finally by the possibility of obstructive hydrocephalus due to arachnoiditis and ependymitis.

24. TERATOMAS AND TERATOIDS

Teratomas have been reported as curious single cases or have been mentioned because of some special clinical manifestation, such as pubertas praecox. A review of neurosurgically pertinent cases was published by Weber (1939). The pathological literature should be consulted concerning the embryological peculiarities of these tumors. Their occurrence in the central nervous system is most common in childhood. Cases of teratoma, therefore, are most numerous in the neurosurgical services of children's hospitals (Ingraham and Bailey: 15 out of 231 cases). Occasionally these tumors are even present at birth. In general, they comprise about 0.3%–0.5% of intracranial tumors and the incidence in males is higher. We had seven male and four female patients. In Weber's review of pineal teratomas only three out of 30 cases were girls; in a subsequent review of Müller and Wohlfart five out of 84 cases of intracranial teratoma were females. The teratomas in the literature are divided by site between the pineal region (almost half of the cases), hypophysial region (about ⅙), spinal cord (around ⅙), lateral ventricles, and many other locations. They vary in size from a pinhead to a child's fist. Externally, the teratomas are nodular and encapsulated, and the color is brownish-red with dark-colored cysts on the surface. They are hard like cartilage, and occasionally calcified or criss-crossed by bony spicules.

HISTOLOGICAL APPEARANCE

Various epithelial formations can be found: cornified or uncornified squamous epithelium, either simple or stratified; accessory structures of the skin including hairs; simple columnar epithelium in papillary or tubular patterns—especially resembling the medullary tube; blood vessels of all types; osseous, cartilagenous and fatty tissue; lymphoblasts; lymphocytes; and spindle-cells or mesenchymal connective tissue, the latter sometimes undergoing partial mucoid degeneration; a neoplastic proliferation of glia (oligodendroglia) has never been encountered by us. The teratomas grow extremely slowly, and small ones may be discovered only by accident; others, such as those around the pineal and pituitary, are important neurosurgically and operation is usually beneficial when technical considerations permit their total removal (Weber, 1939; Krabbe, 1944). The rupture of squamous-epithelium-lined cysts, containing fatty acids, can produce an intense inflammatory reaction in the ventricular system and subarachnoid space, as it does with the epidermoids (Gaupp, 1942).

Further references: Bailey and Jeliffe; Klapproth; Lichtenstein, 1940; Müller and Wohlfart; Saxer.

CHAPTER XV

VASCULAR TUMORS, VASCULAR MALFORMATIONS AND SPACE-OCCUPYING VASCULAR LESIONS

25. ANGIOMAS AND ANEURYSMS

HISTORICAL NOTE AND DEFINITION

Due to the progress in neurosurgical *diagnostic* methods (arteriographic diagnosis of vascular occlusions and malformations), and operative *treatment* (extirpation of arterio-venous aneurysms, ligation of their feeding vessels, reinforcement of the wall of aneurysms, etc.) the above-listed vascular processes have assumed great practical significance. They are the main source of recurrent subarachnoid hemorrhage. Our anatomical knowledge in this field comes from numerous individual reports, at least some of which were presented as rarities, and from the comprehensive studies of Virchow, who also produced the first workable classification—one that is still accepted virtually unchanged. In the last several decades there have also appeared detailed and exhaustive monographs by Bailey and Cushing (1928); by Bergstrand, Olivecrona and Tönnis (1936), as well as the extensive studies and descriptions of Dandy (1928, 1937, 1938).

The following subdivision seems to us useful for classification purposes:

1. Angiomas and arterio-venous angiomas
2. Angioblastomas (*see* Mesodermal Tumors)
3. Aneurysms and varices

The distinction between vascular malformations and vascular tumors is difficult, especially since we must presume an origin from malformations or embryonic rests in the latter group. The guiding principle here, as in the distinction between hamartomas and blastomas (neoplasms), is that of autonomous growth.

Further references: Van Bogaert (1950); Ectors (1950); Green (1945); Haberland; Jefferson (1953); Lange-Cosack (1948); Manuelidis; Neubuerger and Silcott; Norlén (1949); Peters and Tebelis; Pluvinage; Puusepp; Röttgen (1937, 1943); Russell (1941); Sorgo (1938); Tönnis (1936); Tönnis and Schiefer; Turner and Kernohan (1941); Walker (1953).

See also Olivecrona, H., and Ladenheim, J., Congenital arteriovenous aneurysms of the carotid and vertebral arterial systems. Springer, Berlin, 1957.

The angiomas

In spite of many detailed descriptions, we still know little of the anatomy of vascular malformations, since an accurate anatomical or functional analysis of the angiographic findings has not yet been accomplished. For the time being, therefore, we must be satisfied with a pathological approach. I have—with few changes—employed the classification of Bergstrand, Olivecrona, and Tönnis, which is based on the original one by Virchow. I have eliminated the group of arterial angiomas, since it has not yet been possible to verify them arteriographically.

TABLE 6. PATHOLOGICAL CLASSIFICATION OF ANGIOMAS

Type	Site	
	Meninges and bone	Brain and spinal cord
Cavernous angioma	Skull and vertebral column	Cerebrum and brain stem
Capillary angioma (angioma racemosum capillare ectaticum; telangiectasis)	——	Pons and quadrigeminal plate
Venous angioma	Dura, in vicinity of the sagittal sinus; the leptomeninges of the Sylvian fissure and particularly of the base	——
Sturge-Weber's disease (angioma capillare et venosum calcificans)	Leptomeninges and sometimes the outer layers of the cortex; all lobes of the brain, but with a certain predilection for the parieto-occipital region	
Arteriovenous angioma (congenital arteriovenous aneurysm; angioma arteriovenosum aneurysmaticum)	Leptomeninges and convolutions in the distribution of the middle cerebral artery; rarer in distribution of anterior cerebral artery, very rare in that of the vertebral and middle meningeal arteries	

Specifically, it should be said that the *cavernous angioma* is composed of large vascular spaces with walls that simultaneously border the lumens of several vessels; there is thus no brain parenchyma between them. "While in the skin the cavernous angioma is common and the racemose angioma rare, this relationship is exactly reversed in the central nervous system" (Hamperl). Consequently cavernous angiomas are uncommon in "the central nervous system." They have occurred, however, in all lobes of the cerebrum, in the brain stem, in the bones of the skull, and especially in the vertebral column (*see* Spinal Tumors, p. 76). They are circumscribed blue-red tumors without capsule, and the vessels of the leptomeninges cross over them unchanged. The surrounding tissue can be scarred and calcified.

The *capillary angioma* (angioma racemosum capillare ectaticum, telangiectasis): such vascular malformations are usually discovered accidentally. These angiomas form a tangled knot and lie most frequently in the pons, or less often in the quadrigeminal region (aqueduct). The overlying leptomeningeal vessels are also unchanged. These lesions can be the source of recurrent and ultimately fatal hemorrhages.

The *venous angioma* is not a well-defined entity. At best, cases that show varicocele-like venous masses (as, for instance, in the Sylvian fissure) may be included. Some distinction from simple varices is necessary, particularly from those in the vicinity of the longitudinal sinus and the spinal cord.

Sturge-Weber's disease (angioma capillare et venosum calcificans), when full blown, presents a true syndrome in the same manner as Lindau's disease: glaucoma, nevus flammeus of the face, and calcified angioma of the brain. Other vascular malformations can also occur. Kautzky (1949) has called attention to the parallel nerve supply to both leptomeninges and the skin by branches of the trigeminal nerve ("encephalotrigeminal angiomatosis"). However, "full-blown" cases are rare; the facial nevus alone is most common, followed by the combination of facial and cerebral nevi. There is increased vascularity in the leptomeninges, and a sinuous network of venous and large capillary vessels, no thicker than pins, overlies the cerebral cortex. The brain parenchyma is atrophic, scarred, and grossly calcified (*see* Fig. 82d). Heterotopias are also encountered. The controversy regarding the primary or secondary nature of the parenchymal changes seems to favor their regressive (secondary) origin. The characteristic double-contour shadows on X-ray are explained by the particular projection of the calcified gyri (Lindgren). Calcification on X-ray may be lacking.

The *arteriovenous angioma*[1], earlier called the arteriovenous "aneurysm," has become most important now that it can be specifically diagnosed arteriographically and often removed surgically. In this type, the development of the primitive blood vessels into arteries and veins has failed to take place; instead, the embryónic plexus-like pattern has been retained, even though it has been altered secondarily by the effect of blood pressure. Angiomas manifest themselves between the ages of 20 and 30, by focal signs or a subarachnoid hemorrhage. They accounted for about 1.5% of our patients; the number of male patients is twice that of the females. The site of the angiomas, in order of their preference, is in the distribution

---

[1] We are speaking here of congenital arteriovenous *angiomas*, to avoid confusion with the acquired arteriovenous *aneurysms* which develop post-natally.

of the middle cerebral artery and the anterior cerebral artery, with a few cases occurring in the distribution of the vertebral arteries. The angiomas have a characteristic appearance to the naked eye. A cortical area, varying in size from a quarter to the palm of the hand, is covered by markedly tangled vessels—often in the form of a plexus—which are supplied with blood and drained of it by vessels ranging in thickness from a knitting needle to the size of a little finger. The circumscribed angioma itself can be seen lying either on the surface, or buried in the brain substance. It consists of a congerie of blood vessels in which both thin and thick (aneurysmatically dilated) vessels, filled with bright red blood or with blue-red blood, alternate and loop around one another. Histologically, we find vessel lumens of widely varying caliber and structure: some with a thick, hyalin wall without any elastica; some with normal architecture and with elastica; and lastly, cavities surrounded by a single layer of undifferentiated connective tissue, packed with blood (Fig. 82c). In between there are softened and atrophic remnants of the brain parenchyma, foci loaded with hemosiderin-containing macrophages, round cell infiltrates, and other signs of chronic degeneration. A large hemorrhage often results in a not inconsiderable cystic cavity which may communicate with a ventricle. Calcified blood vessels occasionally show up on X-ray. A large proportion of cases of "varicosis spinalis" really belongs to the arteriovenous angioma group.

The angioblastomas

See Mesodermal Tumors, p. 199.

Aneurysms and varices

Pathological dilatation of vessels in the brain and spinal cord is a matter of some importance. The aneurysms occur in older age groups, with males predominating. They are most apt to occur where the blood vessels branch, especially on the middle cerebral artery, carotid, anterior communicating, posterior cerebral, posterior communicating, and anterior cerebral arteries (*see* McDonald and Korb), perhaps because these particular vessels lie free in the subarachnoid space. In 19% of cases they are multiple, and occur more frequently on the left side. They are often associated with congenital anomalies (Slany, 1938). On the carotids we make a distinction between infra- and supra-clinoid aneurysms, the latter group being more common. The site of origin of the aneurysm is usually a local abnormality in the vessel wall which is caused either congenitally (hypoplasia) or through arteriosclerosis, septic emboli, or rarely through specific inflammations (syphilis). Expansion takes place when the blood pressure exceeds the amount the wall can support. Its rupture is thus one of the most common sources of subarachnoid hemorrhage. Such a hemorrhage can break into the brain substance from without (particularly into the medial temporal lobe).

To the naked eye intracranial aneurysms appear as sac-like or cylindrical enlargements of intracranial vessels. When the aneurysm lies extradurally, a circumscribed bulging of the dura of the base can be seen. Aneurysms are elastic in consistency, or hard if they are thrombosed. Their inside is often filled with laminated thrombi, occasionally to such an extent that the lumen of the expanded vessel has returned to nearly normal size. A certain proportion of aneurysms produce focal neurological signs and symptoms by pressure on the cranial nerves; others manifest themselves only by subarachnoid hemorrhage.

There is a gradual transition from the true venous angiomas (*q.v.*) with their great increase in the number of blood vessels and cirsoid structure to the *varices* (phlebectasias). It is often difficult to know where to draw the line between these two forms. One form of varix seems to occur not infrequently in the neighborhood of the superior sagittal sinus; it is best looked upon as a varicose enlargement of a Pacchionian granulation. Varicosities and cylindrical varices (phlebectasias) are of particular importance in the spinal cord. The veins are dilated, tortuous, and give the impression of a plexus of vessels with some of the lumens ectatic. Angiomas in the spinal cord itself are also encountered. The venous angiomas form a portion of the cases of "varicosis spinalis."

Besides being encountered in the brain and meninges, hemangiomas are also found in the skull (frontal and parietal bones), and in the spinal column.

The acquired *arteriovenous aneurysms* occur intracranially most frequently between the carotids and cavernous sinus (producing the picture of pulsating exophthalmos). The fistula is on the intracavernous portion of the carotid artery and develops because of trauma or disease of the vessel wall. This short-circuit leads to a varicose enlargement of the ophthalmic veins, the pulsations being transmitted to the entire eyeball.

CHAPTER XVI

OTHER SPACE-OCCUPYING PROCESSES

26. UNCLASSIFIED TUMORS

In the series of Bailey and Cushing were 192 unclassified tumors, i.e., approximately 6% of the total. In our collection they comprised 4%. We must expect then that 5–8% of tumors in any series are not classifiable according to the system which we have proposed. This fact may be attributed to the peculiarity of some particular tumors—these are the unclassifiable tumors in the narrower sense—or to inadequate technical requisites for study.

In some instances, due to the nature of the operations, only a small amount of material can be retrieved from the aspiration flask. The neoplastic nature of the specimen can be established but a specific diagnosis of the tumor type cannot be made. This is particularly true of the pituitary tumors, where pronounced autolytic changes take place in the physiological saline solution in the aspiration flask. Cushing also included with the unclassified tumors "gliomas" which were verified only clinically—by demonstrating cyst fluid, for example. Our cases were all histologically confirmed.

It is often impossible to fit a particular specimen into our classification system. Cushing, in 1935, mentioned a series of such tumors in which various diagnoses, such as sarcoma, ependymoma, spongioblastoma, neuroblastoma, and others had been made. After thorough study (*see* p. 82 ff.) we have designated such tumors as "unclassified" and attempted to indicate their kinship or similarity to a known group by the addition of such designations as "ependymoma-like," etc. In no case have we tried to force them into our classification. Furthermore, we have given them a general biological characterization, such as malignant or benign, according to the recognized principles (*see* p. 123). As we have shown (1950), some of these tumors can subsequently be assembled into a new group, along with other tumors, and be classified.

27. METASTASES

HISTORICAL NOTE

In the older literature the secondary spread to the brain of tumors elsewhere in the body received very little attention. Some of the authors clearly recognized the process of metastasis, while others assumed a "co-ordinated" neoplastic degeneration of the brain in the presence of general carcinomatous disease of the body (*see* also Wenzel; and Hasse with the first statistics). Since Virchow, a great number of excellent reports have appeared, but agreement is still lacking on certain controversial points. Detailed contributions have been published in the last decade, especially by Hassin and Singer; Brunner (1936); and Zaaijer.

Further references: Bertha (1955); Elsaesser (1944); Gärtner; Globus and Selinsky; Grant and Sayers; Henschen (1934, 1955); Meagher and Eisenhardt; Minkowski; Overhamm; Putschar (1930); Walther (1948).

INCIDENCE AND SITE

The age incidence of brain metastases corresponds to that of the primary tumors. Studies of the age incidence of brain metastases (as, for example, the study by Gutting) show a peak, as might be expected, between the fifth and sixth decade. Our own curve shows a peak around the age of 45 (Fig. 16). Our youngest patient was 14 years old, the oldest 80. There are certain differences according to the particular tumor; the peak for breast metastases, for instance, is at a slightly younger age than that for bronchogenic carcinomas. The average relative incidence of brain metastases varies more than any other type of brain tumor, and depends upon the clinical material of the author. Among brain tumors, therefore, metastases comprised 3.2% of Cushing's series, 5% of 740 cases of Zaaijer's (Schönbauer), 10% of 945 cases of Lill (1952), 18.7% of 31,698 general pathological autopsies reported by Rudershausen (Heidelberg), 25.9% of similar material from 28,831 autopsies of a hospital in Hamburg as reported by Gutting, and finally 36.81% in Kaufman's series from Basel reported by Krasting (144 brain tumors). On the basis of a large *neurosurgical* series, Tönnis found a 3.7% incidence of metastases among 4,532 verified tumors. Quite apart from the sex-dependency of certain primary tumors, males are three times more commonly affected than females (Zaaijer: 27 males and 10 females); this depends upon the higher incidence of certain carcinomas in one or the other sex (for instance, in Gutting's series of bronchogenic carcinomas there were 17 metastases in males and five in females, corresponding to the sex incidence of bronchogenic carcinomas as given by Oberndorfer of 3:1; more recently, the sex predilection has been given as still higher). We had 89 male and 74 female patients.

The location of metastases should really be determined by the mechanism of hematogenous spread and show a preference for the more vascular regions of the brain. Actually, the location of metastases follows no rule and the assumed left-sided preponderance could not be verified. Lastly, there is the important question of which tumors metastasize most commonly to the brain. Arranging them in order of frequency with their corresponding percentage we arrive at the following: first and foremost come the lung tumors (bronchogenic carcinoma),with an incidence of from 21.6% (Gutting) to 37.8% (Brunner); then come the hypernephromas with 10.8% (Gutting) to 16.1% (Brunner); third, in women, is breast carcinoma with 6.09% (Gutting), corresponding to the findings of Brunner and Störtebecker (Olivecrona's series). Thyroid and uterine cancers metastasize rarely. The sarcomas metastasize to the brain three times more commonly than carcinomas, but their absolute incidence is very small since carcinomas and sarcomas occur in the proportion of 10:1.

APPEARANCE TO THE NAKED EYE

Metastatic brain tumors occur in two forms: a) as a circumscribed intracerebral tumor, and b) diffuse meningeal spread. There are no recognized sites of preference. Metastases are almost always multiple, rarely single. (In about one third of Störtebecker's cases, the metastatic tumor was solitary.) They are often nodular and round, or rather wedge-shaped, with the apex pointing towards the ventricular system (Fig. 83). The size varies from that of a pea to an apple. There are also metastases to the dura which show a superficial similarity to meningiomas. Metastasis to the leptomeninges (carcinomatosis of the meninges) results either in a diffuse, whitish deposition, or a formation of flat patches resembling sugar-icing. Even if the diagnosis were not obvious because of their multiplicity, metastases have a type-specific form and border and can be identified on the surface of the brain as well as on the cut section. Their cut surface is either finely tufted and fibrous, like asbestos (small-cell necrotizing bronchial carcinoma), or smoother (squamous cell carcinoma). Through liquefaction, cysts can be produced (Fig. 83) in which hemorrhages occasionally occur, with the result that such tumors can scarcely be recognized as metastases (hypernephromas). They are very loosely attached to their surroundings and often practically "fall out" of the brain tissue on sectioning. The brain may react to even a small metastasis with a pronounced degree of swelling and enlargement of the white matter (Fig. 83).

HISTOLOGICAL APPEARANCE

It seems superfluous to describe the histology of metastases. Only the reaction of the surrounding brain which shows great variations for which

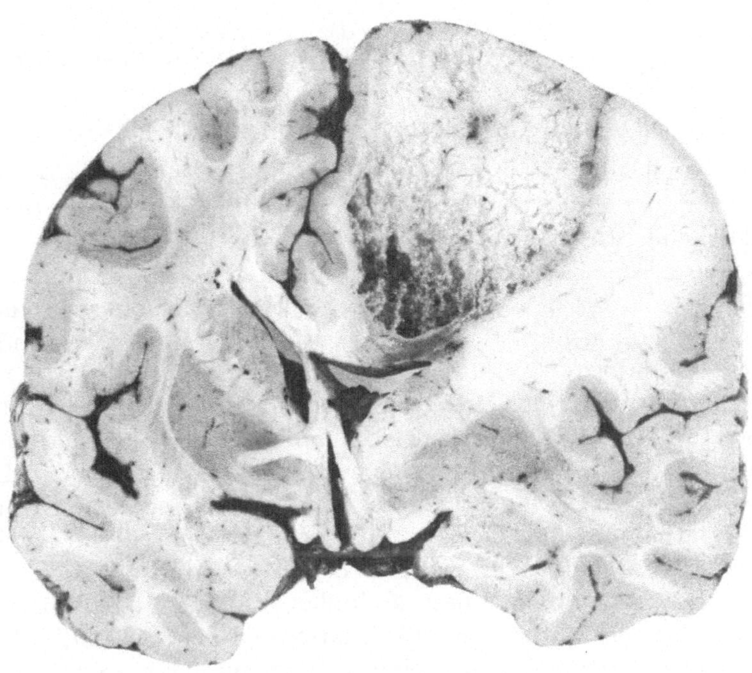

Fig. 83. Metastasis of a small-cell bronchogenic carcinoma with necrotic and cystic degeneration. Marked brain swelling. (Case 1031)

we have no explanation, needs to be described. The brain reacts either "progressively" with astrocytic gliosis, or "regressively" with marked swelling and destruction of both the white and gray matter. It is important, moreover, that blood vessel changes—similar to those occurring in the malignant gliomas—can occur in metastases. Thus, the blood vessels of the marginal zone of the tumor proliferate and expand into a network of sinusoid and lacunar cavities (p. 93) which may show up arteriographically. Metastases cannot be distinguished arteriographically from glioblastomas by the type of vascular changes—which are the same in both—but by the way in which they are circumscribed, assuming of course that the diagnosis was not already obvious from the presence of multiple foci. In diffuse carcinomatosis, there is no visible reaction on the part of the surrounding tissues. In metastases of unknown origin, more attention should be paid to the nuclear vacuoles which could point to the amelanotic form of malignant melanoma[1]. They have frequently helped us settle the diagnosis, e.g., our case (No. 4676) of a 25-year-old woman with amelanotic metastases to the brain in whom a diagnosis of melanotic sarcoma had been made a year previously.

[1] Apitz has made the important diagnostic observation that here the nuclei contain large vacuoles, surrounded by a layer of chromatin.

239

DIFFERENTIAL DIAGNOSIS

Macroscopically it is important to remember that certain metastases do not grow in a circumscribed fashion, but diffusely, so that they look more like meningitis than tumors. These cases are generally rare—perhaps most common after carcinoma of the stomach. It is important to confirm the metastatic nature of a tumor, since the primary tumors are sometimes difficult to diagnose during life and occasionally cannot be found even after a careful autopsy.

The arguments about Mittelbach's cases (*see* Metastases, p. 116 ff.) demonstrate how difficult it often is to make the correct diagnosis. The similarity between the hypernephroma and the angioblastoma of Lindau in its "epithelial" form should be stressed. I myself, together with an experienced pathologist, have once called a Lindau tumor a hypernephroma (*see* p. 202). The 15-year survival period in a case of Olivecrona's makes me think that his may have been a similar situation. It is important to remember, also, that rather unusual situations occur occasionally, like the metastasis of a carcinoma to a benign meningioma (Olivecrona) or to the hypophysis. I, too, have seen such a case. A melanoma can produce an amelanotic metastasis to the brain (*see* footnote, p. 239). The report of a double tumor (glioblastoma and melanosarcoma) suggests a similar situation. Small dural metastases that grow into the brain can, superficially, look like meningiomas, and can be recognized correctly only microscopically. Clinically, it is important to know that a high degree of brain swelling (as shown on ventriculogram) favors a diagnosis of glioblastoma or metastasic tumor (provided that brain abscess or parasites can be excluded). A profound hemiplegia of acute onset also may point to either process ("the acute tumors" of Elsberg). Carcinomatosis is very often indicated by Eberth's syndrome (*see* Fischer-Williams et al.: Brain 77, 82–121, 1954).

28. PARASITES

a) Cysticercus

The most common parasite of man occuring in the brain is the larva of *tinea soleum* which was supposed to have been mentioned as long ago as the Renaissance (Müller, 1558). Parasitism in man with spread to the central nervous system has been exhaustively described by Henneberg in his contributions to Bumke and Foerster's *Handbuch* (1912 and 1936).

Cysticercosis does not single out any particular age group. The occurrence of cysticercosis has varied from one century to another and from country to country, and is steadily decreasing; Virchow (Berlin)—2% of autopsies; Simmonds (Hamburg)—0.025%; Pinheiro and de Mello (1943, South America), up to 1% of autopsies. In cases of generalized cysticercosis the brain is affected in 80%. The cysticerci settle diffusely throughout the brain, while outside the brain proper they infest the leptomeninges, especially in the cisterns. The statement has been made previously (Henneberg, 1936) that cysticercosis is found particularly often in the aqueduct and fourth ventricle. The cysticerci sometimes attach themselves firmly to the neighboring tissue, in which they induce an inflammatory reaction; sometimes they float free. There may be as many as 120–150 cysticerci in a single brain (our own case of a 26-year-old man; E 316).

To the naked eye, the cysticerci appear as floppy, grey-red vesicles the size of lentils or peas, and filled with a clear or cloudy fluid. The watery contents contain either the larvae themselves or whitish, crumbly masses. The cyst wall is often calcified; it is reported to be visible on X-ray in 50% of cases (Wagner and Cosack). In the "racemose" form, the cysts—usually in the cisterns—lie one on top of the other like a bunch of grapes.

HISTOLOGICAL APPEARANCE

The picture is very uniform histologically: on suitable sections the outer membrane of the cyst and the larva within it can be seen. The cyst wall borders immediately upon the encapsulating inflammatory reaction of the brain or leptomeninges. This zone contains giant cells, epithelioid cells, and—farther out—granulation tissue with fibroblasts, lymphocytes and plasma cells, and lastly a capsule, consisting partly of glia and partly of connective tissue. This capsule becomes calcified with time. The condition can be recognized clinically if the cysticerci occur in the skin or eye, or if they are seen on X-ray. Because of their multiplicity, the cystercici are difficult to attack operatively. Nevertheless O. Foerster and many other authors have successfully removed single vesicles from the Rolandic region and the fourth ventricle (Obrador *et al.*, 1951; *see* also Cysticercosis cerebral. F. Isamat de la Riva, Barcelona, 1957).

b) Echinococcus

(*Synonyms: Echinococcus unilocularis or cysticus, Echinococcus multilocularis, hydatid cysts of the older literature.*)

Further references: Arana-Iniguez and San Julian; Schroeder and Medoc; Pinto Pupo and Mattos Pimenta; Posselt.

Echinococcosis is rarer than cysticercosis. The larvae occur in two forms—the unilocular cystic form, or much rarer, the multilocular form. The incidence of tape-worms and their larvae varies geographically. An incidence of 9.8% is reported in Australia (Thomas) and 0.5% for Mecklenburg (Madelung), a region in Germany where tapeworms are most common. They are still very common in South America (Uruguay). They seem to pick out the middle decades, with the cerebral forms occuring in younger individuals as well. In the nervous system they are most common intracranially (incidence of between 2–7.5% of echinococcosis cases), and in the spinal canal (1.94% of cases). The basal ganglia and cerebellum seem most commonly affected. Echinococcosis in the vicinity of the vertebral column characteristically tends to penetrate into the epidural space of the vertebral canal (our own case, reported by Zehnder). Here the vesicles can extend over many segments in the form of long chains. The unilocular cystic type and the multilocular form of echinoccocus are very different in appearance. The former are smooth-walled cysts the size of a cherry or a goose-egg, either single or multiple, with the daughter vesicles lying either inside, outside, or floating free (Posselt; Kaufmann, Fig. 828, p. 1503). In the rarer multilocular form, though, the gelatinous vesicles are compressed and the membrane wrinkled up. The skull may be eroded by underlying cortical vesicles.

In a general way, the histological description given for cysticercosis applies here as well. Between the vesicle septa proliferating glial cells are often present. Clinically, there are complement fixation and skin sensitivity tests for diagnosis. If during ventricular puncture a vesicle happens to be perforated, the specific diagnosis can be made on X-ray. Operative results are only fair, since cerebral echinoccocosis is rarely primary and more commonly represents metastases from infestation elsewhere. Reports indicate that scarcely half of the operated cases have survived for any period of time.

c) Other parasites

Pea- to egg-sized granulomatous lesions occur in Schistosomiasis (Shimidzu; Hunt; Kane and Most) and in coccidiosis (Abbott and Cutler). (*See* also Granulomas.)

29. GRANULOMAS: TUBERCULOMAS[2] AND GUMMAS

a) The tuberculomas

HISTORICAL NOTE

The tuberculomas of the brain previously constituted one of the most common and important space-occupying lesions encountered in neurological practice. Now they are only rarely seen by neurosurgeons. In addition to the contribution by Bruns, we refer here only to the work of recent years, in particular that of Rasdolsky, and van Wagenen (1927),

---

[2] We intend to use the term "tuberculoma" for truly space-occupying lesions and to reserve the name "tubercle" for the smaller, or miliary forms.

and the recently published comprehensive paper of Dott and Levin, describing the cases of cerebral tuberculomas collected by the British Society of Neurological Surgery.

Further references: Asenjo *et al.* (1949); Avendano *et al.;* Bucy and Overhill; Sheps and Simon; and Starr (1894, 1886); Zamora.

INCIDENCE AND SITE

Tuberculomas occur in all age groups but are more common in childhood and adolescence. The youngest case is probably that of the elder Demme, quoted by Bruns, only 23 days old. The increased incidence in certain age groups depends on the way the material is collected, for there is hardly any other type of space-occupying lesion in which the incidence varies as much as in tuberculomas. According to Petersen in 1894, tuberculomas comprised 49.5% of 335 collected cases of brain tumor. There were 32.2% tuberculomas among 600 brain tumor patients, according to Starr, and in this group the incidence was 50.8% in childhood and adolescence, but only 13.6% in patients over 20 years of age. On the other hand, McLean reported an incidence of five to six tuberculomas in 100 brain tumors in 1916, and only 1.4% in 1927; these figures can be related only to the general decrease of tuberculosis. In 1919, according to Eiselsberg, tuberculomas accounted for only 1.6% of brain tumors, and in 1941 for only 1.7%, according to Olivecrona. However, in many countries tuberculomas are still very common, as, for instance, in Spain (10% of brain tumors, Obrador, 1950), and in some South American countries.

Tuberculomas comprised 0.5% of our series. Tuberculomas of the brain are claimed to be about 1/10 as frequent as tuberculous meningitis. Males are affected two to three times more often than females.

According to older reports, tuberculomas are supposed to occur six times more often infratentorially than supratentorially (this preponderance is probably explained by the fact that only the cases with increased intracranial pressure are sent to the hospital). This no longer applies to the current statistics in neurosurgical clinics, where of 17 of van Wagenen's cases only three lay in the cerebellum. Tuberculomas are supposed to begin their growth deep within a sulcus, and usually only a circumscribed meningitis develops, although diffuse spread naturally can also occur. The size of a tuberculoma depends on the location of the affected region and its neurological importance (i.e., the time at which the diagnosis can be made); it can grow as big as an apple. Not infrequently we are dealing with confluent tuberculomas. Occasionally "growth rings" can be recognized on cut sections. Tuberculomas are often multiple—between 24–60% of cases reported earlier. Tuberculomas may be hard, or even completely calcified, but their central caseous necrotic portions can be so softened that on occasion they cannot be distinguished from an abscess, as in our own case No. 6026.

After separation from the brain, tuberculomas sometimes have a coarsely nodular surface. At operation, if there is neither an associated miliary meningeal tuberculosis nor a specific tuberculous meningitis, only the characteristic caseous consistency of the tumor's central necrotic core points to the diagnosis of tuberculoma. Even today the prognosis of tuberculomas is not good, although not as hopeless as before. Of van Wagenen's (1927) cases only five were alive after one year, but the combined statistics of Dott obtained from 17 members of the British Society of Neurological Surgery give a more optimistic impression. Of 94 patients, 16 (17%) died of post-operative tuberculous meningitis—the complication that was so feared previously; 40 patients died ultimately of general tuberculosis. Total removal of cerebral tuberculomas is still the method of choice; a simple decompression has good prospects when followed with conservative therapy, but partial removal of tuberculomas is not to be recommended. Pre- and post-operative protection with Streptomycin should further improve the prognosis.

b) Gummas

(Synonyms: Syphiloma, luetic granuloma.)

Of the various manifestations of lues, only the space-occupying lesions will be dealt with here; the description of luetic meningitis belongs rather to the textbooks of neuropathology and neurology. Gummas, just like tuberculomas, are constantly decreasing in frequency. Indeed, there was a 3.6% incidence of gummas in Starr's statistics (*see* Tuberculomas), but in the most recent data from the U.S. (Cushing, 1932; Grant and Sayers, 1951; and the Mount Sinai Hospital) the incidence dwindles to 0.4–0.5%, i.e., 1/10 of the previous figure. The same objections that were raised above about such statistics apply here as well. According to earlier data, gummas show no special age preference; they are most likely to occur in the central region (or was this simply because these patients came to the clinic more often because of their symptoms?), but there are also infrequent occurrences of gummas in the hypothalamus and pituitary. The gumma of the calvarium that goes on to involve the brain is a real rarity. There are also multiple gummas.

Macroscopically, the gumma can occasionally be identified by the jelly-like infiltration of the leptomeninges, or the chronic circumscribed meningitis. Occasionally, the leptomeninges are stuck to the dura. Gummas are more difficult to separate from the brain than tuberculomas, since they are often fastened to the connective tissue of their surroundings. They are softer in consistency than tuberculomas, and because of the preservation of connective tissue in their necrotic portions, they are "rubbery." Information about the histology of tuberculous and luetic granulomas is provided in neuropathological and pathological textbooks. In a series of 488 cases, the cerebrospinal-fluid Wassermann was positive in 45%, the blood Wassermann in 76%.

Further references: Bechterew, Nonne, Jacob (all cited by Jahnel); Alpers (1939); Bagdasar; Sheps and Simon.

Other granulomas: Of the other granulomas, or granulomatoses, the rarer fungus infections, such as torulosis, must be mentioned; they occur in the form of a chronic meningitis or an inflammation of the perivascular spaces of the brain itself with formation of granulomas (*see* Quodbach; Demme and Mumme; and Dandy, 1938). The most commonly encountered fungus infections in Europe are actinomycosis (Hallervorden, 1931; Elsaesser, 1950; Ley *et al.*), and blastomycosis; 120 cases of this latter condition have already been described (Quodbach; Demme and Mumme). Cerebral actinomycosis can manifest itself as a circumscribed space-occupying process. *Schistosoma japonicum* can produce tangerine-sized granulomas (*see* p. 240). Intradural spinal granulomas can be due to tuberculosis, syphilis, coccidiomycosis, torulosis, and schistosomiasis (Bucy and Overhill).

Furthermore, there are certain rare granulomas that sometimes must be differentiated from true tumors. These include multiple, often diffuse, lesions with chronic inflammatory infiltration, giant cells and frequently eosinophilic elements which in some cases form dense reticulin fiber networks. In the differential diagnosis, encephalomyelitis has to be considered and at times the cases are even reminiscent of multiple sclerosis (H. J. Scherer), or diffuse sarcomatosis of the leptomeninges (*see* p. 205). These are probably specific granulomas (Wilke, 1955)—possibly due to viruses—that may be related to Hodgkin's disease (Schöpe).

The *eosinophilic granulomas* occur in the calvarium; we have observed them frequently. They infiltrate neither the dura, nor the brain. Histologically, the surgical specimen consists of granulation tissue composed of epithelioid cells, single giant cells and foam cells, as well as leukocytes, the majority of which are eosinophils. Biologically, they are benign. Schüller-Christian's lipoid granuloma usually occurs in the skull in multiple form. Its histology is described in pathology textbooks.

30. ARACHNOIDITIS AND EPENDYMITIS
a) Cystic adhesive arachnoiditis

(Synonyms: Leptomeningitis cystica, chronic relapsing meningitis, circumscribed serous meningitis, arachnopathia cystica proliferans, subarachnoid cysts, meningeal cysts.)

The following describes only those processes that have neurosurgical importance. The concept of this disease is historically related to two clinical entities: the so-called serous meningitis described by surgeons, and the local cyst formation of the leptomeninges of the pathologist (as described, for instance, by Stroebe). If we add to this the inflammatory conditions of the leptomeninges—which form a part of Nonne's "pseudotumor cerebri" group—we have a triad as a starting point for our discussion:

1. The acute diffuse meningeal irritation from acute infectious diseases and intoxications.
2. The acute circumscribed meningeal irritation from a neighboring inflammatory process (secondary, "sympathetic" meningitis).
3. The chronic circumscribed adhesive arachnoiditis (cystic?)—the possible end result of condition 1 and 2.

To this is added:

4. The arachnoidal cysts, some of which may be the end result of condition 1 and 2, and others which may be local congenital malformations.

Our knowledge of arachnoiditis has come in part from neurology, and in part from neurosurgery (Oppenheim and Krause; Claude, Bosche and Barré; Petit-Dutaillis; papers by Payr; Pette; E. Scherer, 1935; Zander; Bruetsch). We are also indebted to the numerous contributions of the Paris school (Bollack, David and Puech, 1937; and others), as well as the monograph of D. Russell (1949). Tönnis and Lange; and Zülch have reviewed this subject before the German Neurosurgical Congress in 1949.

Further references: David, Berdet, Guillaumat, and Askenasy; Noetzel; Puech, David, and Brun; Rothman; Vincent, Puech, and David.

INCIDENCE AND SITE

A clear-cut age preference is not yet recognized, except for the well-studied arachnoiditis of the chiasmal region, where a definite increase in incidence has been observed in the third decade. The general incidence varies also and it is impossible to make a definite statement about it. Of 155 space-occupying lesions of the chiasmal region in the series of the Paris authors mentioned above, 71 were arachnoiditis.

The first above-mentioned condition—acute meningeal irritation—has a diffuse distribution. We see chronic arachnoiditis most commonly in the cisterns, usually associated with saccular adhesions. The arachnoidal cysts mentioned under number 4 are located almost exclusively in the region of the large cisterns. Of particular importance here are the cases in the cisterna fossae Sylvii, interhemispherica, and ambiens. Also important are the widespread presence of adhesions and cysts in all the *basal* cisterns (Fig. 84). Rings of adhesions close off the cisternae chiasmatica, basalis,

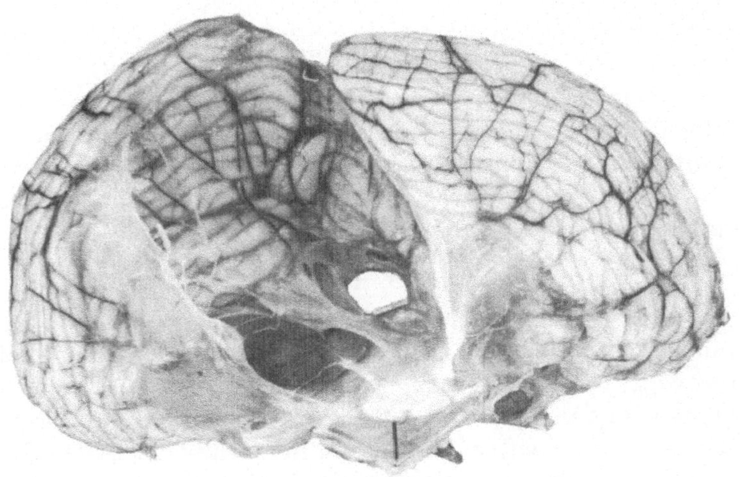

cerebello-medullaris, pontocerebellaris, and magna (our own case No. 1018). If these cisterns are still connected with the foramen of Magendi, they are exposed to the pressure of the ventricular cerebrospinal fluid. Since the latter's pathway to the site of absorption is blocked, obstructive (but "communicating") hydrocephalus of all four ventricles may develop. In the chiasmatic cistern three states can be distinguished according to the Paris school: 1) a heavy feltwork of the arachnoid in which the formation of cicatricial strands and membranes is most prominent; 2) arachnoiditis with cyst formation; 3) predominantly degenerative manifestations in the optic nerve and chiasm, with arachnoiditis in the background. Similar processes are found around the spinal cord where, in addition to the well-recognized cystic arachnoiditis which often develops after operation or trauma, congenital arachnoidal cysts also occur. These often poke through dehiscences in the dura and result in dumbbell shaped cysts that lie partly sub- and partly extra-durally over many segments (the so-called dural cysts).

APPEARANCE TO THE NAKED EYE

In the spinal cord, particularly in the lumbar and cauda regions, the alterations in the arachnoid are in the form of strand-like adhesions of grey-white color, with or without the formation of small cysts containing clear, watery fluid. The large arachnoidal cysts that occur in the cisterns reach the size of a chestnut or a man's fist, have clear, or milky contents, and produce a corresponding displacement of the brain substance and ventricles (Fig. 84). Not infrequently, the bone over the arachnoidal cyst shows a bulge (parasagittaly, in our case No. 25). If a cerebellar pressure

247

cone develops as the result of a space-occupying process with an inflammatory component, the tonsils are kept in the cistern by arachnoidal adhesions, thus setting the stage for chronic recurrent bouts of increased intracranial pressure (Tönnis, 1948).

HISTOLOGICAL APPEARANCE

We see in this condition a thickening of the arachnoid, with beginning fibrosis and increased homogeneity, and infiltration with round cells and single gitter cells. Depending on the stage of development, there are either prominent signs of chronic inflammation, or of cellular proliferation of the arachnoid mesothelium with an increase in fibers but very little infiltration of other cells. Biopsies of cases of the so-called "cured" Streptomycin-treated tuberculosis often disclose membranes still showing the specific histological picture. We found among the large arachnoidal cysts of the cisterns some with different structures (fetal?) that had already been noticed clinically because of their milky and cloudy contents. Their walls consist of a single layer of epithelium which occasionally forms psammoma bodies. It constantly produces new cell layers which swell up, become amorphous, and are finally shed into the cyst as detritus, in a manner similar to the epidermoids (Zülch, 1950). This explains the cloudiness of the cyst fluid.

ETIOLOGY AND PATHOGENESIS

Previous meningitis or meningeal reactions are particularly often implicated, and we can assume that these are most frequent in the first two to three years of life. Most important is meningococcal meningitis, then comes Hemophilus influenzae, hemolytic Streptococcus, and Pneumococci. There are also meningitides caused by B. Coli and the bacillus of Flexner (*see* D. Russell). Spread of infection to the fetal brain during pregnancy has been demonstrated (Eicke, 1943). Arachnoiditis of the chiasmal region is often supposed to be of syphilitic origin. The so-called cured tuberculous meningitis is beginning to play a role again (in the chiasm, cerebello-pontine angle, and particularly the cisterna ambiens). The possibility of curing meningitis with antibiotics will increase the number of patients coming to operation with cysts from cicatricial arachnoiditis.

Diseases of the brain, such as encephalitis (i.e., in its disseminated form), and the acute rheumatic diseases are supposed to produce such conditions locally. Arachnoiditis of traumatic origin is most common in the spinal cord. Some of the arachnoidal cysts described above are probably fetal maldevelopments. Lipiodol, Iodipin, and other contrast media can produce severe arachnoiditis with granuloma formation. There are also cases of arachnoiditis that occur three to five years after spinal operations (Stender, 1939, Davidoff *et al.*, 1947).

b) Ependymitis

Ependymitis during the acute stage of meningitis is only one manifestation of infection of the cerebrospinal fluid spaces. The exudate lying on the ependyma or in the subependymal region causes the development of patchy or wart-like growths of acellular glial tissue (ependymitis granularis sive plastica). However, it should not be assumed that inflammation is the *only* cause of this process. In later stages, islands and tubules of ependyma —lying beneath more superficially placed scar tissue—reveal the previous position of this layer. Cicatricial processes such as these can result in occlusion of the narrow points in the C.S.F. circulation, as has been convincingly demonstrated by the pathology of aqueduct occlusion. On encephalography, we sometimes see the closing off of only one foramen of Monro—probably resulting from a similar process. We have twice seen a block of the inferior one-third of the fourth ventricle. In these two cases adhesions arose as a result of general inflammatory proliferation between the ventricular floor, choroid plexus of the roof, and the meninges of the tonsillar undersurfaces and nodulus—finally forming a cicatricial mass. Obstructive hydrocephalus of the third ventricle and the upper portion of the fourth developed (Zülch, 1950).

Dandy, and Taggart and Walker described a peculiar malformation in the mid-line of the cerebellum, in which there was atresia of the foramina of Luschka and Magendie. As a consequence, a giant sac-like cavity developed between the cisterna magna and the fourth ventricle, with resulting hydrocephalus.

Further references: Hasenjäger and Stroescu; Kautzky and Zülch; Opalski.

Pseudotumor cerebri

Nonne's concept of pseudotumor cerebri is a purely clinical one. It signifies a local or general increase in intracranial pressure not attributable to a tumor. It is related rather to local or general brain swelling or edema, particularly after sinus thrombosis, "otitic hydrocephalus," hemorrhages, post-traumatic or post-hemorrhagic cysts with a tendency to increase in size, arachnoiditis, etc. (*see* Lemke; Nonne; Russell (1949); Tönnis and Lange-Cosack; and Zülch)[3].

[3] 2nd Congress of German Neurosurgeons, Göttingen, 1949, Zbl. Neurochir. **10,** 56–97, 1950.

CHAPTER XVII

METHODS OF
PATHOLOGICAL STUDY

For technique and staining methods, *see* the directions of Romeis, 1940; Schmorl; Spielmeyer, 1927; Masson, 1923; Russell, 1939; Anderson; etc.

The techniques of studying the pathological processes in the nervous system are only slightly different from those used in a general pathological department. Although in the latter the routine study is simple and generally limited to the application of a few methods, in neuropathology it is more diversified. A selective demonstration of the various components of the central nervous system, by using various staining methods, is often necessary. These demands make the course of investigation both longer and more difficult. In a way similar to general neuropathology, we investigate the tumor according to the principles of Spielmeyer—by site, manner of growth, and type. Our study of tumors includes not only the cell type—which, demonstrated by metallic impregnation techniques, was given altogether too much attention in the early contributions of Bailey—but the following as well: manner of growth and spread of the tumor cells; behavior toward the brain tissue (myelin sheath, axis cylinders, ganglion cells); the architecture formed by cell groupings as opposed to the form of individual cells; the degree of cellularity; the life-span of the individual cells; the formation of fibers; the behavior of the connective tissue (free and associated with blood vessels); regressive processes like necrosis, fatty degeneration, calcification, mucoid degeneration, etc. In order to classify a tumor, all of the foregoing points have to be taken into account, and only those tumors will be classified together that agree in a majority of these characteristics. Identical or similar cells alone—with differences in other characteristics—do not constitute a decisive criterion for the classification of a tumor.

It has been shown that no single criterion, such as the bipolar form of a cell, for instance, but rather the sum total of the above listed criteria, is the decisive factor in a tumor's biological behavior.

The value and purpose of pathological studies lies in the setting up of a biologically uniform system in which the tumor's classification and nomenclature indicate the prognosis of the affected patient. Pathological anatomy, in this regard, is a clinical applied science.

Specifically, we begin with an attempt at rough classification on the basis of a survey stain and take into account the opinion of the surgeon. For the neuropathologist such a stain is understandably the Nissl stain or its easily-performed modification with cresyl violet; hemotoxylin and eosin also can be used. If the two impressions agree, further detailed study with special methods, such as gold sublimate, is superfluous unless there is specific scientific interest. If they do not agree, we have to use special stains: in gliomas and paragliomas, for instance, we have to try gold and silver cell impregnation, in connective tissue tumors we try to demonstrate reticulin fibers with silver stains. In any case, it is advisable that the beginner utilize impregnation techniques in addition to the cresyl violet stain in order to verify his diagnosis. With few exceptions, the experienced investigator can recognize and adequately classify brain tumors on paraffin-imbedded material stained with H. & E.—a routine pathological method. The differential-diagnostic value of the different staining methods will be mentioned in the subsequent discussion of individual tumor types.

Fixation

SURGICAL SPECIMENS

The tissue for investigation is usually obtained from operation or autopsy, rarely from a needle biopsy. The fixative of choice is a 10% solution of formalin[1]. One exception to this rule: in the case of gliomas and paragliomas, a piece of the specimen most likely to contain tumor—selected if possible from the marginal growth zone—has to be fixed from the outset in Hortega's solution of formalin ammonium bromide. If immediate fixation in this solution is not possible, experience shows that transfer after two to three days of formol fixation is still adequate. The transfer of autopsy material from formalin after still longer periods of time will be taken up below.

When pituitary adenomas and gliomas are to be removed by suction, the surgeon should also try to secure a solid fragment of the tumor for histological study, removing it preferably with a sharp spoon. Transfer of this tissue into formalin without delay is desirable, particularly with pituitary adenomas, in order to avoid the severe autolytic changes that take place in physiological saline. A sterile dish of formalin or Bouin's or Susa's solution should be kept on the instrument table.

---

[1] This is prepared by diluting the 40% (concentrated) formol solution 1:10, using physiological saline, if possible. Actually such a solution contains 4% formaldehyde.

ASPIRATED MATERIAL[2]

The material from the aspiration flask should always be saved—even if sufficient "tumor tissue" has been removed during the operation—and filtered and fixed in formalin immediately after the operation. Leaving this material in the irrigation fluid leads quickly to autolytic disintegration of the tissue and prevents subsequent study. It is thrown out after adequate histological sections from the operative specimen have been obtained. If the aspirated material must be studied, small bits of suspicious looking tissue are removed with forceps from the now black and crumbly residue. About 1 cc. of tissue is needed, which is then embedded in paraffin.

AUTOPSY MATERIAL

Removal of the brain should be carried out as soon as possible after death, preferably before the general autopsy. When there is no increased intracranial pressure, a certain amount of preliminary fixation of the brain can be achieved by perfusing the subarachnoid space with formalin; this is done with two cannulas, one in the cisterna magna, the other inserted through the cribriform plate. However, this preliminary fixation should be called to the attention of the prosector, since a certain amount of this fluid can run down the esophagus and trachea into stomach and lungs, and can result in rather surprising, and at first inexplainable, changes in these organs.

When the intracranial pressure is raised, preliminary fixation is possible by injecting the formalin into the blood vessels. In such cases generally only the region of the middle cerebral artery and a portion of the region supplied by the anterior cerebral artery are perfused, i.e., after injection of the carotid artery in the neck or after opening the skull and injecting the removed brain. More reliable is injection of the innominate artery and the left carotid and vertebral artery after exposure by a collar-like incision from acromion to acromion. It is particularly difficult to preserve the form of the brain with a high degree of hydrocephalus, especially in children. In these cases the ventricular system may be filled with formalin soon after death, either through previous ventricular puncture sites or through the separated sutures. The removed brain must be carefully protected from any contact with water (because of Nissl's "water artefacts"), and after external inspection and description, should be fixed in ample quantities of formalin with the shape maintained as well as possible. The formalin should be changed after three or five days. Brain-cutting and other procedures—without any significant distortion of the shape of the brain—can be carried out after eight days' fixation at the earliest.

[2] Material remaining after filtration of the contents of the aspiration flask at operation.

The shape of the brain is best preserved by hanging it loosely in a sling of gauze, and at the same time supporting it with a thread under the basilar artery—i.e., base up. Hanging it by a thread alone often results in an ugly distortion of the pons.

If poor fixation of the deeper portions of the brain is suspected, the floor of the third ventricle can be slit open, if no pathological changes in this region are anticipated. This is particularly recommended when there is a high degree of obstructive hydrocephalus with blocking of the aqueduct or beyond. Good fixation can be achieved by exchanging the ventricular fluid with formalin—careful pressure upon the dilated lateral ventricles forces out the C.S.F. and on release draws in the fixative by the natural sucking effect of the ventricles.

On autopsy material, blocks of tissue from the deeper lying portions can be transferred to formalin ammonium bromide even after six to ten days and adequate results obtained with metal impregnations.

Brain cutting

The laying open of the brain after the fashion of Virchow and Zenker destroys the regional relationships of the different parts of the brain, and consequently should have no place in neuropathology. A preference for frontal sections of the brain or a midsagittal cut depends on the site and type of anticipated lesion and the overall alteration in the brain. Tumors of the midline in the third ventricle, aqueduct, and fourth ventricle, as well as certain tumors of the corpus callosum, can be demonstrated by either method. Whereas in general frontal sections are preferred, the method selected should be dictated by the peculiarities of the case, or be in the manner best suited for a display where specimens of certain tumor types are demonstrated in both ways of sectioning so that the clinician can really see the extent of the tumor.

Moreover, the displacements of parts of the brain caused by space-occupying processes (*q.v.*) can be clearly shown by both directions of sectioning. To make a midsagittal section, the medial longitudinal fissure is carefully prepared, the corpus callosum cut with a scalpel, and finally a median cut of the base of the brain is made until all the commissures are divided. Particular care should be exercised in cases where the cingulate gyrus is pressed to one side.

At the time of brain cutting, the external form and changes in it (for instance, through local pressure), changes from fixation, the character of the leptomeninges and blood vessels at the base and over the convexity, the pattern of the gyri and sulci, changes in the regions of the cisterns, etc. have to be recorded.

Usually, frontal sections are made; their descriptions should include the position, extent, growth, color, and consistency of the tumor and the adjacent brain, displacement of the brain with possible enlargement of the white matter from edema and swelling, changes in position and form of the ventricles, metastases, etc.[3]

Histological routine

METHODS OF EMBEDDING

There are three ways of handling the material: supravital squash preparations, frozen sections, and sections of embedded material.

Frozen sections

Frozen sections can be prepared after as little as 24–36 hours of fixation (*see* also Quick Methods). The advantages of this method include dispensing with embedding, better preservation of the tissue, particularly the lessening of shrinkage artefacts, such as one gets in paraffin embedding (which can otherwise be avoided only with time-consuming celloidin imbedding), the opportunity to study fatty substances, and the application of metal impregnation methods. The disadvantages of the method include the difficulty of cutting soft, disintegrating tissue (from necrosis or fatty degeneration, etc.) and the fact that the material from the aspiration flask can not be used. Frozen-section technique is an essential prerequisite for some metal impregnation methods, e.g., the important gold sublimate impregnation. Certain of its disadvantages can be avoided with gelatin embedding.

Gelatin embedding

This method is only rarely used with tumors since the aniline stains work poorly here. It is used only for fat staining of semi-liquid tumors (medulloblastomas), necrotic tumors (glioblastomas), or for the study of brain swelling.

Paraffin embedding

With paraffin embedding each specimen can be quickly and reliably sectioned—especially thin sections—and stained with most methods. It is the method of choice on aspirated material. Its disadvantages include the high degree of shrinkage in material with very much water content (so that the fibers pull apart and spaces are formed around nerve cells and blood vessels), the fact that the sections come apart if cut very thin, and the fact that such material is suitable for only a few metal impregnation

---

[3] There are two ways to do this: one point (e.g., the changes in the ventricular system) can be described over the whole brain on successive sections, and then other items such as brain swelling or edema, etc. can be taken up; or all the points on each individual frontal section are described, without forgetting, however, to localize them (for instance, "in the section at the level of the pituitary stalk one sees . . .").

techniques. The methods of Cajal, Hortega, and Bielschowsky can be carried out on paraffin material only by undependable substitute methods.

Celloidin embedding

Celloidin embedding was previously the only method that allowed the preparation of large sections, i.e., through the whole hemispheres—something which is now possible by using the paraffin method of O. Vogt. It is the method of choice when the original technique of Nissl is to be used. It lends itself particularly well to a study of the growth and spread of a tumor, and the reaction of the surrounding tissue. The different components of the tissue can, on successive sections, be selectively studied (staining of cells, myelinated fibers, glial fibers, connective tissue, or metallic impregnations). Celloidin embedding preserves the tissue best, particularly when it is softened, or has a high fluid content. It is the method of choice in the study of brain edema and swelling. The particular disadvantage of this method is the length of time necessary for embedding, the appreciable thickness of the sections (30–40 μ), and the poor demonstration of the external form of the cells as compared with paraffin material.

SELECTION OF DIFFERENT STAINS

Nuclei

The details of nuclear structure are shown best with the Nissl stain or its modifications (e.g., cresyl violet) on paraffin or frozen sections. Good results are also obtained with other aniline dye methods. Chromatin is also selectively demonstrated by Hortega's metallic method.

Glia

The most beautiful demonstration of astrocytes is accomplished with Cajal's gold sublimate method, particularly with initial fixation in formalin ammonium bromide. If the latter fixation is used only secondarily, it is recommended to warm the frozen sections in formalin ammonium bromide solution before the actual staining. We were unable to obtain good results with Globus' method. Hortega's methods are well described in Calvo's monograph (1954).

When there is special interest in degenerative processes, the microglia in the marginal zone of the tumor can be stained with Hortega's method. However, the method is very sensitive and demands that instructions be followed carefully—i.e., primary fixation in formalin ammonium bromide, and carrying out the stain between the third and sixth day.

The oligodendroglia can be demonstrated with Hortega's or Penfield's methods. The results, however, are not always dependable. For the routine diagnosis of tumors, even for oligodendrogliomas, this method is unnecessary since the tumors can be identified in H. & E. stains, or gold sublimate. In the diagnosis of the polymorphic oligodendrogliomas, however, this method is of value.

If the metallic methods cannot be carried out, Mallory's phosphotungstic acid and hematoxylin for glial fibers can be used on frozen sections as a substitute. However, the results are really satisfactory only with primary or early fixation in Müller's solution. The glial fibers can also be adequately shown by using the Holzer method, or Heidenhain's stain on paraffin material as well. The Golgi method can reveal single tumor cells in their entirety (Klatzo).

Parenchyma

Methods for demonstrating axis cylinders are well known (particularly Bielschowsky; Schultze and Gros), but with the exception of Bodian's method they usually work only on celloidin or frozen sections. Myelin stains can be performed after any method of embedding, including paraffin embedding (where however, staining of glial fibers has to be taken into consideration), or the frozen technique of Spielmeyer.

Fats and Lipids

Fatty or lipid breakdown products can be recognized most clearly and simply with Sudan-black or Scharlach-red staining (fat-Ponceau), but earlier stages of breakdown can be detected with myelin stains. The Marchi method has no place in the study of tumors.

Summary

We use *frozen sections* for quick diagnosis, for demonstration of cells and nuclei, metachromatic substances (using cresyl violet), axis cylinders and myelin sheaths, glial fibers (gold sublimate method), microglia (after Hortega), oligodendroglia (after Hortega and Penfield), and fat. Frozen sections usually suffice for a quick survey of the material. Working with softened tissue is impossible, and in such cases paraffin, celloidin, or gelatin embedding may be substituted.

Paraffin sections are currently the basis for routine work. They are especially suitable for the preparation of thin sections of cellular adenomas, for the rapid survey of blocks larger than those which can be handled as frozen sections, and for the processing of soft, disintegrating material and material filtered from the aspiration flask. The basic methods are survey stains (H. & E., cresyl violet, Van Gieson, Mallory's phosphotungstic acid and hematoxylin, Masson's trichrome), glial methods (Holzer, Mallory), myelin sheath stains (Heidenhain), axons (Bodian) and connective tissue impregnations (Perdrau, Tibor-Pap, Foot, Gomori) or stains (Masson, Van Gieson). For pituitary adenomas we recommend, in addition to H. & E., Masson's stain (with its brilliant demonstration of acidophilic and basophilic cells), or the more difficult techniques of ethyl violet-orange G, neutral violet and fuchsin red, as well as Gomori's chrome-alum-hematoxylin and phloxine.

Celloidin material is suitable for preparation of large blocks when time is not a factor, and for serial and interval sections. With this method of embedding, the natural structure of the tissue is best preserved, and staining with the original Nissl method is most successfully carried out. Various stages of a disease process, e.g., a tumor, can best be contrasted with one another by applying different staining methods to successive sections (nerve cells according to Nissl, myelin sheaths according to Pal and Kulschitzky, glia to Holzer, connective tissue to Klarfeld and Achuccaro).

THE BEST STAINS FOR DIFFERENT TUMOR TYPES

1. Medulloblastomas

The histological diagnosis can be made on the basis of the cresyl violet stain; pre-existing astrocytes are shown with gold sublimate, and other parenchymal remnants with cell or myelin stains. Perdrau's method demonstrates the content of leptomeningeal connective tissue engulfed by the tumor.

Routine stain: Cresyl violet[4] on frozen or paraffin material.

2. Spongioblastomas

The tumor cells are best demonstrated with the gold sublimate method, the Rosenthal fibers with Heidenhain's stain, the tumor architecture and the beginnings of mucoid degeneration with metachromatic cresyl violet.

Routine staining: Cresyl violet on frozen or paraffin material; gold sublimate impregnation on frozen material.

3. Oligodendrogliomas

The classical honeycomb architecture is best seen after paraffin embedding and H. & E. staining, but also to some extent on frozen sections. Mucoid degeneration appears particularly well with metachromatic cresyl violet, the calcification with hematoxylin stains. The spindle-cell and large cell regions are best impregnated with gold sublimate. The polymorphic regions should be impregnated with "specific" methods.

Routine staining: H. & E. on paraffin embedded material.

4. Astrocytomas

Classical demonstration of the tumor cells is accomplished with the gold sublimate method; however, identification is generally sufficiently accurate with aniline stains. The astrocytes are also stained by Mallory's method.

Routine staining: Gold sublimate on frozen sections, cresyl violet on frozen and paraffin material.

[4] If the investigator is used to the H. & E. stain, it can be employed instead.

5. Glioblastomas

Histological diagnosis is possible by using routine chromatic stains. More "mature" cell forms and pre-existing glia can be demonstrated with gold sublimate, fatty degeneration with fat-Ponceau and other Scharlach red stains; the content of connective tissue with its abundant vascular component appears particularly clearly when using Perdrau's method. With the Golgi method, individual cells can be completely delineated (*see* also Sarcomas).

Routine stains: Cresyl violet method on frozen sections, or after embedding.

6. Ependymomas

The best demonstration of the architecture (perivascular zones free of nuclei) is achieved with cresyl violet staining of frozen or embedded material. The radiating patterns are best recognized with H. and E. or Masson's stain.

Routine staining: Cresyl violet on frozen or paraffin sections.

7. Plexus papillomas

Cresyl violet on paraffin material.

8. Pinealomas

Cresyl violet and H. & E. stains on paraffin material.

9. Neurinomas

The architecture shows up best on routine chromatic stains, and the fatty degeneration is brought out with Scharlach red. The silver methods show the absence of free reticulin fibers (which may be important in the differential diagnosis between these tumors and the fibromatous meningiomas) but they impregnate the fine specific fibers. After paraffin embedding and H. & E. staining the architecture may be reminiscent of oligodendrogliomas (because of fatty degeneration), Cresyl violet staining of frozen sections is satisfactory only when the sections are left overnight in the incubator in 70% alcohol.

Routine staining: Cresyl violet and H. & E. on paraffin or frozen sections.

10. Gangliocytomas

The prerequisite for reliable cell type identification is the Nissl method, or one of its modifications (cresyl violet). Here, again, it is recommended that the sections be left overnight in the incubator in 70% alcohol.

Routine staining: Cresyl violet on frozen or paraffin material.

11. Meningiomas

Meningiomas can be recognized on any aniline stain. The subtypes can be distinguished best by using silver-reticulin methods, if the architecture in the cresyl violet stained sections was not already sufficiently characteristic.

Routine staining: Cresyl violet on frozen or paraffin material.

12. Angioblastomas

The connective tissue network of blood vessels appears best with reticulin fiber methods, and the fatty degeneration occurring in some by using appropriate fat stains. However, the network-like architecture (angioreticulum) can be demonstrated well enough with chromatic methods.

Routine staining: Cresyl violet on frozen and paraffin sections, or impregnation by Perdrau's method.

13. Fibromas

Cresyl violet stain, and Perdrau's method on frozen or paraffin sections.

14. Sarcomas

In addition to routine chromatic stains, a prerequisite for the study of all sarcomas is the demonstration of the connective tissue according to the methods of Perdrau, Tibor-Pap, Foot, or Gomori. This applies particularly to the differentiation of monstrocellular sarcomas from glioblastomas.

Routine methods: Chromatic stains, and impregnation of reticulin fibers on frozen and paraffin sections.

15–18. Chondromas, lipomas, osteomas, and chordomas

These tumors can be identified after paraffin embedding and routine chromatic staining. Lipomas can also be studied with fat stains on frozen sections; osteomas usually have to be decalcified before embedding.

Routine staining: H. & E., and cresyl violet stains on paraffin sections.

19. Craniopharyngiomas

Decalcification usually unnecessary.

Routine staining: Cresyl violet, or H. & E. stains on paraffin sections.

20. Pituitary adenomas

Thin paraffin sections. Recognition of the subgroups is generally possible on H. & E. stains, but progressive staining methods and special techniques are desirable (Masson's trichrome, ethyl violet-orange G, neutral violet-acid fuchsin, Heidenhain's hematoxylin, Azan, Gomori's chrome-alum-hematoxylin and phloxine, etc.).

Routine staining: H. & E. stain on paraffin sections.

21. Cylindromatous epitheliomas

H. & E. stain.

22. Epidermoids

From the crumbly, scaly material an attempt should be made to obtain the capsular portions for embedding. This is done by squashing the material with a pair of forceps so that ultimately only a delicate membrane of capsule remains. Embedding in paraffin.

Routine staining: H. & E. stain on paraffin material.

23–24. Dermoids and teratomas

Embedding in paraffin and staining with cresyl violet, H. & E., or according to Van Gieson or Masson.

25. Angiomas and aneurysms

Routine methods: Embedding in paraffin or celloidin (better because the blood remains in the vessels) and routine chromatic stains, or connective tissue stains, and metal impregnations.

26. Unclassified tumors

If the classification of a tumor with routine methods is not possible at first, special stains must be employed to reach a diagnosis. In addition to routine chromatic stains, gold sublimate impregnations on frozen sections should be tried, or the other metallic impregnation methods that demonstrate the shape of the cell. An examination also should be made of the formation of fibers by the cells, the content of connective tissue, the type of regressive processes and the reaction of the connective tissue to them, etc., and a characterization of the tissue type on the basis of these observations should be attempted.

27. Metastases

H. & E., and cresyl violet stains on paraffin sections.

28. Parasites

H. & E., and Van Gieson's stain on paraffin sections.

29. Granulomas

Cresyl violet, H. & E., Azan, and reticulin fiber stains on paraffin sections.

30. Cells in the cerebrospinal fluid

For the study of tumor cells in the cerebrospinal fluid, either embed the sediment according to Alzheimer's method, or smear the material on a slide.

HISTOCHEMICAL METHODS

Although histochemical methods may prove to be very useful for the scientific investigation of tumors, their diagnostic value up to now has not been great. Consequently, we have not included them here.

Quick methods

For rapid diagnosis during operation (Eisenhardt and Cushing, 1930; Badt, 1937; Morris; Russell, 1939; Kautzky, 1951; Klatzo and McMillan; Zülch, 1937) we employ the following methods: From the specimen sent by the surgeon a pea-sized piece of the most obviously neoplastic portion is selected—if possible from the growth zone. This is warmed in formol solution until it begins to steam, but is not allowed to boil. Starting with the first section from the freezing microtome (20 μ or more, if necessary) the slices are collected in warm formalin, then transferred into 1% aqueous cresyl violet solution, and again warmed for one minute. Then the sections are taken through distilled water and graded alcohols into 96% alcohol, where appropriate differentiation is carried out, depending on the thickness and cellularity of the sections. The sections are then carried through absolute alcohol, xylol, and mounted in Canada balsam. With skillful differentiation even thick sections (40 μ) can be sufficiently decolorized to obtain an excellent survey picture. (The whole procedure takes about 8–10 minutes.)

The second method of rapid diagnosis consists of the supravital staining of squash or smear preparations. A little piece of tissue is teased on a slide with a dissecting needle and then covered with Loeffler's methylene blue (diluted 1:1 with distilled water), neutral red (1:10,000), or Alzheimer and Mann's methylene blue-eosin solution, or stained with chlorazol black E. The cover glass is then carefully pressed onto the tissue until it is only one cell-layer thick; however, the tissue relations should not be disturbed. The excess stain is drawn off with filter paper. The section is adequately stained in a few minutes. Another way is to squash the tissue and smear it out with a slide, like a blood smear, and stain it appropriately.

Selection of methods for rapid diagnosis

Needle biopsy
> a) if there is enough time, embedding in paraffin
> b) if diagnosis is required immediately, squash preparation

Operative specimen
> Frozen technique: squash preparation only when the tissue cannot even be sectioned at 30–40 μ.

Other methods
> In my experience, the use of the phase contrast method has no advantage over stained sections when rapid diagnosis is needed. However, that method will certainly prove fruitful in further scientific analyses of neoplastic tissue. The electron microscope has recently been applied to the sutdy of brain tumors and Fernández-Morán has obtained excellent results with it.

BIBLIOGRAPHY

ABBOTT, K. H. and C. B. COURVILLE: Notes on pathology of cranial tumors. Bull. Los Angeles Neurol. Soc. **10**, 10, 1945.

ABBOTT, K. H. and O. I. CUTLER: Chronic coccidioidal meningitis. Review of literature and report of seven cases. Arch. Path. **21**, 320, 1936.

ABBOTT, K. H. and B. GLASS: Intracranial extracerebral (leptomeningeal) glioma. Excerpta Med., Neurol. and Psychiat. **8**, 786, 1955.

ABBOTT, K. H. and J. W. KERNOHAN: Primary sarcomas of the brain. Review of the literature and report of twelve cases. Arch. Neurol. Psychiat. **50**, 42–66, 1943.

ADAIR, F. E. and J. McLEAN: Tumors of the peripheral nervous system. Kapitel XVI in: PENFIELDS Cytology of the nervous system, S. 440–464. Hoeber, New York 1932.

ADSON, A. W., J. W. KERNOHAN and H. W. WOLTMAN: Cranial and cervical chordomas. Arch. Neurol. Psychiat. **33**, 247–261, 1935.

ALAJOUANINE, Th. et al: Les formes chirurgicales spinales de torulose. Rev. neurol. **88**, 153–163, 1953.

ALAJOUANINE, T., J. GUILLAUME et R. THUREL: Méningiome suprasellaire. Rev. neurol. **61**, 70, 1934.

ALAJOUANINE, TH., TH. HORNET et R. THUREL: Pinéalome avec métastases multiples; dissémination par le L. C. R. Rev. neurol. **68**, 793 (1937).

ALAJOUANINE, TH. et TH. HORNET: L'oedème cérébrale generalisée. Ann. Anat. Path. med. chir. 16, 1939.

ALAJOUANINE, Th. et R. THUREL: Tubercule cérébral opéré; survie de trois ans. Rev. neurol. 1945.

ALBERTINI, A. v.: Das Malignitätsproblem in histologisch-zytologischer Betrachtung. Verh. Dtsch. Ges. Path. Hannover 1951; Piscator, Stuttgart 1952.

ALBERTINI, A. v.: Histologische Geschwulstdiagnostik. G. Thieme, Stuttgart 1955.

ALEXANDER: A note on the differential diagnosis of experimentally produced brain tumors and their relation to brain tumors in man. Amer. J. Cancer. **37**, 395, 1939.

ALPERS, B. J.: Origin and development of giant cells in gliomas. Arch. Neurol. Psychiat. **25**, 281, 1931.

ALPERS, B. J.: Primary fibroblastoma of the brain. Arch. Neurol. Psychiat. **26**, 1335, 1931.

ALPERS, B. J.: Gumma of the brain. Amer. J. Syph. **23**, 233, 1939.

ALPERS, B. J. and F. C. GRANT: The ganglioneuromas of the central nervous system. Arch. Neurol. Psychiat. **26**, 501, 1931.

ALPERS, B. J. and R. A. GROFF: Parasellar tumors. Meningeal fibroblastomas arising from the sphenoid ridge. Arch. Neurol. Psychiat. **31**, 713, 1934.

ALPERS, B. J. and S. N. ROWE: The astrocytomas. Amer. J. Canc. **30**, 1, 1937.

ALPERS, B. J. and J. YASKIN: Gliomas of the pons. Arch. Neurol. Psychiat. **41**, 435, 1939.

ALTMANN, H. W.: Zur Morphologie der Wechselwirkung von Kern und Zytoplasma. Verh. Ges. Dtsch. Naturf. u. Ärzte, Freiburg, Sept. 1954, S. 60–68, Springer 1955.

AMSTAD, E.: Beitrag zur Klinik und Histopathologie des Gangliozytoms der Medulla oblongata. Schweiz. Arch. Neurol. **39**, 5–25, 1937.

ANDERSON, I.: How to stain the nervous system. Edinburgh 1929.

ANDRÉ THOMAS and J. JUMENTIÉ: Un cas de tumeur du ventricule latéral. Rev. neurol. 1928, II, 202.

ANTONI, N.: Über Rückenmarkstumoren und Neurofibrome. Wiesbaden 1920.

ANTONI, N.: Tumoren des Rückenmarks, seiner Wurzeln und Häute. Handb. Neurol. BUMKE-FOERSTER, Bd. 14, 1936.

ANTONI, N.: Gliomas of the neurohypophysis and hypophysial stalk. J. Neurosurg. **7**, 521–531, 1950.

AOYAGI, T. und K. KYUNO: Über die endothelialen Zellzapfen in der Dura mater cerebri und ihre Lokalisation in derselben nebst ihrer Beziehung zur Geschwulstbildung in der Dura mater. Neurologia (Tokyo) **11**, 1–11, 1912.

APITZ, K.: Über Pigmentbildungen in den Zellkernen melanotischer Geschwülste. Virchows Arch. **300**, 89, 1937.

APITZ, K.: Die Geschwülste und Gewebsmißbildungen der Nierenrinde. Virchows Arch. **311**, 285, 1943.

ARANA-INIGUEZ, R. and J. SAN JULIAN: Hydatid cysts of the brain. J. Neurosurg. **12**, 323–335, 1955.

ARIETI, S.: The vascularisation of cerebral neoplasms studied with the fuchsin staining method of Eros. J. Neuropath. **1**, 375–393, 1942.

ARLT, H. G.: Multiple Meningeome des Gehirns und diffuse Meningeomatosis des Rückenmarks. Zschr. Neurol. **156**, 713–734, 1936.

ARNOLD, A., P. BAILEY, R. A. HARVEY, J. S. LAUGHLIN and L. L. HAAS: Changes in the central nervous system following irradiation with 23 mev. x-rays from the betatron. Radiology **62**, 37–44, 1954.

ARNOLD, H. and H. M. ZIMMERMANN: Experimental brain tumors. III. Tumors produced with Dibenzanthracene. Cancer Res. **3**, 682–685, 1943.

ASENJO, A., H. VALLADARES u. J. FIERRO: Tuberculomas encefalicos (Revision de 152 casos.) Sistema nerv. (Milano) **1**, 1, 1949.

ASENJO, A., H. VALLADARES u. J. FIERRO: Tuberculomas cerebrales (Revisión de 152 casos). Rev. apar. resp. y tuberculosis (Santiago) **4**, 3–32, 1949.

ASKANAZY: Die Zirbel und ihre Tumoren in ihrem funktionellen Einfluß. Frankf. Z. Path. 24, 1921.

AVENDANO, J., C. ISMODES and E. D. ROCCA: Bacteriologia de los tuberculomas cerebrales. IV. Congresso sul americano de neurocirurgia, Porto Alegre/Brasil. 1951, S. 316–322.

BADT: Bericht über 57 nicht diagnostizierte Hirntumoren, zugleich ein Beitrag zur Symptomatologie der Hirntumoren im Senium. Zschr. Neurol. **138**, 610–656, 1932.

BADT, B.: Mikroskopische Schnelldiagnose bei hirnchirurgischen Eingriffen. Zbl. Neurochir. **2**, 123–140, 1937.

BADTKE, B.: Über einen Fall von spiegelbildlichem Einwärtsschielen bei eineiigen Zwillingen. Klin. Mbl. Augenheilk. **105**, 231, 237, 1940.

BAGDASAR, D.: Le traitement chirurgical des gommes cérébrales. Rev. neurol. 1929 II.

BAGGENSTOSS, A. H. and J. G. LOVE: Pinealomas. Arch. Neurol. Psychiat. **41**, 1187–1206, 1939.

BAHRMANN, E.: Über die fibrinoide Degeneration des Bindegewebes. Virchows Arch. **300**, 342–372, 1937.

BAILEY, O. T.: Relation of glioma of the leptomeninges to neuroglia nests. Arch. Path. **21**, 584, 1936.

BAILEY, O. T.: Histology of meningioma. Arch. Path. **30**, 42–69, 1940.

BAILEY, O. T.: The histogenesis of the medulloblastoma. Excerpta medica, Neurology and Psychiatry **8**, 814, 1955.

BAILEY, O. T. and E. C. CUTLER: Malignant adenomas of the chromophobe cells of the pituitary body. Arch. Path. **29**, 368, 1940.

BAILEY, P.: Cruveilhier's „tumeurs perlées“. Surg. Gynecol. Obstetr. **31**, 390–401, 1920.

BAILEY, P.: A study of tumors arising from ependymal cells. Arch. Neurol. Psychiat. **11**, 1–27, 1924.

BAILEY, P.: Quelques nouvelles observations de tumeurs épendymaires. Ann. Anat. path. méd. chir. **2**, 481–512, 1925.

BAILEY, P.: Further remarks concerning tumors of the glioma group. Bull. Johns Hopkins Hosp. **40**, 354–389, 1927.

BAILEY, P.: Intracranial sarcomatous tumors of leptomeningeal origin. Arch. Surg. (Chicago) **18**, 1359–1402, 1929.

BAILEY, P.: Tumors of the hypophysis cerebri. Kapitel XXVI in: PENFIELDS Cytology and cellular pathology of the nervous system, S. 1133–1144. New York, Hoeber 1932.

BAILEY, P.: Cellular types in primary tumors of the brain. In: PENFIELDS Cytology and cellular pathology of the nervous system, S. 905–951. Hoeber, New York 1932.

BAILEY, P.: Intracranial tumors. Baillière, Tindall and Cox, London 1933. – Die Hirngeschwülste. Enke, Stuttgart 1936 und 1951.

BAILEY, P. and D. BAGDASAR: Intracranial chordoblastoma. Amer. J. Path. **5**, 439–449, 1929.

BAILEY, P. and A. BRUNSCHWIG: Erfahrungen mit der Röntgenbehandlung der Hirngliome. Zschr. Neurol. **161**, 214–217, 1938.

BAILEY, P., D. BUCHANAN and P. BUCY: Intracranial tumors of infancy and childhood. Chicago 1939.

BAILEY, P. and P. C. BUCY: Oligodendrogliomas of the brain. J. Path. Bact. **32**, 735–751, 1929.

BAILEY, P. and P. C. BUCY: Astroblastomas of the brain. Acta Neurol. Psychiatr. Scand. **5**, 439–461, 1930.

BAILEY, P. and P. C. BUCY: The origin and nature of meningeal tumors. Amer. J. Cancer **15**, 15–54, 1931.

BAILEY, P. and H. CUSHING: Medulloblastoma cerebelli. Arch. Neurol. Psychiat. **14**, 192–223, 1925.

BAILEY, P. and H. CUSHING: Tumors of the glioma group. Lipincott, Philadelphia 1926.

BAILEY, P. and H. CUSHING: Die Gewebsverschiedenheit der Gliome und ihre Bedeutung für die Prognose. G. Fischer, Jena 1930.

BAILEY, P. and H. CUSHING: Blood vessel tumors of the brain. Ch. C. Thomas, Springfield 1928.

BAILEY, P. and H. CUSHING: Haemangiomas of cerebellum and retina (Lindau's disease) with report of a case. Arch. Ophthalm. **57**, 447–463, 1928.

BAILEY, P. and H. CUSHING: The microscopic structure of the adenomas in agromegalic dyspituitarism. Amer. J. Path. **4**, 545–563, 1928.

BAILEY, P., H. CUSHING and L. EISENHARDT: Angioblastic meningiomas. Arch. Path. **6**, 953–990, 1928.

BAILEY, P. and N. DOTT: Hypophysial adenomata. Brit. J. Surg. **13**, 314–366, 1925.

BAILEY, P. and L. EISENHARDT: Spongioblastomas of the brain. J. Comp. Neur. **56**, 391–430, 1932.

BAILEY, P. and F. HILLER: The interstitial tissues of the nervous system. J. Nerv. Ment. Dis. **59**, 337–361, 1924.

BAILEY, P. and G. HORRAX: Tumors of the pineal body. Arch. Neurol. Psychiat. **13**, 433, 1925.

BAILEY, P. and G. HORRAX: Pineal pathology: further studies. Arch. Neurol. Psychiat. **19**, 394–415, 1928.

BAILEY, P. and JELIFFE: Tumors of the pineal body. Arch. Intern. Med. **8**, 851–880, 1911.

BAILEY, P., M. C. SOSMAN and A. VAN DESSEL: Roentgen therapy of gliomas of the brain. Amer. J. Roentgenol. **19**, 203–264, 1928.

BAKAY jr., L. V.: Das Oligodendrogliom. Confinia neurol. (Basel), **8**, 157, 1948.

BAKAY, L.: The results of 300 pituitary adenoma operations (Prof. H. Olivecronas series). J. Neurosurg. **7**, 240–255, 1950.

BAKER, A. B. and J. M. ADAMS: Primary fibroblastomas of the brain. Amer. J. Path. **13**, 129–137, 1937.

BAKER, A. B. and J. M. ADAMS: Lipomatosis of the central nervous system. Amer. J. Cancer **34**, 214, 1938.

BANNWARTH, A.: Zum Liquorsyndrom des Hirntumors unter besonderer Berücksichtigung der subtentoriellen Geschwülste. Arch. Psychiatr. **104**, 690–709, 1936.

BANNWARTH, A.: Zur Pathologie des Hirntumors. (I) Arch. Psych. **103**, 471–509, 1935; (II) **104**, 292–343, 1935.

BARGMANN, W., W. HILD, R. ORTMANN und TH. H. SCHIEBLER: Morphologische und experimentelle Untersuchungen über das hypothalamisch-hypophysäre System. Acta Neurovegetativa (Wien) **1**, 233–275, 1950.

BARTEL, J. und W. LANDAU: Über Kleinhirnzysten. Frankf. Z. Path. **4**, 372–383, 1910.

BAUDITZ, A.: Über Dermoide und Epidermoide des Gehirns. Zschr. Neurol. **144**, 135–147, 1933.

BAUER, K. H.: Das Krebsproblem. Springer, Berlin, Göttingen, Heidelberg 1949.

BAUER, K. H.: Synkarzinogenese. Klin. Wschr. 1949, 118.

BAUMGARTEN: Über gummöse Syphilis des Gehirns und des Rückenmarks, namentlich der Hirngefäße und über das Verhältnis dieser Erkrankung zu den tuberkulösen Affektionen. Arch. Anat. Physiol. **86**, 179, 1881.

BECK, E.: Ein Beitrag zur Neurofibromatose. Zschr. Neurol. **162**, 426, 1938.

BECK, D. J. K. and D. S. RUSSEL: Oligodendrogliomatosis of the cerebrospinal pathway. Brain **65**, 352–372, 1942.

BECKMANN, J. W. and L. S. KUBIE: Tumor of the hypophyseal stalk. Brain 52, 127–170, 1929.

BECKMANN, O.: Gliom und Trauma. Inaug.-Diss. Kiel 1930.

BELEZKY, W. K.: Ein Fall von Mesogliom. Virchows Arch. 290, 450–459, 1933.

BENDA, C.: Hypophysis cerebri. Handb. inn. Sekretion, Bd. 1. Kabitzsch, Leipzig 1932.

BENDER, W. und FR. PANSE: Familiäres Gliom (Zur Genetik der Gliome). Mschr. Psychiatr. 83, 253–285, 1932.

BENEDEK, L.: Über die autochthonen Dysembryome (Pinealome) des Gehirns. Zschr Neurol. 156, 677–693, 1936.

BENEDEK, L. und A. JUBA: Die Gewebsstruktur der Gliome mit besonderer Berücksichti gung der Einteilungsmöglichkeit. Arch. Psychiatr. 113, 233–283, 1941.

BENEDEK, L. und A. JUBA: Über die diffuse zentrale Schwannose und das zentrale Neurinom. Dtsch. Z. Nervenhk. 152, 274, 1941.

BENEDEK, L. und A. JUBA: Über das Mikrogliom. Dtsch. Z. Nervenhk. 152, 159, 1941

BENEDEK, L. und A. JUBA: Über den histologischen Aufbau und die systematischei Beziehungen der Ependymome. Dtsch. Z. Nervenhk. 155, 65, 1943.

BENEDEK, L. und A. JUBA: Über die Gewebskultur der Meningeome. Zschr. Neurol. 176, 472, 1943.

BENEDICT, W. L.: Retinoblastoma in homologous eyes of identical twins. Arch. of Ophthalm. 1929, 545.

BENEKE, R.: Beitrag zur traumatischen Ätiologie der Geschwülste des ZNS. und ihrer Häute. Erg. allg. Path. 23, 893, 1932.

BENNETT, W. A.: Primary intracranial neoplasms in military age group – world war II. Mil. Surgeon 99, 594–652, 1946.

BERBLINGER, W.: Zur Kenntnis der Zirbelgeschwülste. Zschr. Neurol. 95, 741–761, 1925.

BERBLINGER, W.: Kurze Bemerkung zu der Arbeit von A. SCHUBACK über die Angiomatosis des ZNS (LINDAUsche Krankheit) in Bd. 110, H. 3/4 ds. Z. Zschr. Neurol. 112, 315–316, 1928.

BERBLINGER, W.: Physiologie und Pathologie der Zirbel. Erg. Inn. Med. 14, 245–312, 1930.

BERBLINGER, W.: Die Adenome der Hypophyse. Nervenarzt 9, 329–340, 1936.

BERBLINGER, W.: Zur Kenntnis der Pinealozytome nebst Bemerkungen über die cerebrogene Frühreife. Schweiz. Z. Path. Bakt. 7, 107–128, 1944.

BERGSTRAND, H.: On gliomas of the cerebral hemispheres. Acta path. microbiol. Scand. Suppl. 11, 100, 1932.

BERGSTRAND, H.: Über das sogenannte Astrozytom des Kleinhirns. Virchows Arch. 287, 538, 1932.

BERGSTRAND, H.: Über das Gliom in den Großhirnhemisphären. Virchows Arch. 287, 797 bis 822, 1933.

BERGSTRAND, H.: Das Kleinhirnastrozytom. Zbl. Neurochir. 2, 359, 1937.

BERGSTRAND, H.: Weiteres über sogenannte Kleinhirnastrozytome. Virchows Arch. 299, 725–739, 1937.

BERGSTRAND, H. und H. OLIVECRONA: Angioblastic meningeomas. Amer. J. Cancer 24, 522, 1935.

BERGSTRAND, H., H. OLIVECRONA und W. TÖNNIS: Gefäßmißbildungen und Gefäßgeschwülste des Gehirns. Thieme, Leipzig 1936.

BERNSTEIN, S. A.: Über das Verhalten des Schädelknochens beim Duraendotheliom. Virchows Arch. 290, 501–539, 1933.

BERTHA, H.: Morphologische Studien der Gefäße bei einem sogenannten „apoplektischen Gliom". Zschr. Neurol. 169, 617–636, 1940.

BERTHA, H.: Die Spiegelschrift der linken Hand. Zschr. Neurol. 175, 68–96, 1942.

BERTHA, H.: Zur Gefäßmorphologie bei Hirntumoren. Acta Neurochir. (Suppl.) 1955.

BERTHA, H. und W. SORGO: Über einen operativ geheilten Fall eines Plexuspapilloms. Chirurg 12, 714–718, 1940.

BERTRAND, I. and R. BERNARD: Dégénérescence maligne d'une tumeur Schwannique du nerf radial dans un cas de maladie de Recklinghausen. Rev. neurol. 1930, II, 66.

BESOLD, G.: Über 2 Fälle von Gehirntumor (Hämangiosarkom oder sog. Periutheliom) in der Gegend des 3. Ventrikels bei zwei Geschwistern. Dtsch. Z. Nervenhk. 8, 49–74, 1895/96.

BICKERSTAFF, E. R., P. C. P. CLOAKE, B. HUGHES and W. T. SMITH: The racemose form of cerebral cysticercosis. Brain 75, 1–18, 1952.

BIELFELD, K.: Über ein metastasierendes Zylindrom. Zbl. Path. u. Path. Anat. **93**, 353–357, 1955.

BIELSCHOWSKY, M.: Über tuberöse Sklerose und ihre Beziehungen zur Recklinghausenschen Krankheit. Zschr. Neurol. **26**, 133, 1914.

BIELSCHOWSKY, M.: Das multiple Ganglioneurom des Gehirns und seine Entstehung. J. Psychol. Neurol. **32**, 1–20, 1925.

BIELSCHOWSKY, M.: Neuroblastic tumors of the Sympathetic-System. Kapitel XXIV in: PENFIELDS Cytology of the nervous system. New York, Hoeber 1932.

BIELSCHOWSKY, M. und GALLUS: Über tuberöse Sklerose. J. Psychol. Neurol. **20**, 307, 1913.

BIELSCHOWSKY, M. und R. HENNEBERG: Über Bau und Histogenese der zentralen Ganglioglioneurome. Mschr. Psychiatr. **68**, 21–51, 1928.

BIELSCHOWSKY, M. und L. PICK: Über das System der Neurome usw. Zschr. Neurol. **6**, 391, 1911.

BIELSCHOWSKY, M. und M. ROSE: Zur Kenntnis der zentralen Veränderungen bei Recklinghausenscher Krankheit. J. Psychol. Neurol. **35**, 42, 1927.

BIELSCHOWSKY, M. und A. SIMON: Über diffuse Hamartome (Ganglioneurome) des Kleinhirns und ihre Genese. J. Psychol. Neurol. **41**, 50–75, 1930.

BIELSCHOWSKY, M. und E. UNGER: Zur Kenntnis der primären Epithelgeschwülste der Adergeflechte des Gehirns. Arch. Klin. Chir. **81**, 61, 1902.

BIRKMAYER, W. und TH. HASENJÄGER: Ventilverschluß des vierten Ventrikels durch ein Epidermoid. Zbl. Neurochir. **5**, 177–184, 1940.

BITTORF, V.: Beiträge zur pathologischen Anatomie der Gehirn- und Rückenmarksgeschwülste. Beitr. path. Anat. **35**, 169, 1904.

BIZZOZERO und BOZZOLO: Studi sui tumori primitivi della dura madre. Riv. Clin. Bol. **4**, 1874.

BLACK, B. K. and D. E. SMITH: Nasal glioma. Arch. Psychol. and Neur. **64**, 614–630, 1950.

BLACK, B. K. and J. W. KERNOHAN: Primary diffuse tumors of the meninges (so-called meningeal meningiomatosis). Cancer **3**, 805–819, 1950.

BLAND, J.: The growth of human meningiomata in culture. Arch. exper. Zellforschg. **22**, 1939.

BLAND, J. and D. RUSSELL: Histological types of meningioma. J. Path. **47**, 291–309, 1938.

DE BLASI, A.: Su di un tumore vascolare della pia madre cerebellare. Pathologica **23**, 1–5, 1931.

BOCHNIK, H. J.: Nekrosekalk und kalzifierende Organisation im Gehirn. Dtsch. Z. Nervenhk. **169**, 358–382, 1953.

BODECHTEL, G.: Ein Neuroepitheliom unter dem klinischen Bild eines Meningeoms der Olfactoriusrinne. Arch. Psychiatr. **101**, 617, 1934.

BODECHTEL, G. und G. DÖRING: Zerebrale Zirkulationsstörungen bei Hirngeschwülsten. Zschr. Neurol. **161**, 166–177, 1938.

BODECHTEL, G. und K. SCHÜLER: Zur Klinik und Pathologie der Liquormetastasen bei Gliomen. Dtsch. Z. Nervenhk. **142**, 85–119, 1937.

BOEMKE, FR. und W. JOEST: Chordome im Bereich des Schädels. Virchows Arch. **297**, 351 bis 367, 1936.

BÖHMIG, R.: Gehirntumor bei zwei Geschwistern. Arch. Psychiatr. **59**, 527, 1918.

BÖHRINGER, H. R.: Neurofibromatose mit maligner Entartung. Schweiz. med. Wschr. **76**, 366–371, 1946.

BOGAERT, L. VAN: Tumeurs bilatérales de l'acoustique et neurofibromatose. Anat. path. méd.-chir. **11**, 353, 1934.

BOGAERT, L. VAN: Pathologie des angiomatoses. Acta neurologica et psychiatrica Belgica **50**, 526–610, 1950.

BOLLACK, J., M. DAVID et P. PUECH: Les arachnoidites opto-chiasmatiques. Masson, Paris 1937.

BONKÁLO, A.: Die Bedeutung der Geschwulstart und des Geschwulstsitzes für die Entstehung der Hirnschwellung. Dtsch. Z. Nervenhk. **149**, 243–253, 1939.

BORCK, W. F. und K. J. ZÜLCH: Über die Erkrankungshäufigkeit der Geschlechter an Hirngeschwülsten. Zbl. Neurochir. **11**, 333–350, 1951.

BORMANN, H.: Artdiagnose der seltenen Schädelbasisgeschwülste. Zbl. Neurochir. **11**, 33–45, 1951.

BORMANN, H. und W. SCHIEFER: Krampfanfälle bei Tumoren des Großhirns. Dtsch. Z. Nervenhk. **166**, 1–16, 1951.

BORST, M.: Allgemeine Pathologie der malignen Geschwülste. In ZWEIFFEL-PAYR: ,,Die Klinik der bösartigen Geschwülste", S. 1–180. Hirzel, 1924.

BORST, M.: Die Lehre von den Geschwülsten. Wiesbaden 1902.

BOSTROEM, A. und H. SPATZ: Über die von der Olfactoriusrinne ausgehenden Meningeome. Nervenarzt 2, 1929.

BOSTROEM, E.: Über die pialen Epidermoide, Dermoide und Lipome etc. Zbl. Path. 8, 1–98, 1897.

BOUWDIJK, B. VAN: Primäres metastasierendes Gehirncarcinom. Zschr. Neurol. 27, 96, 1914.

BOYKIN, F. C., D. COWEN, CH. A. J. IANNUCCI and A. WOLF: Subependymal glomerate astrocytomas. J. Neuropath. 13, 30–49, 1954.

BRADFORD, F. K.: Hemangioblastoma of the posterior fossa (Lindaus Disease). Report of two cases with familial history. J. Neurosurg. 5, 196, 1948.

BRADFORD, F. K. and D. MILLER: Meningeoma showing sarcomatous degeneration. Arch. Neurol. Psychiat. 43, 778, 1940.

BRAUNMÜHL, A. V.: Zur histologischen Differentialdiagnose primärer Gehirncarcinome. Zschr. Neurol. 107, 622, 1926.

BRESSLER, H.: Die Krankheiten des Gehirns und der äußeren Kopfbedeckungen. Berlin 1839.

BRICKNER, R.M.: Brain of patient ,,A" after bilateral frontal lobectomy. Arch. Neurol. Psychiat. 68, 293, 1952.

BRICKNER, R. M.: Intellectual functions of the frontal lobes. The MacMillan Company, New York 1936.

BRILMAYER, C., H. CRAMER und K. SCHÜRMANN: Die Bedeutung bestimmter Farbstoffe in der Diagnostik der Hirntumoren. Zbl. Neurochir. 12, 210–218, 1952.

BROAGER, B.: Multiple cerebellar angioreticulomas. Discussion of high protein contents of the cysts and of the enclosed subarachnoid space. Acta psychiatr. (København.) 24, 317–332, 1949.

BRONFMAN, S. et M. REUMONT: La sarcomatose méningée primitive. J. Belg. Neur. et Psych. 12, 1–31, 1947.

BROUGHAM, M., A. P. HEUSNER and R. D. ADAMS: Acute degenerative changes in adenomas of the pituitary body — with special reference to pituitary apoplexy. J. Neurosurg. 7, 421–439, 1950.

BROUWER, B., J. VAN DER HOEVE and W. MALONEY: A fourth type of phakomatosis: STURGE-WEBER-Syndrome. Kon. Akad. Wet. Verhandl. (Tweede Sectie) 36, I, 33, 1937.

BRUETSCH, W. L.: Etiology of optochiasmatic arachnoiditis. Arch. Neurol. Psychiat. 59, 215–228, 1948.

BRÜTT, H.: Intrakranielles Chondrom als Hirntumor. Dtsch. Z. Chir. 231, 497, 1931.

BRUGGER, G.: Über ein riesiges Meningeom mit intra- und extracraniellem Wachstum. Zbl. Neurochir. 15, 223–225, 1955.

BRUNNER, H.: Zur Pathologie und Klinik der Akustikustumoren. Klin. Wschr. I, 383–387, 1935.

BRUNNER, W.: Über die Häufigkeit von Gehirnmetastasen bösartiger Geschwülste, besonders des primären Lungentumors und ihre Bedeutung für die Klinik. Zschr. Neurol. 154, 793–798, 1936.

BRUNS, L.: Hirngeschwülste und Hirnparasiten. In Handb. d. path. Anat. d. Nervensystems. I. Karger, Berlin 1904.

BRUNS, L.: Geschwülste des Nervensystems. Karger, Berlin 1908.

BUCHSTEIN, H. F. and A. W. ADSON: Tuberculoma of the brain. Arch. Neurol. Psychiat. 43, 635, 1940.

BUCHTALA, V.: Die Strahlentherapie der Hirntumoren. Strahlentherapie 91, 528, 1955.

BUCKLEY, R. C.: Tissue culture studies of the glioblastoma multiforme Amer. J. Path. 5, 467, 1929.

BUCKLEY, R. C. and L. EISENHARDT: Study of a meningioma in supravital preparations, tissue culture and paraffin sections. Amer. J. Path. 5, 659, 1929.

BUCY, P. C.: Tumors of the central nervous system. Tice's System of Medicine. W. F. Prior, 1942.

BUCY, P. C.: Intrinsic tumors of the cerebellum and brainstem. In BANCROFT: ,,Surgical treatment of the nervous system". Lippincott, Philadelphia 1946.

BUCY, P. C., O. FOERSTER, O. GAGEL and W. MAHONEY: Die Tumoren der Brücke; ein Fall von Astrozytom der Brücke. Zschr. Neurol. 157, 136–146, 1937.

Bucy, P. C. and W. A. Gustafson: Structure, nature and classification of the cerebellar astrozytomas. Amer. J. Cancer 35, 327–353, 1939.
Bucy, P. C. and W. A. Gustavson: Gangliocytomas. Amer. J. Cancer 35, 5, 1939.
Bucy, P. C. and W. S. Muncie: Neuroepithelioma of the cerebellum. Amer. J. Pathol. 5, 157–170, 1929.
Bucy, P. C. and H. R. Overhill: Intradural spinal granulomas. J. Neurosurg. 7, 1–12, 1950.
Budde, M.: Zur Kenntnis der bösartigen Hypophysengeschwülste und hypophysärer Kachexie. Frankf. Z. Path. 25, 16–34, 1921.
Büchner, F.: Beiträge zur pathologischen Anatomie und zur allgemeinen Pathologie. G. Fischer, Verlag, Stuttgart 1950.
Büchner, F.: Geschwülste. I. Das Wesen, das Wachstum und die Ursachen der Geschwülste. Lehrb. Allg. Chir. E. Lexer, 2. Bd., 21. Aufl. Enke-Verlag, Stuttgart 1952.
Büchner, F.: Spezielle Pathologie. Urban & Schwarzenberg, München 1955.
Büngeler, W.: Die Definition des Geschwulstbegriffes und die Abgrenzung der Hyperplasien gegenüber den Geschwülsten. Verhandl. d. Dtsch. Ges. f. Path., Hannover 1951; Piscator-Verlag, Stuttgart 1952, S. 10.
Bürki, E.: Über den primären Sehnerventumor und seine Beziehungen zur Recklinghausenschen Neurofibromatose. Bibliotheca Ophthalm. Fasc. 30. Karger 1944.
Busch, E. und E. Christensen: Das Oligodendrozytom der Sehnervenkreuzung. Zbl. Neurochir. 2, 315–320, 1937.
Busch, E. and E. Christensen: Tumors of peripheral nerves with special reference to neurogenous sarcomas. Acta psychiat. et neurol. (Suppl.). Festschrift zu Antonis 60. Geburtstag.
Busch, E. and E. Christensen: The tree types of glioblastoma. J. Neurosurg. 4, 200–220, 1947.
de Buscher, J. and H. J. Scherer: Les gliomes de l'encéphale. L'édition univ. Vromans 1942.
Busse: Aneurysmen und Bildungsfehler der A. communicans ant. Virchows Arch. 229, 178, 1921.
Butenandt, A.: Karzinogene Stoffe und Tumorgenese. Verhandl. d. Dtsch. Ges. f. Path., Hannover 1951; Piscator, Stuttgart 1952, S. 70.
Cagnetto, G.: Neuer Beitrag zum Studium der Akromegalie. Virchows Arch. 187, 197 bis 244, 1907.
Cairns, H.: Spätergebnisse der operativen Behandlung von Hirngeschwülsten. Nervenarzt 9, 401–410, 1936.
Cairns, H.: The ultimate results of operations for intracranial tumours. Yale J. Biol. Med. 8, 421–492, 1936.
Cairns, H. and G. Riddoch: Observations on the treatment of ependymal gliomas. Brain 54, 1931.
Cairns, H. and D. S. Russell: Intracranial and spinal metastases in gliomas of the brain. Brain 54, 377–421, 1931.
Cajal, R. Y.: Nouvelles observations sur l'evolution des neuroblastes. Anat. Anz. 11, 255, 1908.
Calvo, W.: Tumores encefalomedulares. Estudio morfologico y biologico. Arch. Esp. de Morfol. Supl. 5, 1–173, 1954.
Calvo, W. y J. L. Barcia: La malignidad y frecuenzia de los tumores del sistema nervioso en relación con el sexo y la edad de los pacientes. Med. españ. 163, 5–15, 1952.
Calvo, W. y Salorio Barcia: Morbilidad y malignidad de los tumores encefalo-medulares en relación con el ciclo biológico de los pacientes. Rev. Esp. de Oto-Neuro-Oftalm. y Neurocir. 72, 3–14, 1954.
Camerer, J. W.: Hirntuberkulome im Kindesalter. Mschr. Kinderhk. 83, 163, 1940.
Cammann, A.: Histologische Untersuchung an Hirngliomen. Beitr. path. Anat. 90, 1–20, 1932.
Camp, J. D.: Intracranial calcification and its roentgenological significance. Amer. J. Roentgenol. 23, 615–624, 1930.
Campbell, A. C. P., L. Alexander and T. J. Putnam: Vascular pattern in various lesions of the tumors of the CNS. Arch. Neurol. Psychiat. 39, 1150–1202, 1938.
Canti, R. G., J. O. W. Bland and D. S. Russell: Tissue culture of gliomata. The Proc. of the Assoc. f. Res. in Nerv. and Ment. Dis. 16, 1–24, 1935. Williams u. Wilkins, Baltimore 1935.

CARBONE, F., J. BRIHAYE et P. DROCHMANS: Spongioblastome pariéto-occipital et ganglio-cytome dysplasique du cervelet chez le même malade. Acta neurol. psychiatr. Belg. **55**, 568–580, 1955.

CARILLO, R.: Histologia y evolucion clinica de los gliomas. Arch. Neurocir. (Buenos Aires) **4**, 153, 1947.

CARILLO, R. et al: Contribucion clinica y anatomo-patologica sobre 50 tumores de la serie astrocitica-astroblastica del sistema nervioso. Arch. Neurocir. (Buenos Aires) **8**, 64, 1951.

CARMICHAEL, F.: Cerebral gliomata. J. Path. Bact. **31**, 493–510, 1928.

CARMICHAEL, F. A. jr. and H. S. COWLEY: Schistosomiasis of the brain. J. Neurosurg. **9**, 620–634, 1952.

CASPER, J.: Über neurogene Geschwülste im Hinterlappen der Hypophyse. Zbl. path. Anat. **56**, 404–411, 1933.

CASSIRER, R. und F. H. LEWY: Die Formen der Glioblastose und ihre Stellung zur diffusen Hirnsklerose. Zschr. Neurol. **81**, 290, 1923.

CASTELLANO, F., B. GUIDETTI and H. OLIVECRONA: Pterional meningiomas „en plaque". J. Neurosurg. **9**, 188–196, 1952.

CHIOVENDA: I gliomi dell'encephalo. Bologna 1933.

CHRISTENSEN, E.: Über Ganglienzellgeschwülste im Gehirn. Virchows Arch. **300**, 567–581, 1937.

CHRISTENSEN, E.: Two cases of primary intracranial melanoma. Acta chir. Scand. (Stockh.) **85**, 90–98, 1941.

CHRISTENSEN, E.: Chronic adhesive spinal arachnoiditis. Acta psychiatr. (Kobenh.) **17**, 23–38, 1942.

CHRISTENSEN, E.: Medulloblastomas. Excerpta medica, Neurology and Psychiatry, Vol. 8, S. 815, 1955; Ref. Zbl. Neurochir. **16**, 44, 1956.

CHRISTENSEN, E. und E. BUSCH: Die extraduralen Knochengeschwülste des Spinalkanals. Acta psychiatr. (Kobenh.) **12**, 4, 1937.

CHRISTENSEN, E. and D. E. LARA: Intracranial sarcomas. J. Neuropath. **12**, 41–56, 1953.

CHUSID, J. G. and GUTIÉRREZ-MAHONEY, G.: Glioblastoma multiforme of septum pelluci-dum. J. Neurosurg. **11**, 251–257, 1954.

CIMBAL, W.: Beiträge zur Lehre von den Geschwülsten im 4. Ventrikel. Virchows Arch. **166**, 289–316, 1901.

CLAUDE, H., G. BOSCHE et J. A. BARRÉ: Referate über Arachnitis auf dem Internat. Neurol.-Kongreß 1933, Paris. Rev. neurol. **1933**, 825–918.

COENEN, H.: Das Chordom. Bruns' Beitr. klin. Chir. **133**, 1–77, 1925.

COHEN, H. and J. H. DIBLE: Pituitary basophilism associated with a basophil carcinoma of the anterior lobe of the pituitary gland. Brain **59**, 395–407, 1936.

COHN, A. and H. M. ZIMMERMANN: Growth behavior of chemically induced mouse brain tumors in the chick embryo. Excerpta med. Neurol. a. Psychiatr. **8**, 818, 1955.

CONNOR, C. L. and H. CUSHING: Diffuse tumors of the leptomeninges. Arch. Path. **3**, 374–392, 1927.

COOPER, E. R. A.: The relation of oligocytes and astrocytes in cerebral tumours. J. Path. Bact. **44**, 259–266, 1935.

CORNIL, L. et J. E. PAILLAS: Tumeurs cérébrales metâstasiques. Rev. neurol. **71**, 1939.

CORRADINI, W. and J. BROWDER: Angioblastic neoplasms of the brain. J. Neuropath. **7**, 299–308, 1948.

COSTERO, I. and C. M. POMERAT: Standard cellular morphology of gliomas in vitro as compared with explanted normal brain cells. Excerpta medica, Neurol.Psych. **8**, 821, 1955.

COURVILLE, C. B.: Ganglioglioma. Tumor of the central nervous system; review of the literature and report of two cases. Arch. Neurol. Psychiat. **24**, 439–491, 1930.

COURVILLE, C. B.: Cell types in gliomas etc. Arch. Path. **10**, 649, 1930.

COURVILLE, C. B.: Multiple primary tumors of the brain. Amer. J. Cancer **26**, 703, 1936.

COURVILLE, C. B. and K. H. ABBOTT: The angioblastic group of meningiomas. Bull. of the Los Angeles Neurol. Soc. **5**, 47–72, 1940.

COURVILLE, C. B., C. MARSH and P. DEEB: Massive deforming meningiomatous hyper-ostosis. Bull. of the Los Angeles Neurol. Soc. **17**, 177–191, 1952.

COX, L. B.: Studies on the tissue culture of intracranial tumors. Amer. J. Path. **9**, 1933.

COX, L. B.: The cytology of the glioma group with special reference to the inclusion of cells derived from invaded tissue. Amer. J. Path. **9**, 939–998, 1933.

COX, L. B. and M. L. CRANAGE: Studies on the tissue culture of intracranial tumors. J. Path. **45**, 477–499, 1937.

CRAMER, F. and M. W. KINSEY: The cerebellar hemangioblastomas. Arch. Neurol. Psychiat. 67, 237–252, 1952.

CRITCHLEY, M. and F. R. FERGUSON: The cerebrospinal epidermoids (cholesteatomata). Brain 51, 334–384, 1928.

CRITCHLEY, M. and R. N. IRONSIDE: The pituitary adamantinomas. Brain 49, 437–481, 1926.

CROUZON, O. et CH. OBERLING: Les gliomes protoplasmiques pseudopapillaires. Rev. neur. 1929, I, 1199.

CRUVEILHIER, L. J. B.: Anatomie pathologique du corps humain. Baillière, Paris 1829/1835.

CUNEO, H. M. and C. W. RAND: Brain tumors of childhood. Thomas, Springfield (Ohio) 1952.

CUSHING, H.: The pituitary body and its disorders. Philadelphia 1912.

CUSHING, H.: Tumors of the nervus acusticus. Philadelphia 1917.

CUSHING, H.: Experiences with the cerebellar medulloblastomas. Acta path. et microbiol. Scand. 7, 1–86, 1930.

CUSHING, H.: Experiences with the cerebellar astrocytomas. Surg. Gynecol. Obstetr. 52 129–204, 1931.

CUSHING, H.: Pituitary body, hypothalamus and parasympathetic nervous system. Thomas, Springfield 1932.

CUSHING, H.: Dyspituitarism etc. Arch. Int. Med. 51, 487–557, 1933.

CUSHING, H.: Intracranial tumors. Thomas, Springfield 1932. — Intrakranielle Tumoren. Springer, Berlin 1935.

CUSHING, H. and P. BAILEY: Tumors arising from the blood vessels of the brain. Thomas, Springfield 1928.

CUSHING, H. and P. BAILEY: Hemangiomas of cerebellum and retina. Arch. Ophthalm. 57, 447–463, 1928.

CUSHING, H. and L. DAVIDOFF: Pathological findings in acromegaly. Monograph of the Rockefeller Inst. 22, 1927.

CUSHING, H. and L. EISENHARDT: Meningiomas (their classification, regional behavior, life history and surgical end results). Thomas, Springfield u. Baltimore 1938.

DANDY, W. E.: Diagnosis and treatment of hydrocephalus. Surg. Gynecol. Obstetr. 31, 340, 1920: 32, 112, 1921.

DANDY, W. E.: Venous abnormalities and angiomas of the brain. Arch. Surg. 17, 715–793, 1928.

DANDY, W. E.: Brain tumors — general diagnosis and treatment. Practice of Surgery (Lewis) Prior 12, 443–674, 1932.

DANDY, W. E.: Benign tumors in the 3rd ventricle. Thomas, Springfield 1933.

DANDY, W. E.: Benign encapsulated tumors in the lateral ventricles of the brain. Baillière, London 1934.

DANDY, W. E.: Carotid-cavernosus aneurysms. Zbl. Neurochir. 2, 165–206, 1937.

DANDY, W. E.: Hirnchirurgie. J. A. Barth 1938.

DANIS, P. et M. VAN EYCK: Volumineux myxo-chondrome du carrefour pterygomaxillaire à symptomatologie réduite (Névrite optique retrobulbaire). Acta Neur. Psych. Belg. 55, 581–585, 1955.

DANY, A., G. STOLL, L. SINGER, Y. Le GALL et L. HOLDERBACH: Épithéliome de l'hypophyse. Particularités cliniques et postopératoires. Neurochir. (Paris) 1, 197–206, 1955.

DARQUIER et P. SCHMITE: Contribution à l'étude des tumeurs de l'angle ponto-cérébelleux. Rev. neurol. 64, 257–312, 1935.

DAVID, M.: Les méningiomes de la petite aile du sphénoide. Étude radiologique (radiographie et ventriculographie). Paris: Vigot 1933.

DAVID, M. et H. ASKENASY: Les méningiomes olfactifs. Rev. neurol. 68, 489, 1937.

DAVID, M., F. R. BERDET, L. GUILLAUMAT et H. ASKENASY: Arachnoidite syphilitique de la grande cîterne. Rev. neurol. 66, 12, 1936.

DAVID, M., L. GUILLAUMAT et H. ASKENASY: Méningiome intraventriculaire. Rev. neurol. 67, 504, 1937.

DAVID, M., A. LACROIX, S. THIÉFFRY et M. BRUN: Cholestéatome suprasellaire. Rev. neurol. 65, 379–390, 1936.

DAVID, M., G. LOISEL, C. RAMIREZ-CORRIA et M. BRUN: Tumeur angiomateuse et calcifiée sur le plancher du 4. ventricle. Rev. neurol. 1934, 426–434.

DAVIDOFF, C. M.: A thirteen year follow — up study of a series of cases of verified tumors of the brain. Arch. Path. 44, 1246, 1940.

DAVIDOFF, C. M. and A. FERRARO: Intracranial tumors among mental hospital patients. Amer. J. Psych. 8, 1929.

DAVIDOFF, L. M. and J. MARTIN: Hereditary combined neurinomas and meningiomas. J. Neurosurg. 12, 375–384, 1955.

DAVIS, E. W.: Gliomatous tumors in the nasal region. J. Neuropath. 1, 312–319, 1942.

DAVIS, F. A.: Primary tumors of the optic nerve (a phenomenon of Recklinghausen's disease). Arch. Ophthalm. 23, 735–821/957–1018, 1940.

DAVIS, L.: Spongioblastoma multiforme of brain. Ann. Surg. 87, 8–14, 1928.

DAVIS, L. and H. CUSHING: Papillomas of the chorioid plexus with a report of six cases. Arch. Neurol. Psychiat. 13, 681, 1925.

DAVIS, L. and ST. L. GOLDSTEIN: Diagnosis and localization of organic lesions of the central nervous system using radioactive diiodofluorescein. Radiology 59, 514–520, 1952.

DAVIS, L., J. MARTIN, ST. L. GOLDSTEIN and M. ASKENAZY: A study of 211 patients with verified glioblastoma multiforme. J. Neurosurg. 6, 33, 1949.

DAVIS, L., J. MARTIN, F. PADBERG and R. K. ANDERSON: A study of 182 patients with verified astrocytoma, astroblastoma and oligodendroglioma of the brain. J. Neurosurg. 7, 299–312, 1950.

DAVIS, L. F. and A. WEIL: Effect of radiation therapy upon intracranial gliomata. Ann. Surg. 106, 599–618, 1937.

DAVISON, C. M., S. BROCK and C. G. DYKE: Retinal and central nervous hemangioblastosis with visceral changes (von Hippel-Lindau's disease). Bull. Neurol. Inst. New York 5, 72, 1936.

DEERY, E. M.: Some features of glioblastoma multiforme. Bull. Neurol. Inst. New York 2, 157–193, 1932.

DEERY, E. M.: Histologic features of glioblastoma multiforme. Arch. Neurol. Psychiat. 31, 212, 1934.

DEMME, H. und C. MUMME: Blastomykose des Zentralnervensystems. Dtsch. Z. Nervenhk. 127, 1, 1932.

DERMANN, G. L.: Zur Kenntnis der Kleinhirnbrückenwinkelneurinome. Virchows Arch. 261, 39, 1926.

DESCUNS, P., H. GARRÉ and C. PHÉLINE: Tuberculomas of the brain and cerebellum. J. Neurosurg. 11, 243–250, 1954.

DIAS, A.: Pinealtumor mit multiplen Gliomen. Mschr. Psychiatr. 76, 9, 1930.

DIETRICH, A.: Krebs im Gefolge des Krieges. Urban & Schwarzenberg 1950.

DIETRICH, A. und H. SIEGMUND: Die Nebenniere und das chromaffine System. In: Henke-Lubarsch, Handb. d. spez. path. Anat., Bd. 8, S. 1039.

DIEZEL, P. B.: Die Geschwülste der Hirnhäute. Ein Beitrag zur formalen Genese der Meningeome. Virchows Arch. 325, 441–454, 1954.

DIVRY, P. et J. BOBON: Tumeurs encéphaliques et gravidité. Acta Neurol. Psychiatr. Belg. 49, 2, 1949.

DIVRY, P. et L. CHRISTOPHE: Gliome cérébral. J. Belge Neurol. Psychiatr. 31, 509, 1931.

DIVRY, P. et E. EVRARD: Oligodendrogliome de la base du cerveau. J. Belge Neurol. Psychiatr. 1, 39–48, 1936.

DÖRING, G.: Zur Histologie der Umgebung unreifer Hirngeschwülste. Dtsch. Z. Nervenhk. 149, 201–221, 1939.

DÖRING, G.: Histologische Veränderungen des Hirnstamms bei Kleinhirnbrückenwinkeltumoren. Zschr. Neurol. 165, 256–266, 1939.

DÖRING, G.: Über Retothelsarkome des Nasenrachenraumes mit neurologischen Komplikationen. Zschr. Neurol. 168, 432–447, 1940.

DOERNBACH, J.: Über zystische und zellige Geschwülste der Hirnventrikel. Virchows Arch. 316, 51–75, 1949.

DONAT, R.: Pseudoverkalkung des Gehirns bei tumorähnlicher, chronischer encephalitischer Gliaproliferation. Virchows Arch. 312, 726, 1944.

DOTT, N. M. and P. BAILEY: A consideration of the hypophyseal adenomata. Brit. J. Surg. 13, 314–366, 1925.

DOTT, N. M. and E. LEVIN: Intracranial tuberculoma. Edinburgh Med. J. 46, 36–41, 1939.

DREW, J. H. and F. C. GRANT: Benign cysts of the brain. An analysis with comparison of results of operative and non-operative treatment in thirty cases. J. Neurosurg. 5, 107–123, 1948.

DRIGGS, M. und H. SPATZ: Pubertas praecox bei einer hyperplastischen Mißbildung des Tuber cinereum. Virchows Arch. 305, 567, 1940.

DÜRCK, H.: Über traumatisch entstandene gliogene Geschwulstbildungen. 17. Verhandl. Dtsch. Path. Ges. 1914.

DÜRCK, H.: Pathologisch-anatomische Erfahrungen bei Unfallbegutachtung. Beitr. path. Anat. 84, 667, 1930.

DUFFY, W.: Hypophysial duct tumors. Ann. Surg. 72, 537, 1920.

DYES, O.: Die Hirnkammerformen bei Hirntumoren. Fortschr. Röntgenstr. (Erg.-Bd.) 52, 1937.

DYKE, C. G. and L. M. DAVIDOFF: Roentgen treatment of diseases of the nervous system. Lea & Febiger, Philadelphia 1942.

EARNEST, F., J. W. KERNOHAN and W. McK. CRAIG: Oligodendrogliomas. Arch. Neurol. Psychiat. 63, 964–976, 1950.

EBBERS, H.: Über das gleichzeitige Vorkommen von Syringomyelie mit Recklinghausen-scher Erkrankung und Hirntumor. Arch. Psychiatr. 113, 605–617, 1941.

ECHLIN, F.: Cranial osteomas and hyperostoses produced by meningeal fibroblastomas. A clinical and pathologic study. Arch. Surg. 28, 357, 1934.

ECHOLS, D. H.: Giant cell tumors of the cranial bones. Amer. J. Cancer 26, 155, 1936.

ECHOLS, D. H.: Spongioblastoma polare. Arch. Neurol. Psychiat. 39, 494–512, 1938.

ECHOLS, D. H.: Multiple meningeomas – removal of ten tumors from a patient. Arch. Neurol. Psychiat. 46, 440, 1941.

ECKART, G.: Über Lipombildungen im Gehirn und Rückenmark. Allg. Z. Psychiatr. 103, 330–344, 1935.

ECKER, A.: Upward transtentorial herniation of the brain stem and cerebellum due to tumor of the posterior fossa. With special note on tumors of the acoustic nerve. J. Neurosurg. 5, 51, 1948.

ECTORS, L.: Les méningiomes de la 3ème frontale. Desoer, Liège – Masson, Paris 1945.

ECTORS, L.: Anatomo- et physiopathologie des anévrismes intracrâniens. Acta Neurol. Psychiatr. Belg. 50, 403–461, 1950.

ECTORS, L. et L. VAN BOGAERT: Ablation d'un méningiome du trou occipital chez un frère et une soeur. Acta Neurol. Psychiatr. Belg. 53, 193–204, 1953.

EHNI, G. J. and A. W. ADSON: Lipoma of the brain. Arch. Neurol. Psychiat. 53, 299 bis 304, 1945.

EHNI, G. J. and J. G. LOVE: Intraspinal lipomas. Report of cases; review of the literature and clinical and pathological study. Arch. Neurol. Psychiat., 53, 1–29, 1945.

EICKHOFF, W.: Intraneurales Wachstum eines Glioms (N. opticus). Virchows Arch. 302, 222–227, 1938.

EICKE, W. J.: Zur Frage der fetalen Encephalitis, Meningitis und ihrer Folgeerscheinungen. Arch. Psychiatr. 116, 568, 1943.

EICKE, W. J.: Bindegewebige Substitution eines Oligodendroglioms nach Röntgen-bestrahlung. Dtsch. Z. Nervenhk. 169, 273–288, 1952.

EINARSON, L. and A. V. NEEL: Notes on diffuse sclerosis, diffuse gliomatosis and diffuse glioblastomatosis of the brain with a report of two cases. Acta Jutlandica 12, 1–56, 1940.

EISENHARDT, L.: Diagnosis of tumors by supravital technique. Arch. Neurol. Psychiat. 28, 299, 1932.

EISENHARDT, L.: Long postoperative survivals in cases of intracranial tumor. Proc. Assoc. Res. Nervous and Ment. Disease 16, 390–416, 1935.

EISENHARDT, L. and H. CUSHING: Diagnosis of the intracranial tumors by supravital technic. Amer. J. Path. 6, 541, 1930.

EKSTRÖM, G. und G. H. LINDGREN: Gehirnschädigungen nach cerebraler Arteriographie mit Thorotrast. Zbl. Neurochir. 3, 227–248, 1938.

ELSAESSER, K.-H.: Beitrag zur Klinik und pathologischen Anatomie des Meningeoms. Nieft, Bleicherode am Harz 1939.

ELSAESSER, K.-H.: Zur Symptomatologie, Diagnostik und Therapie der Hirnzystizerkose. Zschr. Neurol. 177, 323–362, 1944.

ELSAESSER, K.-H.: Zur Klinik der metastatischen Hirngeschwülste. Zbl. Neurochir. 9, 150–183, 1949.

ELSAESSER, K.-H.: Über die Aktinomykose und ihre Lokalisation im Zentralnervensystem. Dtsch. Z. Nervenhk. 164, 123–142, 1950.

ELSBERG, C. A.: Tumors of the spinal cord. Pathology, symptomatology, diagnosis, treatment. Hoeber, New York 1925.

ELSBERG, C. A. and J. K. GLOBUS: Tumors of the brain with acute onset and rapidly progressive course. Arch. Neurol. Psychiat. 21, 1044, 1929.

ELSBERG, C. A. and N. GOTTEN: Cerebellar medulloblastomas. Bull. Neur. Inst. New York 3, 33–52, 1932.

ELSBERG, C. A. and C. C. HARE: The blood supply of the gliomas. Bull. Neur. Inst. New York 2, 210–246, 1932.

ELVIDGE, E. L., W. PENFIELD and W. CONE: The gliomas of the central nervous system. Proc. Assoc. Res. Nerv. and Ment. Dis. 16, 107–181, 1935.

ENGELBRETH-HOLM, J., G. TEILUM and E. CHRISTENSEN: Eosinophil granuloma of bone: Schüller-Christian's disease. Acta med. Scand. 118, 292–312, 1944.

ERDHEIM, J.: Zur normalen und pathologischen Histologie der Glandula thyreoidea, parathyreoidea und Hypophysis. Beitr. path. Anat. 33, 158–236, 1903.

ERDHEIM, J.: Über Hypophysenganggeschwülste und Hirncholesteatome. Sitzungsberichte der Kaiserlichen Akademie der Wissenschaften Wien 113, 537–726, 1904.

ERDHEIM, J.: Pathologie der Hypophysengeschwülste. Erg. allg. Path. 21, 482, 1926.

ERDHEIM, J.: Über das maligne osteoplastische Duraendotheliom. Fschr. Röntgenstr. 55, 155–174, 1937.

ERNST: Mißbildungen des Nervensystems. Schwalbes Handb. d. Morphologie der Mißbildungen usw., 2. Abt., 2. Kap. Fischer, Jena 1909.

ERNSTING, J.: Choroid plexus papilloma causing spontaneous subarachnoid haemorrhage. J. Neurol. 18, 134–136, 1955.

ESSBACH, H.: Die Meningeome vom Standpunkt der organoiden Geschwulstbetrachtung. Erg. allg. Path. 36, 185, 1943.

EULER, H. V. und B. SKARZINSKY: Biochemie der Tumoren. Urban & Schwarzenberg 1942.

EVANS, J. P. and I. M. SCHEINKER: Diffuse cerebral glioblastosis. J. Neuropath. 2, 178–189, 1943.

EWING, J.: Neoplastic diseases. Saunders, Philadelphia 1922.

FABRITIUS, H.: Ein Fall von zystischem Kleinhirntumor. Beitr. path. Anat. 51, 1911.

FAHR, TH.: Beiträge zur Pathologie der Hypophyse. Dtsch. med. Wschr. 1918, 206.

FAHR, TH.: Kurzer Beitrag zur Frage des meningealen Sarkoms. Zbl. Pathol. 65, 289–291, 1936.

FALKENBERG, K.: Chondrom des Kleinhirnbrückenwinkels. Mschr. Ohrenhk. (Ö) 75, 343–350, 1941.

FANKHAUSER, R.: Gliome beim Rind. Schweiz. Arch. Tierheilk. 89, 438, 1947.

FASIANI, G. M. e G. B. BELLONI: Chirurgia delle vie ottiche intracraniche. Relazione presentata al XLIII Congresso della Società Italiana di Chirurgia, Rom, Okt. 1936/XIV.

FEIRING, E. H.: Multiple intracranial expanding lesions of diverse origin. Neurology 5, 535–541, 1955.

FEIRING, E. H. and L. M. DAVIDOFF: Two tumors, meningioma and glioblastoma multiforme, in one patient. J. Neurosurg. 4, 283, 1947.

FEIRING, E. H., L. M. DAVIDOFF and H. M. ZIMMERMANN: Primary carcinoma of the pituitary. J. Neuropath. 12, 205–223, 1953.

FERNÁNDEZ-MORÁN, H.: Examination of gliomas with the electron microscope. Proc. of the 6. Intern. Congr. of Exper. Cytol. S. 53–59.

FERNÁNDEZ-MORÁN, H.: Examination of brain tumor tissue with the electron microscope. Arkiv för Zoologi 40 A, 1–15, 1948.

FERNER, H.: Untersuchungen über die „zelligen Knötchen" (Epithelgranulationen) und die Kalkkugeln in den Hirnhäuten des Menschen. Z. mikrosk.-anat. Forsch. 48, 592, 1940.

FEYRTER, F.: Über die Neurinome und Neurofibromatose nach Untersuchungen am menschlichen Magen-Darmschlauch. Verlag Med. Wissensch. W. Maudrich, Wien 1948.

FINCHER, E. F.: Intraventricular tumors of the cerebrum. Arch. Neurol. Psychiat. 22, 19–44, 1929.

FINCHER, E. F. and G. P. COON: Ependymomas. Arch. Neurol. Psychiat. 22, 19–44, 1929.

FINDEISEN, L. und W. TÖNNIS: Über intrakranielle Epidermoide. Zbl. Neurochir. 2, 301–315, 1937.

FISCHER, A.: Biology of cells in tissue culture. Carlsberg Foundation, Kopenhagen 1946.

FISCHER, A. W. and H. HOLFELDER: Lokales Amyloid im Gehirn. Eine Spätfolge von Röntgenbestrahlungen. Dtsch. Z. Chir. 227, 475–483, 1930.

FISCHER, E. (s. a. FISCHER-BRÜGGE, E.): Die arteriographische Diagnostik der Stirnhirn- und oralen Stammgangliengeschwülste. Zbl. Neurochir. 4, 72–98, 1939.

FISCHER, W.: Zur Kenntnis der Sarkome. Virchow Arch. 310, 100–105, 1943.

FISCHER, W.: Die Krebsforschung in den letzten 100 Jahren. Fischer, Jena 1947.

FISCHER, W.: Über die bösartigen Geschwülste im hohen Alter. Z. ges. inn. Med. 2, 121, 1947.

FISCHER-BRÜGGE, E.: Erscheinungsformen und diagnostische Bedeutung der Zisternenverquellungen im Hirngefäßbild. Arch. klin. Chir. 200, 1940.

FISCHER-BRÜGGE, E.: Das „Klivuskantensyndrom". Acta Neurochirurgica 2, 36–68, 1951.

FISCHER-WASELS, B.: Allgemeine Geschwulstlehre. In: Handb. der norm. u. path. Anatomie. Bd. XIV/2, Springer, Berlin 1927.

FISCHER-WASELS, B.: Regenerationsgeschwülste. Verhandl. Dtsch. path. Ges. 22. Tagung Danzig 1927, 69, sowie mit W. BÜNGELER: Arch. Entw.mechan. 112, 184, 1927.

FISCHER-WASELS, B.: Die traumatische Entstehung der Gliome und Piatumoren nach R. BENEKE. Mschr. Unfallhk. 39, 489–527, 1932.

FISCHER-WASELS, B.: Die Erblichkeit in der Geschwulstentwicklung. Fschr. Erbpath. 2, 221–261, 1938.

FISCHER-WASELS, B.: Über die Ätiologie der Geschwulstbildung und das Wesen der Malignität. Kolloid-Z. 89, 1939.

FISCHER-WILLIAMS, M., F. D. BOSANQUET and P. M. DANIEL: Carcinomatosis of the meninges. A report of 3 cases. Brain 78, 42–58, 1955.

FLETCHER, E. M., H. W. WOLTMAN and A. W. ADSON: Sacrococcygeal chordomas. A clinical and pathologic study. Arch. Neurol. Psychiat. 33, 283–299, 1935.

FOERSTER, O.: Ein Fall von Vierhügeltumor, durch Operation entfernt. Arch. Psychiatr. 84, 515/516, 1928.

FOERSTER, O.: Diagnostik und Behandlung der Geschwülste des Großhirns. Klin. Wschr. 13, 1737–1742, 1934.

FOERSTER, O.: Motorische Felder und Bahnen. In: Bumke-Foerster, Handb. d. Neur. Bd. VI. Springer 1936.

FOERSTER, O.: Thyreogene intrarhachideale Geschwülste. Zbl. Neurochir. 4, 198–214, 1939.

FOERSTER, O. and P. BAILEY: A contribution to the study of gliomas of the spinal cord with special reference to their operability, S. 9–67. Volume for Davidenkow, Leningrad 1936.

FOERSTER, O. und O. GAGEL: Ein Fall von sog. Gliom des Nervus opticus – Spongioblastoma multiforme ganglioides. Zschr. Neurol. 136, 335–366, 1931.

FOERSTER, O. und O. GAGEL: Ein Fall von Recklinghausenscher Krankheit mit fünf nebeneinander bestehenden verschiedenartigen Tumorbildungen. Zschr. Neurol. 138, 339 bis 360, 1932.

FOERSTER, O. und O. GAGEL: Ein Fall von Gangliozytom der Oblongata. Zschr. Neurol. 141, 797–823, 1932.

FOERSTER, O. und O. GAGEL: Ein Fall von Gangliogliom des Bodens des dritten Ventrikels. Zschr. Neurol. 145, 29–37, 1933.

FOERSTER, O. und O. GAGEL: Ein Fall von Gangliocytoma dysplasticum des Kleinhirns. Zschr. Neurol. 146, 792–803, 1933.

FOERSTER, O. und O. GAGEL: Ein Fall von Ependymcyste des 3. Ventrikels. Zschr. Neurol. 149, 312–344, 1934.

FOERSTER, O. und O. GAGEL: Ein Fall von Ependymoma polycysticum des Kleinhirns. Zschr. Neurol. 150, 515–527, 1934.

FOERSTER, O. und O. GAGEL: Zentrale diffuse Schwannose bei Recklinghausenscher Krankheit. Zschr. Neurol. 151, 1–16, 1934.

FOERSTER, O. und O. GAGEL: Das Ependymom des filum terminale. Zbl. Neurochir. 1, 5–18, 1936.

FOERSTER, O. und O. GAGEL: Astrozytome der Oblongata, Brücke und des Mittelhirns. Zschr. Neurol. 166, 497–528, 1939.

FOERSTER, O. und O. GAGEL: Das umschriebene Arachnoidalsarkom des Kleinhirns. Zschr. Neurol. 164, 565–580, 1939.

FOERSTER, O., O. GAGEL und W. MAHONEY: Die encephalen Tumoren des Mittelhirns, der Brücke und des verlängerten Markes. Arch. Psychiatr. 110, 1–74, 1939.

FOERSTER, O., A. J. McLEAN und O. GAGEL: Ein Fall von Ganglioneuroma amyelinicum des Hirnstammes. Zschr. Neurol. 143, 635–650, 1933.

FOERSTER, O., A. J. McLEAN und O. GAGEL: Ein Fall von Gangliogliom der Regio hypothalamica. Zschr. Neurol. 145, 17–28, 1933.

FOLTZ, E. L., J. B. HOLYOKE and H. L. HEYL: Brain necrosis following X-ray therapy. J. Neurosurg. 10, 423–429, 1953.

FOOT, N. CH.: Peripheral neurogenic tumors. Am. J. Clin. Path. **6**, 1, 1936.
FOOT, N. CH.: Histology of tumors of the peripheral nerves. Arch. Path. **30**, 772—808, 1940.
FOOT, N. CH.: Meningioma. Arch. Path. **30**, 198—211, 1940.
FOOT, N. CH. and I. COHEN: Report of a case of retothelial sarcoma of the cerebral hemispheres. Amer. J. Path. **9**, 123, 1933.
FORD, F. R. and W. M. MIRROR: Primary "sarcomatosis" of the meninges. Bull. Johns Hopkins Hosp. **35**, 65—75, 1924.
FORD, F. R. and W. MUNCIE: Malignant tumors within the third ventricle. Arch. Neurol. Psychiat **39**, 82—95, 1938.
FORSTER, E.: Die Bedeutung des Liquorzellbildes für die Diagnostik der Tumoren des ZNS. Zschr. Neurol. **126**, 683, 1930.
FRANCINI: Richerche istologiche sulla struttura dei neuromi. Atti Accad. Fisiocritici Siena **20**, 837, 1918.
FRANKL-HOCHWART, L.: Über Diagnose der Zirbeldrüsentumoren. Dtsch. Z. Nervenhk. **37**, 455—465, 1909.
FRAUCHIGER, E. und R. FANKHAUSER: Die Nervenkrankheiten unserer Hunde. Huber, Bern 1949.
FRAUCHIGER, E.: Problèmes de la neurologie comparée. Acta Neurol. et Psychiatr. Belg. **1**, 52—60, 1954
FRAZIER, C. H.: A series of pituitary pictures. Arch. Neurol. Psychiat. **23**, 656, 1930.
FRAZIER, C. H.: A clinical and pathological review of parahypophyseal lesions. Surg. etc. **62**, 158—166, 1936.
FRAZIER, C. H. and B. J. ALPERS: Adamantinoma of the craniopharyngeal duct. Arch. Neurol. Psychiat. **26**, 905—965, 1931.
FRAZIER, C. H. and B. J. ALPERS: Meningeal fibroblastomas of the cerebrum. Arch. Neurol. Psychiat. **29**, 935, 1933.
FREEDMAN, H. and F. M. FORSTER: Bone formation and destruction in hyperostoses associated with meningeomas. J. Neuropath. **7**, 69—80, 1948.
FREEMAN, W.: Torula infection of the central nervous system. J. Psychol. Neurol. **43**, 236, 1931.
FREEMAN, D. and H. M. ZIMMERMANN: Experimental brain tumors. V. Behavior in intraocular transplants. Cancer Res. **4**, 273—278, 1944.
FRENCH, J. D.: Plasmocytoma of the hypothalamus. J. Neuropath. **6**, 265—270, 1947.
FRENCH, J. D. and P. C. BUCY: Tumors of septum pellucidum. J. Neurosurg. **5**, 433—449, 1948.
FRIED, B. M.: Sarcomatosis of the brain. Arch. Neurol. Psychiat. **15**, 205—217, 1926.
FRIED, B. M. and R. C. BUCKLEY: Primary carcinoma of the lungs; intracranial metastases. Arch. Path. **9**, 483—527, 1930.
FRIEDMAN, N. B.: Germinoma of the pineal. Its identity with germinoma ("seminoma") of the testis. Cancer Res. **7**, 363—368, 1947.
FULTON, J. F. and P. BAILEY: Contribution to the study of tumors in the region of the third ventricle: their diagnosis and relation to pathological sleep. J. nerv. ment. Dis. **69**, 1—25, 145—164, 261—277, 1929.
FURLOW, L. T.: Intracranial chordoma. Arch. Neurol. Psychiat. **34**, 839—943, 1935.
FURTADO, D.: Angiome caverneux du cerveau. Acta Neurol. et Psychiatr. Belg. **51**, 343—356, 1951.
GÄRTNER, J.: Über intrakranielle Geschwulstmetastasen. Zbl. Path. **93**, 171—183, 1955.
GAGEL, O.: Neurofibromatose. Im Handb. der Neurologie Bumke-Foerster, Bd. 16, 1935.
GAGEL, O.: Tumoren der peripheren Nerven. Im Handb. der Neurologie Bumke-Foerster, Bd. 9, 1935.
GAGEL, O.: Über Hirngeschwülste. Zschr. Neurol. **161**, 69—113, 1938.
GAGEL, O.: Eine Granulationsgeschwulst im Gebiete des Hypothalamus. Zschr. Neurol. **172**, 710—722, 1941.
GAGEL, O. und H. KREISSEL: Die Geschwülste des Nervensystems. „Naturforschung und Medizin in Deutschland." Neurologie Bd. 81, Teil II: Dietrich'sche Verlagsbuchhandlung, Wiesbaden 1948.
GAMPER, E.: Zur Kenntnis der zentralen Veränderungen bei M. Recklinghausen. J. Psychol. Neurol. **39**, 39—84, 1929.

GARCIN, R.: Le syndrome paralytique unilatéral global des nerfs crâniens. Amédée Legrand, Paris: 1927.

GARDNER, W. J. and C. H. FRAZIER: Bilateral acoustic neurofibromas: a clinical study and field survey of a family of five generations with bilateral deafness in thirty-eight members. Arch. Neurol. Psychiat. **23**, 266, 1930.

GARDNER, W. J. and O. A. TURNER: Neuroepithelial cysts of the third ventricle. Arch. Neurol. Psychiat. **38**, 1055, 1937.

GARDNER, W. J. and O. A. TURNER: Familial involving of the NS by multiple tumors of the sheath and enveloping membrane. Amer. J. Cancer **32**, 339, 1938.

GARDNER, W. J. and O. A. TURNER: Cranial chordomas. A clinical and pathologic study. Arch. Surg. **42**, 411–425, 1941.

GASS, H. and W. P. VAN WAGENEN: Meningioma and oligodendroglioma adjacent in the brain. J. Neurosurg. **7**, 440–443, 1950.

GAUCHER: Sur un cas de lipome du corps calleux. Schweiz. med. Wschr. **1936**, 1240.

GAUPP, R.: Ein Teratom im Seitenventrikel. Nervenarzt **15**, 363–373, 1942.

GAUPP, R. und H. JANTZ: Zur Kasuistik der Balkenlipome. Nervenarzt **15**, 58–68, 1942.

GEREBTZOFF, M. A. et E. M. NIZET: Étude histopathologique d'un hémangioblastome du cervelet (maladie de Lindau). J. Neurol. et Psychiatr. Belg. **48**, 577–605, 1948.

GERHARDT, M.: Beitrag zur operativen Behandlung der spinalen Arachnitis. Dtsch. Z. Nervenhk. **140**, 28, 1936.

GERHARTZ, H.: Retothelsarkome des Zentralnervensystems. Virchows Arch. **319**, 339–346, 1951.

GESCHICKTER, C. F.: Mesothelial tumors. Amer. J. Cancer **26**, 378, 1936.

GESCHICKTER, C. F.: Primary tumors of the cranial bones. Amer. J. Cancer **26**, 155, 1936.

GESCHICKTER, C. F.: Tumors of the nervous system. Clin. Med. Surg. **43**, 437, 1936.

GESCHICKTER, C. F. and M. M. COPELAND: Tumors of bone. 1. Aufl. 1931, rev. Aufl. 1936.

GEYER, H. und P. PEDERSEN: Zur Erblichkeit der Neubildungen des ZNS und seiner Hüllen. Zschr. Neurol. **165**, 284–294, 1939.

GIAMPALMO, A.: Zur Frage der extraventrikulären Ependymome. Zbl. Neurochir. **2**, 283 –290, 1937.

GIGANTE, D.: Zur Frage des primitiven Spongioblastoms (Neuroepithelioms). Zschr. Neurol. **170**, 672–684, 1940.

GIVRÉ, A. and H. OLIVECRONA: Surgical experiences with acoustic tumors. J. Neurosurg. **6**, 396-407, 1949.

GLASER, M. A.: Tumors of the pineal, corpora quadrigemina and 3d ventricle. — The interrelationship of their syndromes and their surgical treatment. Brain **52**, 226–262, 1929.

GLASS, B. and K. H. ABBOTT: Intracranial tumors in siblings. Bull. of the Los Angeles Neurol. Soc. **18**, 40–47, 1953.

GLOBUS, J. H.: Umwandlung gutartiger Gliome in bösartige. Zschr. Neurol. **134**, 325, 1931.

GLOBUS, J. H.: Meningiomas. Arch. Neurol. Psychiat. **38**, 667–712, 1937.

GLOBUS, J. H.: Glioneuromas und Spongioneuroblastomas. Forms of primary neuroectodermal tumors of the brain. Amer. J. Cancer **32**, 163–220, 1938.

GLOBUS, J. H.: Infundibuloma. A newly recognized tumor of neurohypophysial derivation with a note on the saccus vasculosus. J. Neuropath. **1**, 59–80, 1942.

GLOBUS, J. H.: Brain tumor. Its contribution to neurology in the remote and recent past. J. Neuropath. **5**, 85–105, 1946.

GLOBUS, J. H. and BERGMANN: Atresia and stenosus of aqueduct of Sylvius. J. Neuropath. **5**, 342, 1946.

GLOBUS, J. H. and R. M. CARES: Neuroepithelioma. J. Neuropath. **12**, 311–348, 1953.

GLOBUS, J. H., GERSTLE and MCDONALD: The midline tumors of the brain. Verh. 3. Intern. Neur. Kongr. Munksgaard, Kopenhagen 1939, S. 785.

GLOBUS, J. H. and H. KUHLENBECK: Tumors of the striatothalamic and related regions, their probable source of origin and more common forms. Arch. Path. **34**, 674–734, 1942.

GLOBUS, J. H. and H. KUHLENBECK: The subependymal cell plate (matrix) and its relationship to brain-tumors etc. J. Neuropath. **3**, 1–35, 1944.

GLOBUS, J. H., H. KUHLENBECK and D. WELLER: Tumors of the aqueduct of Sylvius: Blastomatous formations of varied origin, limited to the mesencephalon. J. Neuropath. **1**, 207–223, 1942.

GLOBUS, J. H. and M. SAPIRSTEIN: Massive hemorrhage into brain tumor: its significance and probable relationship to rapidly fatal termination and antecedent trauma. J. A. M. A. **120**, 348–352, 1942.

GLOBUS, J. H. and H. SELINSKY: Metastatic tumors of the brain. Arch. Neurol. Psychiat. 17, 481, 1927.

GLOBUS, J. H. and S. SILBERT: Pinealomas. Arch. Neurol. Psychiat. 25, 937–985, 1931.

GLOBUS, J. H. und I. STRAUSS: Spongioblastoma multiforme. Arch. Neurol. Psychiat. 14, 139–151, 1925.

GLOBUS, J. H., I. STRAUSS und H. SELINSKY: Das Neurospongioblastom, eine primäre Hirngeschwulst bei disseminierter Neurospongioblastose (tuberöse Sklerose). Zschr. Neurol. 140, 1–29, 1932.

GLOBUS, J. H., I. STRAUSS and H. SELINSKY: Glioneuroma and spongioneuroblastoma forms of primary neuroectodermal tumors of the brain. Amer. J. Cancer 32, 163–220, 1938.

GLOBUS, J. H., I. STRAUSS and H. SELINSKY: Pinealomas. Arch. Path. 31, 533, 1941.

GÖMÖRI, G.: Ein Fall von diffuser Sarkomatose der weichen Häute. Virchows Arch. 278, 196–199, 1930.

GOLD: Ependymom am Boden der Rautengrube. Arb. neurol. Inst. Wien 25, 223, 1924.

GOLDMANN: Studien zur Biologie der bösartigen Neubildungen. Bruns' Beitr. klin. Chir. 72, 20–22 1911.

GOLGI, C.: Sulla struttura sullo sviluppo degli psammomi. Morgagni 11, 874–886, 1869.

GOLGI, C.: Über die Gliome des Gehirns; in: Untersuchungen über den feineren Bau des Nervensystems. Jena 1884.

GONZALES-REVILLA, A.: Intracranial tuberculomas. J. Neurosurg. 9, 555–563, 1952.

GORLAND and G. ARMITAGE: Intracranial tuberculomas. J. Path. Bact. 37, 1933.

GOTTSCHEWSKI, G. H. M.: Über die genetischen Ursachen der Geschwulstbildung. Ärztl. Forschung 7, I, 347–360, 1953.

GOUGH, J.: The structure of the blood vessels in cerebral tumours. J. Path. 51, 23–29, 1940.

GRAF, C.: Angiomatous malformations of the Sylvian aqueduct with remarks on management of aqueductal stenosis. J. Neuropath. 5, 43–53, 1946.

GRAF, K.: Geschwülste des Ohres und des Kleinhirnbrückenwinkels. Thieme, Stuttgart 1952.

GRANT, F. C. and M. P. SAYERS: Notes on a series of brain tumors. J. Neurosurg. 8, 510–514, 1951.

GREEN, J. R.: Encephalo-trigeminal angiomatosis. J. Neuropath. 4, 27–42, 1945.

GREEN, M. I. and J. H. CHILDREY: Intracranial chondroma. J. Nerv. Ment. Dis. 89, 650 bis 652, 1939.

GREENE, H. S. N.: The transplantation of tumors to the brains of heterologous species. Cancer Res. 11, 529–534, 1951.

GREENE, H. S. N.: A conception of tumor autonomy based on transplantation studies: A review. Cancer Res. 11, 899–903, 1951.

GREENE, H. S. N. and H. ARNOLD: The homologous and heterologous transplantation of brain and brain tumors. J. Neurosurg. 2, 315–331, 1945.

GREENFIELD, J. G.: The pathological examination of forty intracranial neoplasms. Brain 42, 29, 1919.

GREENFIELD, J. G.: Two cases of medulloepithelioma etc. Amer. J. Path. 38, 11, 1934.

GREENFIELD, J. G. and E. G. ROBERTSON: Cystic oligodendrogliomas of the cerebral hemispheres and ventricular oligodendrogliomas. Brain 56, 247, 1933.

GRINKER, R. R.: Tumors of the retina. Kapitel XII aus: Penfield's Cytology and cellular pathology of the nervous system. New York, Hoeber 1932.

GRINKER, R. R. and E. STEVENS: Mucoid degeneration of oligodendrogliomas. Arch. Path. 8, 171–179, 1929.

GROFF, R. A.: The dissemination of glioma by extension at a distance. Amer. J. Canc. 29, 651–658, 1937.

GROMELSKI: Beitrag zur Lehre von den primären epithelialen Geschwülsten des Zentralnervensystems. Virchows Arch. 261, 933, 1926.

GROSS, S. A. and A. P. FRIEDMAN: Cerebral metastases from a mixed tumor of the parotid gland. Neurology 5, 435–437, 1955.

GRUBER, G.: Über raumbeengende Neubildungen im Schädel. Fortschr. Röntgenstr. 52, 234, 1935.

GRÜN: Die Geschwülste des ZNS und ihrer Hüllen bei unseren Haustieren. Med.-vet. Inaug.-Diss. Berlin 1936.

GUILLAIN, G.: Maladie de Recklinghausen avec tumeurs polymorphes du névraxe. Jb. Psychiatr. 52, 15, 1935.

GUILLAIN, G., J. BERTRAND et J. GRUNER: Les gliomes infiltrés du tronc cérébral. Masson, Paris 1945.

GUILLAIN, G., J. BERTRAND et R. MESSIMY: Sténose de l'aqueduc de Sylvius par une tumeur tres limitée. Rev. neurol. **66**, 533–540, 1936.

GUILLAIN, G., D. PETIT-DUTAILLIS, J. BERTRAND et P. SCHMITE: Chondrome de la dure-mère. Opération et guérison complète. Bull. et mém. Soc. méd. d. hôp. de Paris **54**, 1484–1491, 1930.

GUILLAUME, J., R. ROGÉ et G. MAZARS: Un cas de neurinome géant du ganglion de Gasser. Rev. neurol. **81**, 225–226, 1949.

GULEKE, A.: Chirurgie der Hirngeschwülste. Enke-Verlag, Stuttgart 1936.

GULEKE, A.: Gehäuftes Auftreten mehrfacher Krebsgeschwülste. Dtsch. Gesundheits-wesen **1946**, 200.

GUTMANN, E. und H. SPATZ: Die Meningeome des vorderen Chiasmawinkels. Nervenarzt **2**, 581–591, 1929.

GUTTING, J.: Hirnmetastase und Primärtumor. Diss. Med. Akad., Düsseldorf 1940.

HABERLAND, K.: Über ein spinales Angioma racemosum venosum. Arch. Psychiatr. **184**, 417–425, 1950.

HAENE, A. DE, G. HOFFMANN et J. HOZAY: Sur les gliomes du tronc cérébral. Acta Neurol. et Psychiatr. Belg. **53**, 355–365, 1953.

HÄRTER, O.: Ein Beitrag zum Bild der oral-basalen Großhirnspongioblastome. Zbl. Path. **87**, 209–214, 1951.

HÄUSSLER, G.: Hirndruck — Hirnödem — Hirnschwellung. Zbl. Neurochir. **2**, 247–261, 328–339, 1937.

HÄUSSLER, G. und G. DÖRING: Über eine hämangioblastomatöse Geschwulst der Dura in der linken Parietalgegend. Bruns Beitr. klin. Chir. **169**, 624–634, 1939.

HALDEMAN: Pineal gland tumors. Arch. Neurol. Psychiat. **18**, 724—754, 1927.

HALLERVORDEN, J.: Ein Aktinomykom im 3. Ventrikel. Arch. Psychiatr. **95**, 527, 1931.

HALLERVORDEN, J.: Erbliche Hirntumoren. Nervenarzt **9**, 1–8, 1936.

HALLERVORDEN, J.: Oligodendrogliom nach Hirntrauma. Nervenarzt **19**, 163–167, 1948.

HALLERVORDEN, J.: Bemerkungen zur zentralen Neurofibromatose und tuberösen Sklerose. Dtsch. Z. Nervenhk. **169**, 308–321, 1952.

HAMBÜCHER, D.: Plexuszysten im 3. Hirnventrikel, ihre Herkunft und ihre Lokalisation. Beitr. path Anat. u. allg. Path. **112**, 453–469, 1952.

HAMBY, W. B.: Spongioblastoma multiforme in the region of the hypothalamus. Arch. Neurol. Psychiat. **31**, 1258—1265, 1934.

HAMBY, W. B. and W. J. GARDNER: Ependymal cyst in the quadrigeminal region. Arch. Neurol. Psychiat. **33**, 391, 1935.

HAMPEL, E.: Klinik und Pathologie der chronischen Arachnitis adhaesiva. Dtsch. Z. Nervenhk. **144**, 107, 1937.

HAMPERL, H.: Verimpfende Wirkung von Hirnpunktionen. Wien. klin. Wschr. **1929**, 432.

HAMPERL, H.: Über gutartige Bronchialtumoren (Zylindrome und Carcinoide). Virchows Arch. **300**, 46, 1937.

HAMPERL, H.: Über die Gutartigkeit und die Bösartigkeit von Geschwülsten. Verhandl. Dtsch. Ges. Path., Hannover 1951, 35. Tagg., 29–54. Piscator, Stuttgart.

HARBITZ, F.: Über das gleichwertige Auftreten multipler Neurinome und Gliome. Acta pathol. microbiol. Scand. **9**, 359, 1932.

HARBITZ, H. F.: A case of multiple meningiomas combined with diffuse meningiomatosis. Acta pathol. microbiol. Scand. **12**, 24–37, 1935.

HARDMAN, J.: The angioarchitecture of the gliomata. Brain **63**, 91–118, 1940.

HARDMAN, J. and G. JEFFERSON: Cerebellopontine angle signs produced by ependymo-mata (cyst, tumour). Zbl. Neurochir. **3**, 137–145, 1938.

HARE, C. C. and A. WOLF: Intramedullary tumors of the brain stem. Arch. Neurol. Psychiat. **32**, 1230–1252, 1934.

HARRIS, W. and H. CAIRNS: Diagnosis and treatment of pineal tumors. Lancet 1932, I, 3–8.

HART, K.: Über primäre epitheliale Geschwülste des Gehirns. Arch. Psychiatr. **47**, 739, 1910.

HASENJÄGER, TH.: Über seitenventrikelnahe Gliome als eine besondere Gruppe unter den Großhirngeschwülsten. Arch. Psychiatr. **110**, 570–605, 1938.

HASENJÄGER, TH.: Über die Ependymitis blastomatosa bei ventrikelnahen Gliomen. Arch. Psychiatr. **110**, 605–632, 1939.

HASENJÄGER, TH. und H. SPATZ: Über örtliche Veränderungen der Konfiguration des Gehirns beim Hirndruck. Arch. Psychiatr. **107**, 193–222, 1938.

HASENJÄGER, TH. und G. STROESCU: Über den Zusammenhang zwischen Meningitis und Ependymitis. Arch. Psychiatr. **109**, 46–81, 1938.

HASS, G. M.: Chordomas of the cranium and cervical portion of the spine. Review of the literature with report of a case. Arch. Neurol. Psychiat. **32**, 300–327, 1934.

HASSE, K. E.: Krankheiten des Nervenapparates. Virchows Handb. d. spez. Path. u. Ther. Bd. IV/1. Erlangen 1855.

HASSELBACH, H. v.: Ependymäres Gliom des 4. Ventrikels. Beitr. path. Anat. **86**, 120–134, 1931.

HASSIN, G.: Histopathology of peripheral and central nervous system. W. Wood & Co., Baltimore 1933.

HASSIN, G. B. and H. D. SINGER: Histopathology of cerebral carcinoma. Arch. Neurol. Psychiat. **8**, 155–171, 1922.

HAUSMANN, L. and L. STEVENSON: Astrocytomas of the cerebellum. Arch. Neurol. Psychiat. **30**, 1100, 1933.

HAYMAKER, W. and M. H. YENERMAN: Pathological features of colloid cysts of the 3rd ventricle. A consideration of 60 cases. Excerpta medica, Neurol. Psych. **8**, 788, 1955.

HEINE, J.: Über die Vielgestaltigkeit und Kriechbewegungen der Sarkomzellen. Virchows Arch. **280**, 122, 1931.

HEINE, J.: Beitrag zur Verknöcherung der Meningeome. Gazeta Médica Portuguesa **4**, 817–823, 1951.

HEINLEIN, H. and K. FALKENBERG: Beitrag zur Kasuistik der Ganglioneurome des Kleinhirns. Zschr. Neurol. **166**, 128–135, 1939.

HELD: Die Entwicklung des Nervengewebes bei den Wirbeltieren. Leipzig 1909.

HENDERSON, W. R.: The pituitary adenomata. A follow-up study of the surgical results in 338 cases (Dr. Harvey Cushing's series). Brit. J. Surg. **26**, 809–921, 1939.

HENNEBERG, R.: Über einen Fall von Tumor und Zyste im Großhirn. Berl. klin. Wschr. **1902**, 13.

HENNEBERG, R.: Über Geschwülste der hinteren Schließungsrinne des Rückenmarks. Berl. klin. Wschr. **1921**, 1289.

HENNEBERG, R.: Die tierischen Parasiten des Zentralnervensystems. In: BUMKE-FOERSTER, Handb. d. Neur., Bd. 14, S. 286. Springer 1936.

HENNEBERG, R. und G. KOCH: Über „zentrale" Neurofibromatose und die Geschwülste des Kleinhirnbrückenwinkels. Arch. Psychiatr. **36**, 251, 1903.

HENSCHEN, F.: Über die Geschwülste der hinteren Schädelgrube, insbesondere des Kleinhirnbrückenwinkels. G. Fischer, Jena 1910.

HENSCHEN, F.: Referat über Gliome. Verh. 27. Kongr. d. Dt. Ges. f. Path., Rostock; Z. Path. **60**, Erg.-H. 27, 8, 1934.

HENSCHEN, F.: Die Tumoren des Lateralrecessus. Eine besondere Form der Kleinhirnbrückenwinkeltumoren. Arch. Psychiatr. **185**, 640–656, 1950.

HENSCHEN, F.: Tumoren des ZNS und seiner Hüllen in: Hdb. Spez. pathol. Anat. u. Histol., Bd. XIII, 3, Springer, Berlin 1955.

HERRMANN, G.: Periphere Nervenverletzung und Gliombildung. Med. Klin. **25**, 703–706, 1929.

HERXHEIMER, G.: Über Tumoren des Nebennierenmarks etc. Beitr. path. Anat. **57**, 112–167, 1914.

HERXHEIMER, G. und ROTH: Zum Studium der Recklinghausenschen Neurofibromatose. Beitr. path. Anat. **58**, 1914.

HERZOG, G.: Primäre Knochengeschwülste. Im Handb. d. path. Anat., Henke-Lubarsch, Bd. IX, 5. Berlin 1944.

HEUYER, G., J. LHERMITTE, TH. DE MARTEL and C. VOGT: Un cas de macrogénitosomie précoce liée à un épendymogliome de la région mamillo-tubérale. Rev. neurol. **1931**, II, 194.

HEYCK, H.: Glioblastom nach Leukotomie. Mschr. Psychiatr. **128**, 180–188, 1954.

HILDEBRANDT, K.: Zur Kenntnis der gliomatösen Neubildungen des Gehirns mit besonderer Berücksichtigung der ependymären Gliome. Virchows Arch. **185**, 1906. — Inaug.-Diss. Berlin 1906.

HIRSCH, E. F. und E. OLDBERG: Neuroepitheliom des Kleinhirns. Zbl. Path. **69**, 113–115, 1938.

HIRSCH, O. and K. ELLIOT: Ependymomas of the lateral ventricles of the brain. Amer. J. Path. **1**, 627, 1925.

His, W.: Die Entwicklung des menschlichen Gehirns. Hirzel, Leipzig 1904.

Hoelzer, H.: Über einen Fall von Varix des Sinus rectus. Zbl. Neurochir. 5, 152–157, 1940.

Hoeve, J. van der: Les phacomatoses de Bourneville, de Recklinghausen et de von Hippel-Lindau. J. Belge Neurol. Psychiatr. 33, 752–762, 1933.

Hoff, H. und L. Schönbauer: Hirnchirurgie. Deuticke, Leipzig u. Wien 1933.

Hoppe, H. J.: Diskordantes Auftreten von Hirntumoren bei erbgleichen Zwillingen. Zbl. Neurochir. 12, 34–36, 1952.

Horrax, G.: Meningiomas of the brain. Arch. Neurol. Psychiat. 41, 140, 1939.

Horrax, G.: The role of pinealomas in the causation of diabetes insipidus. Ann. Surg. 126, 725–739, 1947.

Horrax, G.: The diagnosis and treatment of pineal tumors. Radiology 52, 186–192, 1949.

Horrax, G.: A comparison of results after intracapsular enucleation and total extirpation of acoustic tumors. J. Neurol. Neurosurg. Psychiat. 13, 268–270, 1950.

Horrax, G.: Treatment of tumors of the pineal body. Arch. Neurol. Psychiat. 64, 227–242, 1950.

Horrax, G.: Diagnostic studies and survival statistics in a series of meningiomas of the brain. Arch. Neurol. Psychiat. 67, 204, 1952.

Horrax, G. and W. Q. Wu: Postoperative survival of patients with intracranial oligodendroglioma with special reference to radical tumor removal. A study of 26 patients. J. Neurosurg. 8, 473–479, 1951.

Horrax, G. and J. P. Wyatt: Ectopic pinealomas in the chiasmal region. J. Neurosurg. 4, 309–326, 1947.

Hortega, Del Rio P.: Estructura y systematisacion de los gliomas y paragliomas. Arch. Espan. Oncol. 2, 411–677, 1932.

Hortega, Del Rio P.: Contribucion al conocimiento citologico de los oligodendrogliomas. Arch. de histol. normal y patol. 2, 267–305, 1944.

Hortega, Del Rio P.: Contribucion al conocimiento citologico de los tumores del nervio y quiasma optiquos. Arch. de histol. normal y patol. 2, 307–358, 1944.

Hortega, Del Rio P.: Nomenclatura y clasificacion de los tumores del sistema nervioso. Buenos Aires 1945.

Hortega, Del Rio P., J. M. Prado y M. Polak: Sincitio y diferenciaciones citoplasmicas de los meningoexoteliomas. Arch. de histol. normal y patol. 21, 125–170, 1944.

Hosoi, K.: Meningiomas, with special reference to the multiple intracranial type. Amer. J. Path. 6, 245–260, 1930.

Hosoi, K.: Multiple intracranial angiomas. Amer. J. Path. 6, 235–260, 1930.

Hosoi, K.: Teratoma and teratoid tumors of the brain. Arch. Path. 9, 1207–1219, 1930.

Hosoi, K.: Multiple neurofibromatosis (von Recklinghausen's disease). With special reference to malignant transformation. Arch. Surg. 22, 258–281, 1931.

Hsü, J. K.: Primary intracranial sarcomas. Arch. Neurol. Psychiat. 43, 901–924, 1940.

Hueck, W.: Über die zelluläre und organoide Betrachtungsweise der Geschwülste. Arch. klin. Chir. 1941, 202.

Hug, O.: Krebsbildung in einem pialen Epidermoid. Virchows Arch. 308, 679–689, 1942.

Hunt, W. E., W. Abramson and T. A. Weaver: Cerebral schistosomiasis. Report of a case simulating cerebral neoplasm. J. Amer. Med. Assoc. 136, 686–690, 1948.

Ihlberg, G.: Ein Fall von Gliosarkom des Mittelhirns. Zschr. Neurol. 122, 747–755, 1929.

Imperatori, Ch. I.: Chordomas of the cervical region. Ann. Otol. etc 56, 271, 1947.

Ingraham, F. D.: Medulloblastoma cerebelli: diagnosis, treatment and survivals, with report of 56 cases. New England J. Med. 238, 171, 1948.

Ingraham, F. D. and O. T. Bailey: Cystic teratomas and teratoid tumors of the central nervous system in infancy and childhood. J. Neurosurg. 3, 511–532, 1946.

Ingraham, F. D. and Scott: Craniopharyngiomas in children. J. Pediatr. 29, 95, 1946.

Insausti, T.: Contribucion al estudio anatomoclinico de los glioepiteliomas (ependimomas). Neuropsiquiatria 2, 185–209, 1951.

Insausti, T., R. F. Matera, J. Prado y E. Franke: Epidermoides craneanos y espinales. Arch. Neurocir. (Buenos Aires) 9, 56–91, 1952.

Ironside, R. and M. Guttmacher: The corpus callosum and its tumors. Brain 52, 442 bis 484, 1929.

Jacob, H.: Die diffuse Markdestruktion im Gefolge eines Hirnödems. Zschr. Neurol. 168, 322, 1940.

JAHNEL, F.: Allgemeine Pathologie und pathologische Anatomie der Syphilis des Nervensystems in: Hdb. d. Haut- u. Geschlechtskrankh. Bd. 17, S, 1, Springer, Berlin 1929.

JAMES, T. G. I. and W. PAGEL: Oligodendroglioma with extracranial metastases. Brit. J. Surg. 39, 56–65, 1951.

JEFFERSON, G.: The tentorial pressure cone. Arch. Neurol. Psychiat. 40, 937, 1938.

JEFFERSON, G.: Compression of chiasma, optic nerve and optic tracts by intracranial aneurysm. Brain 60, 444, 1942.

JEFFERSON, G.: The Bowman lecture. Concerning injuries, aneurysms and tumours involving the cavernous sinus. Transact. Ophthalm. Soc. 73, 117–152, 1953.

JEFFERSON, G.: The invasive adenomas of the anterior pituitary. In: The Sherrington Lectures III, 1–63. Eaton Press, Liverpool 1954.

JELIFFE, S. E. und J. H. LARKIN: Über ein malignes Chordom mit Symptomen von seiten des Gehirns und Rückenmarks. Zschr. Neurol. 5, 590–604, 1911.

JENTZER, A.: Tumeurs cérébrales. Classification anatomo-pathologique. Helvet. med. acta 1938, 5.

JENTZER, A.: Glioblastomes traités par le cobalt. Neurochir. (Paris) 1, 153–162, 1955.

JEQUIER-DOGE, M.: A propos de la classification des tumeurs cérébrales. Schweiz. Arch. Neur. 48, 1941.

JORDAN: Über die Entstehung von Tumoren, Tuberkulomen etc. Münchn. Med. Wschr. 48, 174, 1901.

JOSEPHY, H.: Ein Fall von Porobulbie mit solitärem zentralem Neurinom. Zschr. Neurol. 93, 62–82, 1924.

JOUGHIN, I. L.: Coincident tumor of the brain in twins. Arch. Neurol. Psychiat. 19, 948–950, 1928.

JUBA, A.: Geschwülste des Zentralnervensystems (Meningeom, Neurinom) in der Gewebekultur. Mschr. Psychiatr. 113, 321–336, 1947.

JUHÁSZ, P.: Über ein diffuses Kleinhirnoligodendrogliom und das Oligodendrogliom der hinteren Schädelgrube. Zschr. Neurol. 174, 701–714, 1942.

JUHÁSZ, P.: Ein knotiges Kleinhirnoligodendrogliom. Zschr. Neurol. 175, 745, 1945.

JUNG, R.: Über die Angiome Lindaus als eine charakteristische Gruppe unter den Kleinhirntumoren. Arch. Psychiatr. 103, 580–626, 1935.

JUNGHERR, E. and A. WOLF: Gliomas in animals. Amer. J. Cancer 37, 493–509, 1939.

JUROW, H. N.: Psammomatous dural endothelioma (meningioma) with pulmonary metastasis. Arch. Path. 32, 222–226, 1941.

KALBFLEISCH, H. H.: Spätveränderungen im menschlichen Gehirn nach intensiver Röntgenbestrahlung. Strahlentherapie 76, 584, 1947.

KALBFLEISCH, H. H. und H. GREBE: Über das Einwachsen der Schädelmeningeome in das umgebende Gewebe, namentlich in das Gehirn. Arch. klin. Chir. 188, 118–137, 1937.

KALM, H.: Über die Metastasierung von Geschwülsten in die Liquorräume. Dtsch. Z. Nervenhk. 159, 397–407, 1948.

KALM, H.: Ein malignes Tentoriummeningeom mit Metastasierung in die Oblongata und in die subarachnoidalen Liquorräume. Dtsch. Z. Nervenhk. 163, 131–140, 1950.

KALM, H. und R. MAGUN: Beitrag zur Klinik und pathologischen Anatomie der Pinealome. Dtsch. Z. Nervenhk. 164, 453–468, 1950.

KANE, CH. A. and H. MOST: Schistosomiasis of the central nervous system. Arch. Neurol. Psychiat. 59, 141, 1948.

KARITZKY, B.: Nekrosen und Blutungen in Hirngeschwülsten. Virchows Arch. 289, 1933.

KAUFMANN, E.: Lehrbuch der speziellen Pathologischen Anatomie. W. de Gruyter, Berlin 1922.

KAUTZKY, R.: Das gefäßreiche parietale Glioblastom. Dtsch. Z. Nervenhk. 159, 57–74, 1948.

KAUTZKY, R.: Die Bedeutung der Hirnhaut-Innervation und ihrer Entwicklung für die Pathogenese der Sturge-Weberschen Krankheit. Dtsch. Z. Nervenhk. 161, 506–525, 1949.

KAUTZKY, R.: Die Schnelldiagnose intrakranialer Erkrankungen mit Hilfe des supravital gefärbten Quetschpräparates. Virchows Arch. 320, 495–550, 1951.

KAUTZKY, R. und N. VIERDT: Ein Angioblastom des Großhirns. Zbl. Neurochir. 13, 158–163, 1953.

KAUTZKY, R. und K. J. ZÜLCH: Neurol.-Neurochir. Röntgendiagnostik und andere Methoden zur Erkennung intrakranialer Erkrankungen. Springer, Heidelberg 1955.

KELLER, H.: Sogenannte „hyperplastische Capillarangiome" (Lindau) und Großhirncyste, zugleich ein Beitrag zur Tumorcysten-Frage. Virchows Arch. 289, 151–181, 1933.

KERNOHAN, J. W.: Primary tumors of the spinal cord and intradural filum terminale. In: Cytology and cellular pathology of the nervous system. Hoeber, New York 1932.

KERNOHAN, J. W. and A. ADSON: Simplified classification of gliomas. In: Proc. of the Mayo Clin. 24, 71–75, 1949.

KERNOHAN, J. W. and E. M. FLETCHER-KERNOHAN: Ependymomas. A study of 109 cases. In: Tumors of the nervous system, WILLIAMS-WILKINS 1937. Proc. Res. Nerv. Ment. Dis. 16, 182–209, 1935.

KERNOHAN, J. W., J. R. LEARMONTH and J. B. DOYLE: Neuroblastomas and gangliocytomas of the central nervous system. Brain 55, 278–310, 1932.

KERNOHAN, J. W., R. F. MABON, H. J. SVIEN and A. W. ADSON: A simplified classification of the gliomas. Proc. Staff Meet. Mayo-Clinie. 24, 71–75, 1949.

KERNOHAN, J. W. and G. P. SAYRE: Tumors of the central nervous system. Armed forces Institute of Path., Washington 1952.

KERNOHAN, J. W., H. W. WOLTMAN and A. W. ADSON: Intramedullary tumors of the spinal cord. Arch. Neurol. Psychiat. 25, 679–699, 1931.

KERNOHAN, J. W., H. W. WOLTMAN and A. W. ADSON: Gliomas arising from the region of the cauda equina. Clinical, surgical and histologic considerations. Arch. Neurol. Psychiat. 29, 287–305, 1933.

KERNOHAN, J. W., H. W. WOLTMAN and A. W. ADSON: Gliomas of the cerebellopontine angle. J. Neuropath. 7, 4, 1948.

KERSHMAN, J.: The medulloblast and the medulloblastomas. Arch. Neurol. Psychiat. 40, 937–967, 1938.

KESSEL, F. K. und H. OLIVECRONA: Über Foramen-Monroi-Zysten (sog. Kolloidzysten des 3. Ventrikels). Zbl. Neurochir. 1, 18–38, 1936.

KHERSONSKY, R. A., B. G. ROUBINSTEIN et K. S. WINER: Sur les tumeurs de la base du cerveau chez les enfants. Arch. méd. enf. 39, 707–720, 1936.

KINO, F.: Über das Verhalten der Glia bei Gliomen. Frankf. Z. Path. 50, 1937.

KINO, F.: Über ein subependymäres, multiples, malignes Glioblastom. Zschr. Neurol. 160, 297–305, 1937.

KLAPPROTH, W.: Teratom der Zirbel kombiniert mit Adenom. Zbl. Path. 32, 618–630, 1922.

KLAR, E., BECKER u. SCHEER: Eine kombinierte chirurgisch-radiologische Behandlung bei Glioblastoma multiforme mit Co 60. Langenbecks Arch. 55, 280, 1954.

KLATZO, I.: A study of glioblastoma multiforme by the Golgi method. Amer. J. Path. 28, 357–367, 1952.

KLATZO, I. and C. G. McMILLAN: A new technic for the rapid diagnosis of brain tumors using Chlorazol Black E., Laboratory Investigation 1, 24–29, 1952.

KLEBS, E.: Beitrag zur Geschwulstlehre. Vjschr. prakt. Heilkd., Prag 1877, 34; Allgemeine Pathologie 1889, 720.

KLINGLER, M.: Über Knorpelgeschwülste der Schädelbasis mit intrakranieller Ausdehnung. Acta Neurochir. (Wien) 1, 337–380, 1951.

KLOSS, K.: Hirntumoren höherer Altersstufen. Acta Neurochir. (Wien) 2, 217–232, 1952.

KOCH, G.: Beitrag zur Erblichkeit der Hirngeschwülste (vorläufige Mitteilung). Acta geneticae medicae et gemellologicae 3, 169–191, 1953.

KÖHLMEIER, W.: Zur Frage der Metastasierung der Gliome. Virchows Arch. 308, 51–59, 1941.

KÖHLMEIER, W.: Über multizentrisch entstandene Oligodendrogliome. Zschr. Neurol. 175, 385, 1943.

KÖHLMEIER, W.: Zur Kenntnis der metastasierenden Hypophysengeschwülste. Virchows Arch. 312, 26–34, 1944.

KOELLA, W.: Das Angioblastom. Schweiz. Arch. Neurol. 59, 208–238, 1947.

KÖRNYEY, ST.: Eine sich entlang den Gefäßwandungen ausbreitende Hirngeschwulst (adventitielles Sarkom). Zschr. Neurol. 149, 50, 1933.

KÖRNYEY, ST.: Diagnostische Bedeutung röntgenologisch darstellbarer Kalkherde in den Großhirnhemisphären usw. Zbl. Neurochir. 2, 224–242, 1937.

KOOPMANN: Weiterer Beitrag zur Frage des Hirntraumas und seiner tödlichen Folgen. Mschr. Unfallheilk. 31, 97–99, 1924.

KORBSCH, H.: Zur Morphologie und Genese des Neurinoms. Arch. Psychiatr. 92, 183 bis 278, 1930.

KORBSCH, H.: Die sogenannte Meningitis tumorosa. Nervenarzt 5, 67, 1932.

KORBSCH, H.: Die Grundsubstanz der Neurinome. Zschr. Neurol. 165, 337–340, 1939.

KRABBE, K. H.: Facial and meningeal angiomatosis associated with calcifications in the brain cortex. Arch. Neurol. Psychiat. **32**, 737, 1934.

KRABBE, K. H.: Un cas de tératome dans la glande pinéale guéri par intervention opératoire. Acta psychiatr. Belg. **19**, 234, 1944.

KRAINER, L.: Die Hirn- und Rückenmarkslipome. Virchows Arch. **295**, 106, 1935.

KRASTING, K.: Beitrag zur Statistik und Kasuistik metastatischer Tumoren, besonders der Carcinommetastasen im Zentralnervensystem. Z. Krebsforschg. **4**, 315–379, 1906.

KRAUS, H.: Multiple Gehirntumoren. Wien. med. Wschr. **1949**, 174–176.

KRAUS, J. E.: Neoplastic diseases of the human hypophysis. Arch. Path. **39–40**, 343, 1945.

KRAUS, R.: Die Hypophyse. Im Handb. d. spez. path. Anat. Henke-Lubarsch Bd. 8, 1926.

KRAUSE, F.: Chirurgie des Gehirns. URBAN & Schwarzenberg 1908.

KRAYENBÜHL, H.: Spontane spinale Subarachnoidalblutung und akute Rückenmarkskompression bei intraduralem, spinalem Neurinom. Schweiz. med. Wschr. **77**, 25, 1947.

KRAYENBÜHL, H. und F. LÜTHY: Das spinale Neurinom und sympathische Ganglioneurom im Kindesalter. Z. Pathol. u. Bakteriol. **10**, 51–65, 1947.

KRAYENBÜHL, H. und A. E. SCHMID: Zur Lokalisation intrakranieller orbitaler Dermoide. Ophthalmologica **106**, 251–270, 1943.

KRAYENBÜHL, H. und G. WEBER: Diagnostik und Grundzüge der Therapie der Hirntumoren im Kindesalter. Acta helvetica paed'atrica **2**, 115–153, 1947.

KREDEL, F. E.: Tissue culture of intracranial tumors with a note on the meningiomas. Amer. J. Path. **4**, 337, 1928.

KREDEL, F. E.: Intracranial tumors in tissue culture. Arch. Surg. **18**, 2002, 1929.

KRIEG, W.: Aseptische Meningitis nach Operation von Cholesteatomen des Gehirns. Zbl. Neurochir. **1**, 79–86, 1936.

KRIEG, W.: 164 Fälle von Cholesteatomen des Gehirns. Zbl. Chir. **1936**, 3047.

KRÜCKE, W.: Über Nachweis, Wirkung und Wanderung von Thorotrast im menschlichen Organismus. Naturw. **37**, 284–286, 1950.

KRUMBEIN: Über die Band- oder Palisadenstellung der Kerne, eine Wuchsform des feinfibrillären mesenchymalen Gewebes. Zugleich eine Ableitung der Neurinome (Verocay) vom feinfibrillären Bindegewebe (Fibroma tenuifibrillare). Virchows Arch. **255**, 309–331, 1925.

KRYNAUW, R. A. and C. JACKSON: Presence of parasitic agent in various intracranial tumors of man. Nature (London) **162**, 147–148, 1948.

KÜSTER, H.: Über Gliome der Nebenniere. Virchows Arch. **180**, 117–130, 1905.

KUFS, H.: Kritische Betrachtungen über die Frage der primären Krebsentwicklung im Gehirn usw. Arch. Psychiatr. **78**, 663, 1926.

KUFS, H.: Klinik, Histopathologie und Vererbungspathologie der v. Hippel-Lindauschen Erkrankung. Zschr. Neurol. **138**, 414–427, 1932.

KUFS, H.: Multiple Cystizerken im Gehirn und Entwicklung von unbefruchteten Bandwurmeiern in den Cystizerkenmembranen. Arch. Psychiatr. **186**, 361–370, 1951.

KUHLENBECK, H.: Vorlesungen über das Zentralnervensystem der Wirbeltiere. Fischer, Jena 1927.

KUHLENBECK, H.: Neoplastic transformation of the subependymal cell plate in the floor of the fourth ventricle (subependymal spongioblastoma). J. Neuropath. **6**, 139–151, 1947.

KUHLENBECK, H. and W. HAYMAKER: Neuroectodermal tumors containing neoplastic neuronal elements: Ganglioneuroma, spongioneuroblastoma and glioneuroma. Mil. Surg. **99**, 4, 1946.

KUNTZMANN, J., C. M. GROS et J. MEYER: A propos de deux cas de thorotrastome à manifestation clinique tardive. J. d. Chir. **66**, 201–212, 1950, Ref. Zbl. Neurochir. **11**, 297, 1951.

KUX, E.: Über ein bösartiges Pinealom und bösartiges fötales Adenom der Hypophyse. Ziegl. Beitr. **87**, 59, 1931.

KWAN, S. T. and B. J. ALPERS: The Oligodendrogliomas. Arch. Neurol. Psychiat. **26**, 279–322, 1931.

LAAS, E.: Über die sog. Endotheliome der Hirnhäute. Beitr. path. Anat. **95**, 431–449, 1935.

LANDAU, W.: Das diffuse Gliom. Frankf. Z. Path. **5**, 469–514, 1910.

LANDAU, W.: Über Rückbildungsvorgänge in Gliomen. Frankf. Z. Path. **7**, 351, 1911.

LANGE, J.: Hirnchirurgie und Lokalisationslehre. Mschr. Psychiatr. **99**, 130 144, 1938.

LANGE-COSACK, H.: Gefäßmißbildungen des Gehirns und seiner Häute. In: KIRSCHNER-NORDMANN, Die Chirurgie, Bd. III, S. 613–660, 1948.

LANGE-COSACK, H.: Verschiedene Gruppen der hypothalamischen Pubertas praecox. Dtsch. Z. Nervenhk. **166**, 499–545, 1951.

LAPRESLE, J., M. G. NETSKY and A. ZIMMERMAN: The pathology of meningiomas. A study of 121 cases. Amer. J. Path. **28**, 757–791, 1952.

LAUCHE, A.: Über rhythmische Strukturen in menschlichen Geweben. Virchows Arch. **257**, 751, 1925.

LAUCHE, A.: Ungewöhnlich lokalisierte Melanoblastommetastasen im ZNS. Münch. med. Wschr. **1938**, 194.

LAWRENCE, E. A. and E. J. DONLAN: Neoplastic diseases in infants and children. Cancer Res. **12**, 900, 1952.

LAYMON, C. W. and F. T. BECKER: Massive metastasizing meningioma involving the scalp. Arch. Dermatol. **59**, 626–635, 1949.

LEARMONTH, J. R.: On leptomeningeomas of the spinal cord. Brit. J. Surg. **14**, 397, 1927.

LEARMONTH, J. R. and J. D. CAMP: Multiple tumor implants in the ventricles revealed by ventriculography. Report of case. Amer. J. Roentgenol. **29**, 3, 1933.

LEARMONTH, J. R. and J. W. KERNOHAN: Tumour of the Gasserian ganglion: sheath neuroma. Brain **53**, 1–6, 1930.

LEARMONTH, J. R. and A. VERBRUGGEN: Chondroma of the falx. J. Nerv. Ment. Dis. **76**, 463–466, 1932.

LEAVITT, F. H.: Cerebellar tumors occuring in identical twins. Arch. Neurol. Psychiat. **19**, 617–623, 1928.

LEBERT: Über Krebs und die mit Krebs verwechselten Geschwülste im Gehirn und seinen Hüllen. Virchows Arch. **3**, 461, 1851.

LE BLANC: Beitrag zur pathologischen Anatomie der Hirntumoren. Inaug.-Diss. Bonn 1868.

LEHOCZKY, T. v.: Zur Frage der primären Gehirnkarzinome. Arch. Psychiatr. **82**, 527–567, 1928.

LEHOCZKY, T. v.: Über die Anatomie und Klinik der Epidermoidzysten des Gehirns. Zschr. Neurol. **122**, 756, 1929.

LEHOCZKY, T. v.: Hemangioendotheliomatous meningioma simulating cerebral arteriosclerosis. Neurology **3**, 737–743, 1953.

LEMKE, R.: Über Hirnzysten. Dtsch. Z. Nervenhk. **162**, 70–89, 1950.

LENČE, P.: Über seltene primäre Lokalisationen melanotischer Tumoren. Erg. allg. Path. **32**, 48, 1937.

LENHOSSÉK, M. v.: Der feinere Bau des Nervensystems. Berlin 1895.

LESSE, ST. and M. G. NETSKY: Metastasis of neoplasms to the central nervous system and meninges. Arch. Neurol. Psychiat. **72**, 133–153, 1954.

LESZYNSKY, W. M.: Report of a case of intracranial tumor resulting from traumatism. J. Amer. Med. Assoc. **49**, 1361, 1907.

LETTERER, E.: Über heterotype Geschwülste der Aderhäute. Beitr. path. Anat. **67**, 370, 1920.

LETTRÉ, H.: Der Stand der Krebsforschung. Die Medizinische. 1953, 27/28, 897–907.

LEY, A., R. JACAS and C. OLIVERAS: Torula granuloma of the cervical spinal cord. J. Neurosurg. **8**, 327–335, 1951.

LEY, A. and A. G. ROSENDO: Primary sarcomas of the cerebellum. Acta Neurochir. **3**, 1–16, 1952.

LHERMITTE, J. et DUCLOS: Sur un ganglioneurome diffus du cortex du cervelet. Bull. de l'Ass. Franç. pour l'étude du cancer **9**, 99–106, 1920.

LIBER, A. F.: The nature of Rosenthal fibers. J. Nerv. Ment. Dis. **85**, 3, 1937.

LICHTENSTEIN, B. W.: Teratoma of the pineal body. Arch. Neurol. Psychiat. **44**, 153, 1940.

LICHTENSTEIN, B. W.: Multiple primary tumors of the brain. Arch. Neurol. Psychiat. **46**, 59, 1941.

LICHTENSTEIN, B. W. and H. ZEITLIN: Ganglioneuromas of the spinal cord. Arch. Neurol. Psychiat. **37**, 1356, 1937.

LIEBEGOTT, G.: Ein Beitrag zur Klinik und Pathologie der Kleinhirnangiome Lindaus. Nervenarzt **10**, 178–186, 1937.

LILL, H.: Über metastatische Hirntumoren. Wien. med. Wschr. **1952**, 277–278.

LINCK, A.: Chordoma malignum, ein Beitrag zur Kenntnis der Geschwülste an der Schädelbasis. Beitr. path. Anat. u. allg. Pathol. **46**, 573–585, 1909.

LINDAU, A.: Studien über Kleinhirnzysten. Bau, Pathogenese und Beziehungen zur Angiomatosis retinae. Acta path. microbiol. scand. **1926**, Supl. 1, 128 pp.

LINDAU, A.: Zur Frage der Angiomatosis retinae und ihrer Hirnkomplikationen. Acta ophthalm. **4**, 193, 1927.

LINDENBERG, R.: Über ein Plexusepitheliom des 3. Ventrikels mit geschichtetem Platten-epithel und einer Auskleidung der Ventrikelwand mit dem gleichen Epithel. Zbl. Path. 88, 47–51, 1951.

LINDGREN, E.: Röntgenologie einschließlich Kontrastmethoden. In Handb. d. Neurochir. Bd. II. Springer, Berlin 1954.

LINK, K. und H. SCHLEUSSING: Statistische Erhebungen an 248 intrakraniellen Geschwül-sten. Arch. Psychiatr. u. Zschr. Neurol. 184, 646–652, 1950.

LIST, C. F.: Die operative Behandlung der Akustikusneurinome und ihre Ergebnisse. Arch. Klin. Chir. 171, 282, 1932.

LIST, C. F., J. F. HOLT and M. EVERETT: Lipoma of the corpus callosum. Amer. J. Roent-genol. 55, 125, 1946.

LIST, C. F., J. R. WILLIAMS and G. W. BALYEAT: Vascular lesions in pituitary adenomas. J. Neurosurg. 9, 177–187, 1952.

LOELIGER, H. TH.: Über Facialisneurinome. Acta oto-laryng. (Stockh.) 35, 543–555, 1947.

LOEPP, W. und R. LORENZ: Röntgendiagnostik des Schädels. Thieme-Verlag, Stuttgart 1954.

LOEW, F. und W. TÖNNIS: Klinik und Behandlung der Neurinome des Nervus trigeminus. Zbl. Neurochir. 14, 32- 41, 1954.

LOISEL, G.: Les astrocytomes du cervelet de l'enfant. Arnette, Paris 1935.

LORENZ, R.: Differentialdiagnose der arteriographisch darstellbaren, intrakraniellen Ge-schwülste. Glioblastom, Meningeom, Sarkom. Zbl. Neurochir. 4, 30–60, 1940.

LORENZ, R.: Erfahrungen auf dem Gebiete der Röntgenbestrahlung von Hirntumoren. Zbl. Neurochir. 9, 209–215, 1949.

LOTMAR, O.: Beiträge zur Histologie des Glioms. NISSL-ALZHEIMER. Arbeiten 6, 433, 1918.

LOTMAR, F.: Zur Kenntnis der Lindauschen Krankheit. Schweiz. Arch. Neurol. 1935, 36.

LOVE, J. G. and J. W. KERNOHAN: Dermoids and epidermoidal tumors of the CNS. J. A. M. A. 107, 1876–1882, 1936.

LOVE, J. G., C. H. SHELDEN and J. W. KERNOHAN: Tumor of the hypophysial duct. (Rathke's cysts). Arch. Surg. 39, 28, 1939.

LÜERS, TH.: Über diffuse Gliome des Gehirns unter besonderer Berücksichtigung der all-gemeinen Geschwulstfragen. Arch. Geschw.forsch. 5, 220–244, 1953.

LÜTHY, F. und F. J. IRSIGLER: Beitrag zur Klinik und Histologie der Ependymome der Cauda Equina. Acta Neurochir. (Wien) 2, 354--368, 1952.

LÜTHY, F. und M. KLINGLER: Der Tumorettentumor des Hypophysenhinterlappens. Schweiz. Z. Allgem. Path. u. Bakt. 14, 721–729, 1951.

LUMSDEN, C. E.: Observations on the morphogenesis and growth rate of astrocytic gliomas in tissue culture. Excerpta medica, Neurology and Psychiatry, Vol. 8, S. 792, 1955.

LUNDBERG, A.: Über die primären Tumoren des Sehnerven und der Sehnervenkreuzung. Inaug.-Diss. Örebro 1935.

LUYENDIJK, W.: Multiple meningiomas and meningiomatosis. Acta Neurochir. (Wien) 3, 263, 1954.

LUZZATTO, A.: Osservazioni sulla angioarchitettonica dei tumori cerebrali. Riv. pat. nerv. 59, 293–375, 1942.

LYSHOLM, E.: Röntgenologische Diagnostik in der Chirurgie der Gehirnkrankheiten. Neue dtsch. Chir. 50, III, 1941 (Abb. 151)

MABON, R. F., H. J. SVIEN, J. W. KERNOHAN and W. McK. CRAIG: Ependymomas. Proc. of the Staff Meeting of the Mayo Clinic 24, 65–71, 1949.

MABON, R. F., H. J. SVIEN, A. W. ADSON and J. W. KERNOHAN: Astrocytomas of the cerebellum. Arch. Neurol. Psychiat. 64, 74- 88, 1950.

MABON, R. F., H. J. SVIEN, E. GATES and J. W. KERNOHAN: Medulloepithelioma. A criti-cal reevaluation. J. Neuropath. 9, 193, 1950.

MABREY, R. E.: Chordoma, a study of 150 cases. Amer. J. Cancer 25, 501- 517, 1935.

MACDONALD, A. E.: Lindau's disease. Arch. Ophth. 23, 564 –576, 1940.

McDONALD, C. A. and M. KORB: Intracranial aneurysms. Arch. Neurol. Psychiat. 42, 415–429, 1939.

McKENZIE, K. G. and M. C. SOSMAN: The roentgenological diagnosis of craniopharyngeal pouch tumors. Amer. J. Roentgenol. 11, 171, 1924.

McLEAN, A.J.: Die Kraniopharyngealtaschentumoren. Zschr. Neurol. 126, 639–682, 1930.

McLEAN, A. J.: Paraphysial cysts. Arch. Neurol. Psychiat. 36, 485–512, 1936.

McLEAN, A. J.: Intracranial tumors. Handb. d. Neur. BUMKE-FOERSTER, Bd. 14, S. 131. Springer, Berlin 1936.

McLean, A. J.: Pituitary tumors. Handb. d. Neur. Bumke-Foerster, Bd. 14. Springer, Berlin 1936.

McK. Craig, W. and G. Horrax: The occurrence of hemangioblastomas (two cerebellar and one spinal) in three members of a family. J. Neurosurg. 6, 518–529, 1949.

McK. Craig, W., H. M. Keith and J. W. Kernohan: Tumors of the brain occurring in childhood. Acta psychiatr. et neurol. 24, 375–390, 1949.

McK. Craig, W., H. P. Wagener and J. W. Kernohan: Lindau-von Hippel disease. A report of four cases. Arch. Neurol Psychiat. 46, 36–54, 1941.

Maffei, W. E.: Tumores do sistema nervoso. Revista Neur. (São Paulo) 3, 42, 1937.

Mage, J. et H. J. Scherer: Tumeur cérébrale parvicellulaire se propageant dans l'espace de Virchow-Robin. J. Belge Neur. 37, 731–746, 1937.

Mahaim, Ch.: Les tumeurs pinéales et leurs formes malignes avec métastases spinales. Arch. Suisses de Neurologie et de Psychiatr. 71, 1–37, 1953.

Mahoney, W.: Die Epidermoide des Zentralnervensystems. Zschr. Neurol. 416–471, 1936.

Maiss, U.: Zur Klinik und Anatomie des Gangliocytoma dysplasticum des Kleinhirns. Zschr. Neurol. 169, 170–182, 1940.

Majerszky-Sántha, K.: Craniospinale Meningeome. Arch. Psychiatr. 116, 648–657, 1943.

Mallory, F. B.: Three gliomata of ependymal origin: two in the fourth ventricle, one subcutaneous over the coccyx. J. Med. Res. 8, 1, 1902.

Mallory, F. B.: A contribution to the classification of tumors. J. Med. Res. 13, 113, 1904/05.

Mallory, F. B.: The type of cell of the so called dural endothelioma. J. Med. Res. 41, 349, 1920.

Manuelidis, E. E.: Über Hämangiome des Gehirns. Arch. Psychiatr. 184, 601–645, 1950.

Manzini, C.: I gliomi multipli dell'encephalo. Riv. Neurol. 21, 63–67, 1951.

Marburg, O.: Zur Kenntnis der neuroepithelialen Geschwülste. Blastoma ependymale. Arb. neurol Inst. Wien 23, 192, 1921.

Marburg, O.: Zur Kenntnis der sogenannten Medulloblastome. Sphaeroblastoma polymorph. Dtsch. Z. Nervenhk. 289, 117–119, 1931.

Marburg, O.: Unfall und Hirngeschwulst. Springer, Wien 1934.

Marburg, O.: Über Reizgeschwülste und meningeale Tumoren. Virchows Arch. 294, 759–773, 1935.

Marchesani, O.: Untersuchungen über die Glia. II. Mitteilung (Das Glioma retinae). Arch. Augenhk. 103, 484–510, 1930.

Marcos, F.: Über ein hochgradig polymorphes Meningeom mit langsamem Wachstum. Zbl. Neurochir. 14, 304–307, 1954.

Marinesco, T. and M. Goldstein: Sur une forme anatomique, non encore décrite, de médulloblastome: médullomyoblastome. Ann. anat. path., Paris 10, 513–525, 1933.

Markiewicz, T.: Über späte Schädigung des menschlichen Hirns durch Röntgenstrahlen. Zschr. Neurol. 152, 548, 1935.

Marquardt, M.: Über ein umschriebenes Arachnoidalsarkom des Kleinhirns. Zschr. Neurol. 171, 117, 1941.

Martel, Th. de et J. Guillaume: Les tumeurs cérébrales. Doin et Cie., Paris 1931.

Martel, Th. de et J. Guillaume: Les meningeomes chez les enfants. Rev. neurol. 64, 699–702, 1935.

Martel, Th. de et J. Guillaume: Tumeurs de l'amygdale cérébelleuse. Rev. neurol. 64, 776, 1935.

Martin, J.: The transplantation of human brain tumors into animal hosts. J. Neuropath. 10, 40–47, 1951.

Martin, P.: Two cases of oligodendroglioma. Brain 54, 330, 1931.

Martin, P. and H. Cushing: Primary gliomas of the chiasm and optic nerves. Arch. Ophthalm. 52, 209–241, 1923.

Masson, C. B. et R. Dreyfuss: Neurogliocytome embryonaire du vermis. Rev. neurol. 2, 227, 1925.

Masson, P.: Diagnostics de laboratoire: Tumeurs. Maloine, Paris 1923.

Masson, P.: Les naevi pigmentaires, tumeurs nerveuses. Ann. anat. path., Paris 5, 1926.

Masson, P.: Experimental and spontaneous Schwannomas (periph. gliomas). Amer. J. Path. 11, 367, 1935.

Matthes, Th.: Thorotrastschäden und Krebsgefahr. Arch. Geschwulstforsch. 6, 162–182, 1954.

MEAGHER, R. and L. EISENHARDT: Intracranial carcinomatous metastases. Ann. Surg. 1, 132, 1931.

MERZBACHER, L. und UYEDA: Gliastudien. Das reaktive Gliom und die reaktive Gliose. Zschr. Neurol. 1, 285–317, 1910.

MEYER, A.: Herniation of the brain. Arch. Neurol. Psychiat. 4, 387–400, 1920.

MEYER, H. H.: Über Besonderheiten corticaler Gliome und ihre Abgrenzbarkeit gegen Tumoren der Meningen. Virchows Arch. 300, 296–318, 1937.

MEYER, H. H. und H. SCHELLER: Über ein Fibromyxom des Gehirns. Virchows Arch. 300, 473, 1937.

MEYER, O.: Ein besonderer Typ von Riesenzellengliom. Frankf. Z. Path. 14, 1913.

MINKOWSKI, M.: Über metastatische Hirngeschwülste. Zürich-Leipzig 1941.

MITTELBACH, M.: Über Gliome mit Metastasen. Beitr. path. Anat. 95, 538, 1935.

MÖLLER, H. U.: Familial angiomatosis retinae et cerebelli – LINDAUS disease. Acta ophthalm. (Copenh.) 244, 1929.

MOERSCH, F. P., W. McK. CRAIG and J. W. KERNOHAN: Tumors of the brain in aged persons. Arch. Neurol. Psychiat 45, 235–245, 1941.

MONAKOW, C. VON: Gliom und Schädeltrauma. Schweiz. Arch. Neurol. 14, 289, 1924.

MONIZ, E.: Die cerebrale Arteriographie und Phlebographie. In: Handb. d. Neurologie, Erg.-Bd. II. Springer, Berlin 1940.

MOORE, G. E.: Fluorescein as an agent in the differentiation of normal and malignant tissue. Science 106, 130, 1947.

MOORE, M. T. and K. STERN: Vascular lesions in the brain-stem and occipital lobe occuring in association with brain tumors. Brain 61, 70–98, 1938.

MOORE, G. E., W. T. PEYTON, L. A. FRENCH and W. W. WALKER: The clinical use of fluorescein in neurosurgery: the localization of brain tumors. J. Neurosurg. 5, 392, 1948.

MORELLI, E.: Contributo allo studio delle principali classificationi dei tumori del encephalo. Pathologica (Genova) 28, 243, 1936.

MORRIS, A. A.: The use of the smear technique in the rapid histological diagnosis of tumors of the central nervous system. J. Neurosurg. 4, 497, 1947.

MÜLLER, H. R.: Unfall und Hirntumor. Wissenschaftl. Vers. der Hamburger Ärztekammer. Ärztebl. Norddeutschl., Juli 1938. – Zbl. Chir. 1939, 1164–1165.

MÜLLER, R. and G. WOHLFART: Om tumörer i corpus pineale. Särtryck ur Nordisk Medicin 33, 15, 1947.

MÜLLER, R. and G. WOHLFART: Intracranial teratomas and teratoid tumors. Acta psych. (Københ.) 22, 69–95, 1947.

MÜLLER, R. and G. WOHLFART: Craniopharyngiomas. Acta Med. Scand. 138, 121–138, 1950.

MÜLLER, WALTER: Änderung des Gewebscharakters nicht radikal operierter Gliome. Zschr. Neurol. 148, 469–477, 1933.

MÜLLER, WALTER: Weitere Untersuchungen über die Entdifferenzierung von Gliomen nach operativem Eingriff. Erg. Path. 60, 1934

MÜLLER, WILHELM: Zur Frage der hyophysären Tumoren vom Mischtyp. Acta Neurovegetativa 8, 451–465, 1954.

MÜLLER, WILHELM und F. MARCOS: Über das Vorkommen von Ganglienzellen in einem Hypophysentumor. Virchows Arch. 325, 733–736, 1954.

MÜLLER, WILHELM und F. OSWALD: Über das Vorkommen von Zysten in Hypophysentumoren. Zbl. Neurochir. 14, 272–281, 1954.

MÜLLER, WILHELM und H. W. PIA: Zur Klinik und Ätiologie der Massenblutungen in Hypophysenadenomen. Dt. Z. Nervenheilk. 170, 326–336, 1953.

MULLIGAN, R. M., K. T. NEUBUERGER, J. T. LUCAS and W. B. LEWIS: Intracranial neoplasms produced in dogs by methylcholanthrene. Exper. Med. a. Surg. 4, 7–19, 1946.

MURATORIO, A., L. PERRIA and U. SACCHI: On the so-called circumscribed type of glioblastoma multiforme. Pathologica 46, 1954.

MURRAY, M. R.: Comparative data on tissue culture of acoustic neurilemmoma and meningioma. J. Neuropath. 1, 123, 1942.

MUSHETT, CH. W.: Elektive Differenzierungsstörungen des ZNS am Hühnchenkeim nach kurzfristigem Sauerstoffmangel. Beitr. path. Anat. 367–387, 1953.

MUTHMANN, A. und E. SAUERBECK: Über eine Gliageschwulst des 4. Ventrikels. – Neuroepithelioma gliomatosum. Beitr. path. Anat. 34, 445, 1903.

MYERSON, J.: Multiple tumors of the brain of diverse origin. J. Neuropath. 1, 406–415, 1942.

NAESLUND, J.: A study of neuro-epithelioma gliomatosum. Upsala Läkoref. Förh. **31**, 193, 1926.

NAFFZIGER, H. C. and E. B. BOLDREY: Cancer of nervous system (Brain, spinal cord and peripheral nerves). J. Amer. Med. Assoc. **136**, 96–103, 1948.

NATONEK, D.: Zur Kenntnis der primären Epitheltumoren des Gehirns. Virchows Arch. **218**, 170, 1914.

NETSKY, M. G., B. AUGUST and W. FOWLER: The longevity of patients with glioblastoma multiforme. J. Neurosurg. **7**, 261–269, 1950.

NETSKY, M. G. and R. R. J. STROBOS: Neoplasms within the midbrain. Arch. Neurol. Psychiat. **68**, 116–129, 1952.

NEUBÜRGER, K. T.: Über das Auftreten von Gliomen nach Kriegsschußverletzungen. Münch. med. Wschr. **13**, 508, 1925.

NEUBUERGER, K. T. and C. L. DAVIS: Cerebral tumor in a dog resembling human medulloblastoma. Cancer Res. **3**, 243- 247, 1943.

NEUBUERGER, K. T. and W. L. SILCOTT: Angioma simplex of the pons. J. Nerv. Ment. Dis. **94**, 586–592, 1941.

NIEMEYER, P.: Diagnostic angiographique des hernies cérébrales. Acta Neurochir. **4**, 241–260, 1955.

NIEMEYER, P. e A. AKERMAN: Diagnostik und chirurgische Behandlung der arteriovenösen Hirnaneurysmen. Med. Cir. Farm. **1953**, 204.

NISHII, B.: Zur Kenntnis der diffusen Sarkomatose des Nervensystems. Arb. Neur. Inst. Wien **31**, 116–129, 1929.

NOETZEL, H.: Arachnoidalcysten in der Cisterna ambiens. Zbl. Neurochir. **4**, 281–294, 1940.

NOETZEL, H.: Über Meningeome und ihre unterschiedlichen Auswirkungen am Gehirn. Beitr. path. Anat. u. allgem. Path. **111**, 391–406, 1951.

NOETZEL, H.: Vortrag Arbeitsgemeinschaft Hirntraumafragen. Mainz 1953.

NONNE, M.: Über diffuse Sarkomatose der Pia mater des ganzen Zentralnervensystems. Dtsch. Z. Nervenhk. **21**, 396, 1902.

NORDENSTAM, H. and N. RINGERTZ: Cerebellar astrocytoma. J. Neuropath. **10**, 343–367, 1951.

NORLÉN, G.: Arteriovenous aneurysms of the brain. — Report of ten cases of total removal of the lesion. J. Neurosurg. **6**, 475, 1949.

NORLÉN, G.: Papillomas of the choroid plexus. Acta Chir. Scand. **99**, 273–279, 1950.

NORTHFIELD, D. W. C. and D. S. RUSSELL: The fate of thorium dioxide (thorotrast) in cerebral arteriography. Lancet **1**, 377, 1937.

NORTHFIELD, D. W. C.: Acoustic neurinoma. J. Neurol. Neurosurg. (London) **13**, 277–279, 1950.

NOWOTNY, K. und UIBERALL: Zur Kenntnis der Neurinome des Trigeminus. Zschr Neurol. **150**, 75- 99, 1934.

OBERDISSE, K. und W. TÖNNIS: Pathophysiologie, Klinik und Behandlung der Hypophysenadenome. Erg. inn. Med. u. Kinderhk. **4**, 975- 1057, 1953.

OBERLING, CH.: Les tumeurs des méninges. Bull. Assoc. Franç. étude Canc. **11**, 365, 1922.

OBERLING, CH.: A propos des glioses méningées (Gliose méningo-encéphalique) des centres nerveux et du nerf optique. Rev. biol. Canad. **2**, 120, 1943.

OBERLING, CH. et P. GUÉRIN: La production expérimentale de tumeurs hypophysaires chez le rat. C. r. Soc. Biol. Paris, Dec. 1936.

OBRADOR ALCALDE, S.: Case report: Hairy teratomatous cyst in the occipito-cerebellar region. J. Neurol. Psychiat. **17**, 298–299, 1954.

OBRADOR, S. und E. LEY: Personal experience with cerebral cysticercosis. Acta neurochir. (Wien) **1**, 434, 1951.

OBRADOR ALCALDE, S., MORALES PLEGUEZUELO y J. J. VAZQUEZ ANON: Ependimoblastomas de la medula cervical. Rev. Clin. Espan. **45**, 304–310, 1952.

OBRADOR ALCALDE, S. und F. SOTO: Condroma frontal de la hoz del cerebro. Rev. Clin. Espan. **51**, 257–260, 1953.

OLIVECRONA, H.: Zwei Ganglioneurome des Großhirns. Virchows Arch. **226**, 1, 1919.

OLIVECRONA, H.: Die chirurgische Behandlung der Hirntumoren. Springer 1927.

OLIVECRONA, H.: Die Gliome der Großhirnhemisphären. Dtsch. Z. Nervenhk. **128**, 1–44, 1932.

OLIVECRONA, H.: On suprasellar cholesteatomas. Brain **55**, 122, 1932.

OLIVECRONA, H.: Die parasagittalen Meningeome. Georg Thieme-Verlag, Leipzig 1934.

OLIVECRONA, H.: Die spezielle Chirurgie der Gehirnkrankheiten. III. Bd., S. 193–374. Enke-Verlag, Stuttgart 1941.

OLIVECRONA, H.: Cholesteatomas of the cerebello-pontine angle. Acta psychiatr. (Kobenh.) 24, 639, 1949.

OLIVECRONA, H.: Die arteriovenösen Aneurysmen des Gehirns. Dtsch. med. Wschr. 75, 1169–1173, 1950.

OLIVECRONA, H.: The cerebellar angioreticulomas. J. Neurosurg. 9, 317–330, 1952.

OLIVECRONA, H. and H. URBAN: Über Meningeome der Siebbeinplatte. Beitr. klin. Chir. 161, 224, 1935.

OPALSKI, A.: Studien zur allgemeinen Histopathologie der Ventrikelwände. Zschr. Neurol. 150, 42–74, 1934.

OPPENHEIM, H.: Die Geschwülste im Gehirn. Wien 1902 (Nothnagels Spec. Path. u. Therapie, Bd. 9).

OPPENHEIM, H. und F. KRAUSE: Operative Erfolge bei Geschwülsten der Sehhügel und Vierhügelgegend. Berl. klin. Wschr. 50, 2316–2322, 1913.

ORR, T. G.: Actinomycoma of the third ventricle.

ORZECHOWSKI, K. v.: Neurinome. Pathologische Anatomie in: Hdb. Haut- u. Geschlechtskrankh. Bd. XII, 2, S. 161, Springer, Berlin 1932.

ORZECHOWSKI, K. v. und Z. W. KULIGOWSKI: Ein Fall von Neuroblastoma verum des Stirnlappens. Zschr. Neurol. 147, 696–712, 1933.

OSTERTAG, B.: Über raumbeengende Neubildungen im Schädel. Fortschr. Röntgenstr. 52, 329, 1935.

OSTERTAG, B.: Einteilung und Charakteristik der Hirngewächse. Fischer, Jena 1936.

OSTERTAG, B.: Anatomie und Pathologie der raumfordernden Prozesse des Schädelbinnenraumes. In: Spezielle Chirurgie der Gehirnkrankheiten. Neue Deutsche Chirurgie, Bd. 50, III. F. Enke, Stuttgart 1941.

OSTERTAG, B.: Die Onkotopik der Hirngewächse. J. Nerv. Ment. Dis. 116, 726–738, 1952.

OSTERTAG, B. und H. BUSCHMANN: Wieweit kann Wehrdienstbeschädigung bei Geschwülsten angenommen werden? Med. Klin. 37, 351–353, 1941.

OSTERTAG, B., O. STOCHDORPH und G. SCHMIDT: Zur Spongioblastose und Spongioblastomatose des Gehirns, ihrer Charakteristik und pathogenetischen Bedeutung. Arch. Psychiatr. 182, 249–274, 1949.

OSTERTAG, B., O. STOCHDORPH und G. SCHMIDT: Die Gliomtypen des Hirnstammes und des Allocortex: Spongioblastosen, -blastomatosen und spongioblastische Glioblastome. Arch. Psychiatr. 185, 314–325, 1950.

OVERHAMM, G. C.: JACKSON-Epilepsie auf Grund von Gehirnmetastasen eines primären Schilddrüsencarcinoms. Zschr. Neurol. 98, 755, 1925.

PAARMANN, H.-FR.: Das Retinagliom und seine Metastasen. Virchows Arch. 322, 49–65, 1952.

PAPPENHEIMER, A. M.: Über Geschwülste des Corpus pineale. Virchows Arch. 200, 122, 1910.

PARKER, E. F. and J. W. KERNOHAN: The relation of injury and glioma of the brain. J. Amer. Med. Assoc. 97, 535–539, 1931.

PASS, K. E.: Erbpathologische Untersuchungen in Familien von Hirntumorkranken. Zschr. Neurol. 161, 204–211, 1938.

PAUL, F.: Beitrag zur Histopathologie der Ganglioneurome des Zentralnervensystems. Beitr. path. Anat. 75, 221–228, 1926.

PEDERSEN, O. und H. GEYER: Diskordantes Auftreten von Hirntumoren bei erbgleichen Zwillingen. Zbl. Neurochir. 3, 53–63, 1938.

PEERS, J. H.: The occurence of tumors of the CNS in routine autopsies. Amer. J. Path. 12, 911, 1936.

PEERS, J. H.: The response of the central nervous system to the application of carcinogenic hydrocarbons. I. Dibencanthracene. Amer. J. Path. 15, 261–272, 1939.

PENFIELD, W.: Principles of the pathology of neurosurgery. Chapter VI, 303–347. Nelson & Sons, 1927 (Suppl. 1932).

PENFIELD, W.: A paper on the classification of brain tumors and its practical application. Brit. med. J. 1931, 337.

PENFIELD, W.: Tumors of the sheaths of the nervous system. Kapitel 19 in PENFIELDS Cytology and cellular pathology of the nervous system, S. 955–990. Hoeber 1932.

PENNYBACKER, J.: Recurrence in cerebellar haemangiomas. Zbl. Neurochir. 14, 63–73, 1954.

PENNYBACKER, J. and H. CAIRNS: Results in 130 cases of acoustic neurinoma. J. Neurol., Neurosurg., (London) 13, 272–277, 1950.

PENNYBACKER, J. and SP. MEADOWS: Normal ventriculogramms in tumors of the hemispheres. Lancet **1938**, I, 186.

PNNEYBACKER, J. and D. S. RUSSELL: Necrosis of the brain due to radiation therapy. J. Neurol., Neurosurg. (London) **11**, 183–198, 1948.

PERLMUTTER, I., G. HORRAX and J. L. POPPEN: Cystic hemangioblastomas of the cerebellum: Endresults in 25 verified cases. Surg. Gynec. Obstet. **91**, 89–99, 1950.

PERRET, G. E.: Experimentelle Untersuchungen über Massenverschiebung und Formveränderungen des Gehirns bei raumbeengenden Prozessen. Zbl. Neurochir. **5**, 5, 1940; Arch. Psychiatr. **112**, 385–408, 1941.

PERRIA, L. e U. SACCHI: Incidenza del fattore eta e dello stroma tumorale sul decorso del glioblastoma. Sistema nervoso **3**, 176–186, 1950.

PERTHES, P.: Glückliche Entfernung eines Tumors des Plexus chorioideus aus dem Seitenventrikel des Cerebrum. Münch. med. Wschr. **66**, 677–678, 1919.

PETERS, G.: Zur Pathogenese der Sturge-Weberschen Krankheit. Zschr. Neurol. **164**, 365–379, 1939.

PETERS, G.: Beitrag zur Pathologie und Klinik der Meningeome. Dtsch. Z. Nervenhk. **167**, 83–101, 1951.

PETERS, G.: Hirntrauma und Gliom. Fortschr. Neurol. **20**, 403–422, 1952.

PETERS, G. und F. TEBELIS: Beitrag zur Klinik, Anatomie und Pathogenese der Sturge-Weberschen Erkrankung. Zschr. Neurol. **157**, 782–794, 1937.

PETIT-DUTAILLIS, D.: Traitement chirurgical des méningites séreuses. XIIIe Réunion neurol. intern. ann.-Rev. neurol., Juin 1933.

PETIT-DUTAILLIS, D. et S. DAUM: Les méningiomes de la fosse postérieure. Rev. neurol. **81**, 557–572, 1949.

PETTE, H.: Ausbreitungsweise diffuser meningealer Hirn- und Rückenmarksgeschwülste und ihre Symptomatologie. Dtsch. Z. Nervenhk. **109**, 155, 1929.

PETTE, H.: Zum Problem der Allgemeinerscheinungen beim Tumor cerebri. Dtsch. Z. Nervenhk. **130**, 1–4, 1933.

PETTE, H.: Die verschiedenen Formen der Meningitis serosa. Zbl. Neurochir. **1**, 86–98, 1936.

PETTE, H.: Pachymeningitis und Leptomeningitis. Handb. d. Neurol. BUMKE-FOERSTER, Bd. 10, S. 268–412. Springer, Berlin 1936.

PETTE, H.: Klinik der Hirngeschwülste. Zschr. Neurol. **161**, 10–68, 1938.

PETTE, H.: Die bösartigen Geschwülste des Zentralnervensystems. Münch. med. Wschr. **1951**, 1–6 u. 67–74.

PETTE, H. und ST. KÖRNYEY: Zur Kenntnis der Rückenmarksgliome mit Ausgang in Syringomyelie. Dtsch. Z. Nervenhk. **117, 118, 119**, 371–408, 1931.

PFLEGER, L.: Beobachtungen über Hetertopie grauer Substanz im Mark des Kleinhirns. Zbl. med. Wissenschaften **26**, 468–469, 1880.

PIA, H. W.: Die Verquellung der Cisterna basalis und ambiens im Hirngefäßbild. Acta Neurochir. (Wien) **3**, 315–328, 1953.

PIA, H. W.: Klinik und Syndrome der Schläfenlappengeschwülste. Fortschr. Neurol. **21**, 555–595, 1953.

PICK, L. und M. BIELSCHOWSKY: Über das System der Neurome und Beobachtung an einem Ganglioneurom des Gehirns nebst Untersuchung über die Genese der Nervenfasern in „Neurinomen". Zschr. Neurol. **6**, 391–437, 1911.

PILCHER, C.: Spongioblastoma polare of the pons. Arch. Neurol. Psychiat. **32**, 1210–1230, 1934.

PIMENTA, DE MATTOS, A. und W. E. MAFFEI: Neuroepitelioma cerebral. J. Brasil. Neurol. **2**, 21–29, 1950.

PIMENTA, DE MATTOS, A., F. DE BASTOS OLIVEIRA und W. E. MAFFEI: Die BOECKsche Krankheit. Acta Neurochir. (Wien) **4**, 261–276, 1955.

PINHEIRO, J. y A. R. DE MELLO: Consideracões sobre a cisticercose encefalica. Arch. serv. nac. doenças mentais **1943**, 773.

PINTO, F.: Ein Meningeom mit 22jährigem Wachstum. Zbl. Path. **90**, 403, 1953.

PINTO, F.: Sôbre o problema do edema e da tumefaçao cerebral. Medicina Cirurgia Farmacia **208**, 337–353, 1953.

PINTO PUPO, P. y A. MATTOS PIMENTA: Cisticercose do IV ventriculo; consideracões anatomo-clinicas e sobre a terapeutica cirurgica. Arquivos de Neuro-Psiquiatria **7**, 274–291, 1949.

PLUVINAGE, R.: Teleangiectasies et angiomes caverneux cérébraux. Semaine Hôp. 859, 1948.

POLMETEER, F. E. and J. W. KERNOHAN: Meningeal gliomatosis: Study of 42 cases. Arch. Neurol. Psychiat. 57, 593–616, 1947.

POLZER-HODITZ, CHR. v.: Wert und Möglichkeiten der sogenannten histologischen Schnelldiagnosen. Inaug.-Diss. Basel 1952. – Mikroskopie (Wien) 6, 339–352, 1951.

POMERAT, C. M.: Dynamic neuropathology. J. Neuropath. 14, 28–38, 1955.

POPPEN, J. L. and A. B. KING: Chordoma: Experience with thirteen cases. J. Neurosurg. 9, 139–163, 1952.

PORTUGAL, J. R. and A. AKERMAN: Tumor do lobo frontal esquerdo (astroblastoma). Hemiplegia homolateral. J. Brasil. Neur. 1, 317–327, 1949.

PORTUGAL, J. R., P. ELEJALDE and N. COSTA: Meningeomas supra-selares. J. Brasil. Neurol. 1, 455–505, 1949.

POSSELT, A : Die vielkammerige Blasenwurmgeschwulst außerhalb der Leber (extrahepat. Alveolarechinokokkus). Erg. allg. Path. 26, 423–611, 1932.

PRADO, J. M.: Contribucion al estudio de los hemangioblastomas del cerebelo. Arch. histol. normal y patol. 1, 207–231, 1942.

PRADO, J. M., T. INSAUSTI y R. F. MATERA: Gliomas mixtos. Astroblastoma-Oligodendrocitoma, relato de un caso. Arch. Neurocir. (Buenos Aires) 7, 439–445, 1950.

PRIESEL, A.: Über Gewebsmißbildungen in der Neurohypophyse und am Infundibulum des Menschen. Virchows Arch. 238, 423–440, 1922.

PRYM, P.: Über das Endotheliom der Dura. Virchows Arch. 215, 212–216, 1914.

PUECH, P.: Les tumeurs de l'hypophyse, leur diagnostic précoce et les indications therapeutiques. Masson & Cie., Paris 1934.

PUECH, P., M. DAVID et M. BRUN: Contribution à l'étude des arachnoidites opto-chiasmatiques. Rev. d'Oto-Neuro-Ophthalm. 11, 641–649, 1933.

PUECH, P. et L. STUHL: Adénomes de l'hypophyse. Presse Méd. Nr. 55, 1934.

PUTSCHAR, W.: Pathologie und Symptomatologie der Carcinommetastasen im ZNS. Zschr. Neurol 126, 129–148, 1930.

PUTSCHAR, W.: Über Angiomatosis des Zentralnervensystems. Münch. med. Wschr. 1935, 1084.

PUUSEPP, L.: Die Tumoren des Gehirns, ihre Symptomatologie, Diagnostik und operative Behandlung. Dorpat (Tartu) 1927/1929.

QUARTI, M.: Considerazioni anatomoradiologiche sull'adenoma dell'ipofisi. Chir. (Milano) 8, 387–391, 1953.

QUODBACH, K.: Ein Beitrag zur Pathologie der Blastomykosen des Zentralnervensystems. Zbl. Path. 69, 227–231, 1938.

RAAF, J. E. and J. W. KERNOHAN: Relation of abnormal collections of cells in posterior medullary velum of cerebellum to origin of medulloblastomas. Arch. Neurol. Psychiat. 52, 163–169, 1944.

RADERMECKER, R.: A propos du rapport entre traumatisme cérébral et gliome. J. Belge Neurol. 35, 699–708, 1935.

RAND, C. W.: Hemangioma of the spinal cord. Arch. Neurol. Psychiat. 18, 755, 1927.

RAND, C. W.: Multiple primary tumors compromising the central nervous system. Bull. of the Los Angeles Neurol. Soc. 19, 128–134, 1954.

RAND, C. W. and D. L. REEVES: Dermoid and epidermoid tumors (cholesteatomas) of the central nervous system. Report of twenty-three cases. Arch. Surg. 46, 350–376, 1943.

RANKE, O.: Histologisches zur Gliomfrage. Zschr. Neurol. 5, 690, 1911.

RAPP: Über die Häufigkeit der Hirntumoren unter dem Sektionsmaterial d. Path. Inst. Tübingen. Diss. Tübingen 1924.

RASDOLSKY, J.: Tuberkel des Gehirns. Zschr. Neurol. 154, 18, 1935.

RASMUSSEN, T. B., J. W. KERNOHAN and A. W. ADSON: Pathologic classification, with surgical consideration, of intraspinal tumors. Ann. Surg. 111, 513–530, 1940.

RATZENHOFER, M.: Beitrag zur Kenntnis des Lipoidgehaltes der Neurinome. Virchows Arch. 306, 193–227, 1940.

RAUCH, H. J.: Die Ausbreitungsart der Gliome und ihr Einfluß auf den Gewebsaufbau. Arch. Psychiatr. 117, 479–540, 1944.

v. RECKLINGHAUSEN, F.: Über die multiplen Fibrome der Haut und ihre Beziehung zu den multiplen Neuromen. Festschrift f. Virchow. A. Hirschwald, Berlin 1882.

REICHARDT, M.: Hirnschwellung. Allg. Z. Psychiatr. 75, 34, 1919.

REICHL, L. u. BIRKMAYER, W.: Zwei vom Clivus Blumenbachii ausgehende Meningeome. Nervenarzt 12, 508, 1939.

REINHARDT, G.: Trauma-Fremdkörper-Hirngeschwulst. Münch. med. Wschr. **1928**, 399.

RETTELBACH, E. und SCHUTZBACH: Über Sehnerventumoren, ihre Beziehungen zur Neurofibromatosis Recklinghausen und ihr klinisches Krankheitsbild. v. Graefes Arch. Augenhk. **145**, 179—241, 1941.

REYMOND, A.: Classification anatomo-pathologique des tumeurs cérébrales. Ophthalmologica **125**, 204—230, 1953.

REYMOND, A.: Méningites tumorales. Oncologia **6**, 85—91, 1953.

REYMOND, A. et N. RINGERTZ: L'oligodendrogliome. Arch. Suisses Neurol. **65**, 221—254, 1950.

RHOADS, C. P. und W. P. VAN WAGENEN: Observations on the histology of the tumors of the nervus acusticus. Amer. J. Path. **4**, 145, 1928.

RIBBERT, H.: Über das Endotheliom der Dura. Virchows Arch. **200**, 141, 1910.

RIBBERT, H.: Über das Spongioblastom und das Gliom. Virchows Arch. **225**, 195, 1918.

RICH, Th A. R.: The pathogenesis of tuberculosis. Thomas, Springfield 1944.

RIESSNER, D. und K. J. ZÜLCH: Über die Formveränderungen des Hirns (Massenverschiebungen, Zisternenverquellungen bei raumbeengenden Prozessen). Dtsch. Z. Chir. **253**, 1—61, 1939.

RINGERTZ, N.: ,,Grading" of gliomas. Acta path. microbiol. Scand. **27**, 51—64, 1950.

RINGERTZ, N.: On the question of different histologic types of medulloblastoma. Excerpta med. Neurol. Psychiat. **8**, 820, 1955.

RINGERTZ, N. und EHRNER: Über Sarkombildung bei Recklinghausenscher Neurofibromatose. Zschr. Neurol. **177**, 297, 1944.

RINGERTZ, N. and FLYGER, G.: Tumors of the pineal region. J. Neuropath. **13**, 540—561, 1954.

RINGERTZ, N. and H. NORDENSTAM: Cerebellar astrocytoma. J. Neuropath. **10**, 343—367, 1951.

RINGERTZ, N. and A. REYMOND: Ependymomas and choroid plexus papillomas. J. Neuropath. **8**, 355—380, 1949.

RINGERTZ, N. and J. H. TOLA: Medulloblastoma. J. Neuropath. **9**, 354—372, 1950.

RINKE, H. W.: Zur Kenntnis der Ependymome. Zschr. Neurol. **148**, 736—752, 1933.

ROBERTSON, H. E.: Das Ganglioneuroblastom, ein besonderer Typus im System der Neurome. Virchows Arch. **220**, 147, 1914.

ROBERTSON, H. E.: Ein Fall von Ganglioneuroma am Boden des dritten Ventrikels mit Einbeziehung des Chiasma opticum. Virchows Arch. **220**, 80, 1915.

ROCA DE VINALS, R.: Citodiagnóstico clinico. Anales del Hospital de la Santa Cruz y San Pablo.

ROCHAT, G. F.: Großhirnangiom bei der Lindauschen (v. Hippelschen) Erkrankung. Klin. Mschr. f. Augenhk. **86**, 23, 1931.

RÖSSLE, R.: 2 Fälle von Gliomen auf traumatischer Basis. Münch. med. Wschr. 2530, 1911.

RÖSSLE, R.: Das Retothelsarkom der Lymphdrüsen. Beitr. path. Anat. **103**, 385, 1939.

RÖSSLE, R.: Stufen der Malignität. Sitz.ber. Dtsch. Akad. Wissensch. Berlin 1949, Akademie-Verlag 1950 u. Dtsch. med. Wschr. **75**, 1950.

RÖTTGEN, P.: Weitere Erfahrungen an kongenitalen arteriovenösen Aneurysmen des Schädelinneren. Zbl. Neurochir. **2**, 18—34, 1937.

RÖTTGEN, P.: Über arterio-venöse Rankenangiome des Kleinhirns. Zbl. Neurochir. **8**, 161—171, 1943.

RÖTTGEN, P. und G. PETERS: Über Massenblutungen in Hypophysenadenomen. Zbl. Neurochir. **12**, 65—73, 1952.

ROMAN, B.: Zur Kenntnis des Neuroepithelioma gliomatosum. Virchows Arch. **211**, 126, 1913.

ROMEIS, B.: Blutgefäß- und Lymphgefäßapparate — 6. Bd. im Handb. d. mikrosk. Anat. d. Menschen. Springer, Berlin 1940.

ROMEIS, B.: Mikroskoipsche Technik. Leibniz, München 1948.

ROSENHAGEN, H.: Zur Klinik des Angioma racemosum arteriovenosum der Rückenmarkshäute. Zschr. Neurol. **147**, 216—229, 1933.

ROSENTHAL, W.: Über eine eigentümliche, mit Syringomyelie komplizierte Geschwulst des Rückenmarks. Beitr. path. Anat. **23**, 111, 1898.

ROTHMANN, A.: Eine ungewöhnlich große Arachnoidalcyste. Zbl. Path. **73**, 5, 1939.

ROULET, F.: Über das Verhalten der Bindegewebsfasern unter normalen und pathologischen Bedingungen. Erg. allg. Path. **32**, 1, 1937.

ROULET, F.: Die ausgesprochen blastomatösen Retikulosen. Verh. d. Dtsch. Ges. f. Path. 37. Tagg., Marburg 1953. — Stuttgart, G. Fischer 1954, S. 105–126.

ROUSSY, G. et L. CORNIL: A propos de la classification des tumeurs des méninges. Rev. neurol. 49, 122, 1928.

ROUSSY, G., R. LEROUX et CH. OBERLING: Précis d'Anatomie Pathologique. Masson, Paris 1950.

ROUSSY, G., J. LHERMITTE et L. CORNIL: Essai de classification des tumeurs cérébrales. Ann. Anat. path. 1, 333–378, 1924.

ROUSSY, G. et CH. OBERLING: Les tumeurs angiomateuses des centres nerveux. Presse méd. 11, 1–32, 1930.

ROUSSY, G. et CH. OBERLING: Atlas du cancer. Felix Alcan 1931.

ROUSSY, G. and CH. OBERLING: Histologic classification cf tumors of the central nervous system. Arch. Neurol. Psychiat. 27, 1281–1289, 1932.

ROUSSY, G. et CH. OBERLING: Contribution à l'étude des tumeurs hypophysaires. Presse méd. 1933, 1799.

ROUSSY, G., CH. OBERLING et C. RAILEANU: Les neurospongiomes. Presse méd. 977–981, 1931.

ROWBOTHAM, G. F.: The hyperostoses in relation with the meningiomas. Brit. J. Surg. 26, 593, 1939.

RÜBSAMEN, H.: Mißbildungen durch Sauerstoffmangel im Experiment und in der menschlichen Pathologie. Verh. d. Ges. Dt. Naturf. u. Ärzte, Freiburg, Sept. 1954. Berlin-Göttingen-Heidelberg, Springer 1955, S. 126–132.

RUDERSHAUSEN, V.: Über Häufigkeit und Art der Hirngeschwülste an Hand des Sektionsmaterials des Path. Inst. Heidelberg. Virchows Arch. 285, 318, 1932.

RUF, F. und K. PHILIPP: Die Verwendung radioaktiver Isotope in Diagnostik und Therapie. Röntgen- u. Labor-Praxis 4, 236, 1951.

RUSSELL, D. S.: The occurence and distribution of intranuclear „inclusion bodies" in gliomas. J. Path. Bact. 35, 625–634, 1932.

RUSSELL, D. S.: Histological technique for intracranial tumors. Oxford University Press 1939.

RUSSELL, D. S.: Angiectasias y angiomas de cerebro y medula espinal. Actas Espanolas de Neurologia y Psiquiatria 2, 133–152, 1941.

RUSSELL, D. S.: The pinealoma: its relationship to teratoma. J. Path. Bact. 56, 145–150, 1944.

RUSSELL, D. S.: Meningeal tumours: a review. J. Clin. Path. 3, 191–211, 1950.

RUSSELL, D. S.: Observations on the pathology of hydrocephalus. Her Majesty's Stationary Office, London 1949/1952.

RUSSELL, D. S.: „Ectopic pinealoma": its kinship to atypical teratoma of the pineal gland. Report of a case. J. Path. Bact. 68, 125, 1954.

RUSSELL, D. S.: Polar spongioblastomas: their place in the glioma series. Excerpta Med., Neur. Psych. 8, S. 818, 1955.

RUSSELL, D. S. and J. O. W. BLAND: A study of tumors by tissue culture. J. Path. Bact. 36, 273, 1933.

RUSSELL, D. S. and J. O. W. BLAND: Further notes on the tissue culture of gliomas with special reference to BAILEYs spongioblastoma. J. Path. Bact. 39, 375, 1934.

RUSSELL, D. S. and R. W. B. ELLIS: Circumscribed cerebral tumors in young infants. Arch. dis. Childh. 8, 329, 1933.

RUSSELL, D. S., C. W. WILSON and K. TANSLEY: Experimental radio-necrosis of the brain in rabbits. J. Neurol., Neurosurg. (London) 12, 187, 1949.

RUSSELL, W. O and E. SACHS: Pinealoma. A clinicopathologic study of seven cases with a review of the literatur. Arch. Path. 35, 240–261, 1943.

SACCHI, U.: I tumori cerebrali sperimentali. Sistema Nervoso 3, 209–222, 1953.

SACCONE, A. and J. A. EPSTEIN: Granuloblastoma, primary neuroectodermal tumor of cerebellum. J. Neuropath. 7, 287–298, 1948.

SACCONE, A. and O. ROSENTHAL: Chorioid papillomas. Arch. Path. 25, 850, 1938.

SACHS, E.: The diagnosis and treatment of brain tumors. C. V. Mosby Co., St. Louis 1931.

SACHS, E.: The problem of the glioblastomas. J. Neurosurg. 7, 185–189, 1950.

SAGER, O. et J. BAZGAN: Oligodendroblastome intéressant le corps calleux. Rev. neurol. 72, 32–40, 1939/1940.

SALUS, F.: Zur Kenntnis der malignen Hypophysenadenome. Zschr. Neurol. 148, 574 bis 583, 1933.

Sántha, K. v.: Diffuse Lemmoblastose des ZNS. Zschr. Neurol. **154**, 763, 1936.

Santos, R. dos: Arteriography in bone tumours. J. Bone Joint Surg. **32**, 15–29, 1950.

Santos, J. and W. Pagel: Oligodendroglioma with extracranial metastasis. Brit. J. Surg. **39**, 56, 1951.

Sans and Alexander: Vascular pattern of certain intracranial neoplasmas. Arch. Neurol. Psychiat. **42**, 44, 1939.

Saxer, F.: Ein Beitrag zur Kenntnis der Dermoide und Teratome. Beitr. path. Anat. **31**, 452, 1902.

Saxer, F.: Ependymepithel, Gliom und epitheliale Geschwülste. Beitr. path. Anat. **32**, 316, 1902.

Schade, H.: Über Quellungsphysiologie und Ödementstehung. Erg. inn. Med. **32**, 425–463, 1927.

Schär, W. und E. Christensen: Mißbildungstumoren des Großhirns. Zbl. Neurochir. **4**, 142–154, 1939.

Schaffer, K.: Bemerkungen zur Histopathologie des Hirnglioms. Mschr. Psychiatr **65**, 208, 1927.

Schaltenbrand, G.: Sobre una familia con enfermedad de Recklinghausen. Prensa méd. argent. **20**, 2011, 1933.

Schaltenbrand, G.: Hirngeschwulst und Lebensalter. Zbl. Neurochir. **3**, 169–188, 1938.

Schaltenbrand, G.: Die Nervenkrankheiten. II. (Röntgenschäden: S. 576). Thieme 1951.

Schaltenbrand, G. und P. Bailey: Die perivasculäre Gliamembran des Gehirns. J. Psychol. u. Neurol. **35**, 251, 1928.

Schaper: Die frühesten Differenzierungsvorgänge im ZNS. Arch. Entw.mechan. **5**, 81–130, 1897.

Scheid, P.: Über Geschwulstbildung nach Schußverletzung. Frankf. Z. Path. **51**, 446, 1938.

Scheidegger, S.: Die extramedullären pialen Lipome des Rückenmarks. Zschr Neurol. **154**, 507, 1936.

Scheinker, I. M.: Beitrag zur Frage der diffusen Sklerose (diffuse Glioblastose des ZNS). Dtsch. Z. Nervenhk. **139**, 253, 1936.

Scheinker, I. M.: Beitrag zur Frage der zentralen Neurinome. Zschr. Neurol. **155**, 1936.

Scheinker, I. M.: Über die Umwandlung gutartiger Hirngliome in bösartige Glioblastome. Dtsch. Z. Nervenhk. **145**, 54–69, 1938.

Scheinker, I. M.: Zur Frage der Pathogenese und Pathologie der Medulloblastome. Mschr. Psychiatr. **101**, 103–113, 1939.

Scheinker, I. M.: Subependymoma: A newly recognized tumor of subependymal derivation. J. Neurosurg. **2**, 232–240, 1945.

Scheinker, I. M.: Neurosurgical pathology. Ch. C. Thomas, Springfield 1948.

Scheinker, I. M. and I. P. Evans: Diffuse cerebral glioblastosis. J. Neuropath. **2**, 178–189, 1943.

Schellenberg, W.: Eigenartiger Tumor des Schädeldaches als Folge eines Schädeltraumas. Frankf. Z. Path. **38**, 319–324, 1929.

Scheller, H.: Liquorbefunde bei Hirngeschwülsten. Mschr. Psychiatr. **95**, 257-324, 1937.

Scherer, E.: Über Zystenbildung der weichen Häute der Sylviischen Furche mit hochgradiger Deformation des Gehirns. Zschr. Neurol. **152**, 787, 1935.

Scherer, E.: Über die pialen Lipome des Gehirns. Zschr. Neurol. **154**, 45–61, 1935.

Scherer, H. J.: Gliomstudien I: Die Bedeutung des Mesenchyms in Gliomen. Virchows Arch. **291**, 321–340, 1933.

Scherer, H. J.: Untersuchungen über den geweblichen Aufbau der Geschwülste des peripheren Nervensystems. Virchows Arch. **292**, 479–553, 1934.

Scherer, H. J.: Gliomstudien II. Virchows Arch. **294**, 795, 1935.

Scherer, H. J.: Influence des tumeurs méningées sur le tissu cérébral. Rev. neurol. **66**, 307–322, 1936.

Scherer, H. J.: Structural development in gliomas. Amer. J. Cancer **34**, 333, 1938.

Scherer, H. J.: The frequency of gliomas having variable histological structure. J. Belge Neurol. **38**, 1, 1938.

Scherer, H. J.: A critical review: the pathology of cerebral gliomas. J. Belge Neurol. **3**, 147–177, 1940.

Scherer, H. J.: The forms of growth in gliomas and their practical significance. Brain **63**, 1–112, 1940.

Scherer, H. J.: Vergleichende Pathologie des Nervensystems der Säugetiere. Thieme, Leipzig 1944.

SCHIEFER, W.: Über Sellaveränderungen bei gesteigertem Schädelinnendruck. Zbl. Neurochir. **14**, 281–283, 1954.

SCHIEFER, W. und G. UDVARHELYI: Das Glioblastoma multiforme im Serienangiogramm. Acta Neurochir. (Wien) **4**, 76–105, 1954.

SCHLEUSSING, H.: Zur Histogenese der tuberkulösen Käseherde im Gehirn. Zbl. ges. Neurol. **116**, 340–341, 1952.

SCHMID, R. und R. GAUPP: Zur Frage der Angioblastomatose des Rückenmarks. Nervenarzt **16**, 290–309, 1943.

SCHMIDT, M. B.: Über die Pacchionischen Granulationen und ihr Verhalten zu den Sarkomen und Psammomen der Dura mater. Virchows Arch. **170**, 429, 1902.

SCHMINCKE, A.: Beitrag zur Lehre der Ganglioneurome: Ein Ganglioneurom des Gehirns. Beitr. path. Anat. **47**, 354–371, 1909/10.

SCHMINCKE, A.: Ein Ganglioglioneurom des Gehirns. Zbl. Path. Erg.-Bd. **25**, 1914; Verh. Dtsch. Path. Ges. **17**, 537, 1914.

SCHMINCKE, A.: Zur Kenntnis der diffusen, meningealen Gliome des Kleinhirns. Zschr. Neurol. **93**, 109, 1924.

SCHMINCKE, A.: Durale Implantationsmetastasen bei Kleinhirnneurinomen. Beitr. path. Anat. **73**, 511, 1925.

SCHMINCKE, A.: Zur Kenntnis der Zirbelgeschwülste. Ein Ganglioneurom der Zirbel. Beitr. path. Anat. **83**, 279–288, 1930.

SCHMORL, G.: Die pathologisch-histologischen Untersuchungsmethoden. Vogel, Berlin 1934.

SCHNITKER, M. T. and D. AYER: The primary melanomas of the leptomeninges. A clinicopathologic study with a review of the literature and the report of an additional case. J. Nerv. Ment. Dis. **87**, 45, 1938.

SCHÖNBAUER, L.: Über das gehäufte Vorkommen von Karzinomen bei Geschwistern, die Beziehungen der kranken zu den gesunden Geschwistern, gegebenenfalls zur Ascendenz. Wien. klin. Wschr. **65**, 386–389, 1953.

SCHÖPE, M.: Zur Frage Blastom-Encephalitis. Zschr. Neurol. **161**, 177–183, 1938.

SCHÖPE, M.: Über ein Gangliogliom des Occipitallappens mit psychischen Veränderungen. Zschr. Neurol. **174**, 522, 1942.

SCHÖPE, M.: Zur Pathogenese des Meningeoms und des zentralen Neurinoms bei der v. RECKLINGHAUSENschen Krankheit. Arch. Psychiatr. u. Zschr. Neurol. **186**, 603–622, 1951.

SCHOLZ, W.: Über die Einwirkung von Röntgenstrahlen auf das Hirngewebe. Dtsch. Z. Nervenhk. **166**, 133, 1935.

SCHOLZ, W. and Y. K. HSÜ: Late damage from Roentgen irradiation of the human brain. Arch. Neurol. Psychiat. **40**, 928–936, 1938.

SCHROEDER, A. y J. MEDOC: Quiste hidatico del cerebro. Anais do IV. Congr. Sul-Americano de Neurocir., Porte Alegre (Bras.) Mai 1951.

SCHUBACK, A.: Über die Angiomatose des ZNS (LINDAUsche Krankheit). Zschr. Neurol. **110**, 359–371, 1927.

SCHWARTZ, P.: Anatomische Typen der Hirngliome. Nervenarzt **5**, 449–456, 1932.

SCHWARTZ, P.: Anatomische Typen der Hirngliome. Mitt. d. II. intern. Kongr. Krebsforschg., S. 257–260, 1936.

SCHWARTZ, P. and H. R. KLAUER: Diffuse systematische blastomatöse Wucherung des gliösen Apparates im Gehirn. Zschr. Neurol. **109**, 438–452, 1927.

SCOTT, M. and H. T. WYCIS: Intracranial neurinoma of the hypoglossal nerve. J. Neurosurg. **6**, 333–336, 1949.

SEIFARTH, G.: Das Neuroepitheliom des Rückenmarks im Lichte der organoiden Geschwulstbetrachtung. Virchows Arch. **316**, 149–186, 1949.

SELBACH, C. und H.: Die Hirnvolumenvermehrung als Problem der physikalischen Chemie des Hirngewebes. Allg. Z. Psychiatr. **125**, 137–165, 1949.

SELIGMAN, A. M. and SHEAR: Experimental production of brain tumors in mice with methylcholanthrene. Amer. J. Canc. **37**, 364–399, 1939.

SHENKIN, H. A., F. C. GRANT and J. H. DREW: Postoperative period of survival of patients with oligodendroglioma of the brain. Arch. Neurol. Psychiat. **58**, 710–715, 1947.

SHEPS, J. G. and J. L. SIMON: Solitary cerebral gumma. J. Neuropath. **2**, 353–364, 1943.

SHIMIDZU, K.: Ein Operationsfall von Schistosomiasis cerebri. Arch. klin. Chir. **182**, 401 bis 407, 1935.

SILVER, M. L. and G. HENNIGAR: Cerebellar hemangioma (hemangioblastoma). J. Neurosurg. **9**, 484–494, 1952.

SIMON, Th.: Das Spinnenzell- und Pinselzellengliom. Virchows Arch. **61**, 90–100, 1874.

SINGER, L. und J. SEILER: Untersuchungen über die Morphologie der Gliome. Virchows Arch. **287**, 823, 1933; Klin. Wschr. **12**, 20, 1933.

SKILLIKORN, S. A. and R. W. GARRITY: Intracranial Boeck's sarcoid tumor resembling meningioma. J. Neurosurg., **12**, 407–413, 1955.

SLANY,: Anomalien des Circ. art. Villisi in ihrer Beziehung zu Aneurysmenbildung an der Hirnbasis. Virchows Arch. **301**, 62, 1938.

SMITT, W. G. S : Über intracranielle Chondrome. Dtsch. Z. Nervenhk. **109**, 170–177, 1929.

SMYTH, G. E. and STERN: Tumours of the thalamus. Brain **61**, 339, 1938.

SORGO, W.: Weitere Mitteilungen über Klinik und Histologie des kongenitalen arteriovenösen Aneurysmas des Gehirns. Zbl. Neurochir. **3**, 64–87, 1938.

SORGO, W.: Kontrastmitteldiagnostik cerebraler Erkrankungen, Abb. 36/37. Deuticke 1940.

SORGO, W.: Die Liquorveränderungen beim raumbeengenden Prozeß des Gehirns mit besonderer Berücksichtigung der Liquorpassagestörungen. Zbl. Neurochir. **5**, 135–151, 1940.

SORGO, W.: Über Hirntumoren des Kindesalters. Wien. med. Wschr. I, 259–261, 1940.

SORGO, W.: Klinik, Histologie und Operation eines Angioma arteriovenosum congenitale der Arteria cerebri posterior. Zbl. Neurochir. **9**, 108–114, 1949.

SPANNER, R.: Zur Anatomie der arterio-venösen Anastomosen. Verh. Dtsch. Ges. Kreislaufforschg. **18**, 258–277, 1952.

SPATZ, H.: Neuere Ansichten über Pathologie und Prognose der Hirngeschwülste. Münch. med. Wschr. 1930, 825.

SPATZ, H.: Über multizentrisch wachsende Gliome und zur Frage des Gliosarkoms. Zschr. Neurol. **161**, 160–161, 1938.

SPATZ, H. und TH. HASENJÄGER: Über örtliche Veränderungen der Konfiguration des Gehirns bei Hirndruck. Arch. Psychiatr. **107**, 193, 1937.

SPIELMEYER, W.: Histopathologie des Nervensystems. Springer, Berlin 1922.

SPIELMEYER, W.: Technik der mikroskopischen Untersuchung des Nervensystems. Springer 1927.

SPILLER, W. G.: Gliomatosis of the pia and metastasis of glioma. J. Nerv. Ment. Dis. **34**, 297–302, 1907.

SPITZ, E. B., H. A. SHENKIN and F. C. GRANT: Cerebellar medulloblastoma in adults. Arch. Neurol. Psychiat. **57**, 417–422, 1947.

STAEMMLER, M.: Hirngeschwulst und Unfall (Narbengliom). Nervenarzt **19**, 427–431, 1948.

STARR, A.: Brain tumors in childhood. Med. News **29**, 1886.

STARR, A.: Hirnchirurgie. Deuticke, Wién 1894.

STENDER, A.: Über das Meningeom des Keilbeinrückens. Zschr. Neurol. **147**, 244, 1933.

STENDER, A.: Über frontoorbitale Dermoidcysten. Zbl. Neurochir. **2**, 114–123, 1937.

STENDER, A.: Apoplektiformer Krankheitsbeginn bei Hirntumoren (Halbseitenlähmung). Zschr. Neurol. **163**, 123–168, 1938.

STENDER, A.: Arachnitis spinalis. Zbl. Neurochir. **4**, 214–233, 1939.

STENDER, A. und K. J. ZÜLCH: Über die Ventrikeltumoren bei tuberöser Sklerose. Zschr. Neurol. **176**, 556–578, 1943.

STEVENSON, L.: Tumors of the cerebellum. Arch. Neurol. Psychiat. **26**, 875–876, 1931.

STEVENSON, L. and F. ECHLIN: Nature and origin of some tumors of the cerebellum. Arch. Neurol. Psychiat. **31**, 93–109, 1934.

STOCHDORPH, O.: Gliomsystematik in topistischer Betrachtung. Z. Forschg. ges. Med. **7**, 32–34, 1953.

STOCHDORPH, O.: Die Gewebsbilder der Hirngewächse und ihre Ordnung. Veröffentlichung a. d. morph. Path., H. 60. Gustav Fischer Verlag, Stuttgart 1955.

STÖRTEBECKER, T. P.: Metastatic tumors of the brain from a neurosurgical point of view. A follow up study of 158 cases. J. Neurosurg. **11**, 84–111, 1954.

STOOKEY, B. and J. SCARFF: Occlusion of the aqueduct of Sylvius by neoplastic and non-neoplastic processes with a rational surgical treatment for relief of the resultant obstructive hydrocephalus. Bull. Neur. Inst. New York **5**, 348–377, 1936.

STORCH, E.: Über die pathologisch-anatomischen Vorgänge am Stützgerüst des ZNS. Virchows Arch. **157**, 127–171, 1899.

STOUT, A. P.: The malignant tumors of the peripheral nerves. Amer. J. Cancer **25**, 1–36, 1935.

STOUT, A. P.: Tumors of the peripheral nervous system. Armed Forces Institute of Pathology. Atlas of tumor pathology II, 6, 1949.

STRADA, F.: Beiträge zur Kenntnis der Geschwülste der Hypophyse und der Hypophysengegend. Virchows Arch. **203** 1, 1911.

STRAUSS, I. and J. H. GLOBUS: Spongioblastoma with unusually rapid growth following decompression. Neurol. Bull. 1918, I, 273–279.

STRAUSS, I. and J. H. GLOBUS: Pinealoma in a child of 20 months. Arch. Neurol. Psychiat. **25**, 213, 1931.

STROEBE, H.: Über Entstehung und Bau der Hirngliome. Beitr. path. Anat. 18, 405–485, 1895.

STROEBE, H.: Krankhafte Veränderungen der knöchernen Kapsel und der Hüllen des Gehirns. Im Handb. d. path. Anat. d. Nervensyst. Berlin 1904.

STUMPF: Histologische Beiträge zur Kenntnis des Glioms. Beitr. path. Anat. **51**, 1, 1911.

SUN KEUN KIM: Cerebral paragonimiasis. J. Neurosurg. **12**, 89–94, 1955.

SUSMAN, W.: The significance of the different types of cells of the anterior pituitary. Endocrinology **19**, 592–598, 1935.

SVIEN, H. J., R. F. MABON, J. W. KERNOHAN and A. W. ADSON: Astrocytomas. Proc. Staff Meet., Mayo-Clin. **24**, 54–64, 1949.

SVIEN, H. J., R. F. MABON, J. W. KERNOHAN and W. McK. CRAIG: Ependymoma of the brain: pathologic aspects. Neurology **3**, 1–15, 1953.

SWEET, W.: A review of dermoid, teratoid and teratomatous intracranial tumors. Dis. Nerv. Syst. **1**, 228–238, 1940.

SWEET, W. and P. BAILEY: Experimental production of intracranial tumors in the white rat. Arch. Neurol. Psychiat. **45**, 1047–1049, 1941.

SYLVÉN, BENGT: Über die Elektivität und die Fehlerquellen der Schleimfärbung mit Mucikarmin im Vergleich mit metachromatischen Färbungen. Virchows Arch. **303**, 280, 1939.

TAGGART, J. K. and E. A. WALKER: Congenital atresia of the foramen of Luschka and Magendie. Arch. Neurol. Psychiat. **48**, 582, 1942.

TANNENBERG, J.: Über die Pathogenese der Syringomyelie; zugleich ein Beitrag zum Vorkommen von Capillarhaemangiomen im Rückenmark. Zschr. Neurol. **92**, 119–174, 1924.

TARLOV, J. M.: The effect of roentgentherapy on gliomas. Arch. Neurol. Psychiat. **38**, 513, 1937.

TARLOV, J. M. and L. DAVIDOFF: Subarachnoid and ventricular implants in ependymal and other gliomas. J. Neuropath. **5**, 213–224, 1946.

TEGERTER and SMITH: A case of diffuse neurofibromatosis etc. Amer. J. Cancer **31**, 212, 1937.

TELTSCHAROW, L. und K. J. ZÜLCH: Das Astrocytom des Großhirns vom pathologisch-anatomischen Standpunkt aus. Arch. Psychiatr. **179**, 691–722, 1948.

THIÉBAUT, F.: Klinik und Histologie der Kraniopharyngeome. Wien. klin. Wschr. 409, 1947.

THIELEN, H.: Beitrag zur Kenntnis der sog. Gliastifte; Neuroepithelioma gliomatosum microcysticum medullae spinalis. Dtsch. Z. Nervenhk. **34**, 390, 1908.

THUMS, K.: Zwillingsforschung in der Neurologie. Zbl. inn. Med. **59**, 2–41, 1938.

THUREL, R.: Tumeurs de la région pinéale; traitement combiné, chirurgical (incision de la lame sousoptique) et radiothérapeutique. Rev. neurol. **73**, 1941.

TITRUD, L. A. and W. T. PEYTON: Nasopharyngeal tumors and their neurological complications. J. Nerv. Ment. Dis. **92**, 727–747, 1940.

TÖNNIS, W.: Hirngeschwülste im Kindesalter. Kinderärztl. Praxis 8, 3, 1936.

TÖNNIS, W.: El diagnostico del glioblastoma multiforme por medio de la arteriografia. Un nuevo ensayo de tratamiento de estos tumores. Rev. méd. Chile **12**, 1938.

TÖNNIS, W.: Über Hirngeschwülste. Zschr. Neurol. **161**, 114–149, 1938.

TÖNNIS, W.: Die Chirurgie des Gehirns und seiner Häute. Kirschner-Nordmann, Bd. III. Urban & Schwarzenberg, Wien 1948.

TÖNNIS, W.: Anzeigestellung zur operativen Behandlung der Geschwülste im Bereich des Türkensattels. Klin. Mbl. Augenheilk. **114**, 1–18, 1949.

TÖNNIS, W.: Die operative Behandlung der das For. opticum überschreitenden Geschwülste des N. opticus. Acta Neurochir. **1**, 52–71, 1950.

TÖNNIS, W. und W. F. BORCK: Großhirntumoren des Kindesalters. Zbl. Neurochir. 13, 72–98, 1953.

TÖNNIS, W. und GRIPONISSIOTIS: Zur operativen Behandlung der posttraumatischen Spätepilepsie. Arch. klin. Chir. 196, 515, 1939.

TÖNNIS, W., W. MÜLLER und H. BRILMAYER: Zur Problematik der „mixed types" der Hypophysenadenome. (Ein Vorschlag zur Aufteilung der chromophoben Adenome.) Acta Endocrin. (Copenh.) 13, 227–230, 1953.

TÖNNIS, W., W. MÜLLER, F. OSWALD und H. BRILMAYER: Kann die Rachendachhypophyse eine vikariierende Funktion ausüben? Klin. Wschr. 32, 912–914, 1954.

TÖNNIS, W., K. OBERDISSE und E. WEBER: Bericht über 264 operierte Hypophysenadenome. Acta Neurochir. 3, 113–130, 1953.

TÖNNIS, W. und W. SCHIEFER: Zur Frage des Wachstums arteriovenöser Angiome. Zbl. Neurochir. 15, 145–150, 1955.

TÖNNIS, W. und K. SCHÜRMANN: Meningeome der Keilbeinflügel. Zbl. Neurochir. 11, 1–13, 1951.

TÖNNIS, W. und K. J. ZÜLCH: Das Ependymom der Großhirnhemisphären im Jugendalter. Zbl. Neurochir. 2, 141–164, 1937.

TÖNNIS, W. und K. J. ZÜLCH: Intrakranielle Ganglienzellgeschwülste. Zbl. Neurochir. 4, 273–307, 1939.

TÖPPICH, G.: Über eine ausreifende Ganglienzellgeschwulst des Schläfenlappens. Zschr. Neurol. 156, 29, 1936.

TÖPPICH, G.: Die Zottenkrebse der Adergeflechte der Rautengrube. Frankf. Z. Path. 33, 1926.

TOLOSA, E.: Gliome der Seitenventrikel. Acta Neurochir. (Wien) 3, 369–388, 1954.

TOMPKINS, V. N., W. HAYMAKER and E. H. CAMPBELL: Metastatic pineal tumors. J. Neurosurg. 7, 159–169, 1950.

TONNING, H. O., R. F. WARREN and H. J. BARRIE: Familial haemangiomata of the cerebellum. J. Neurosurg. 9, 124–132, 1952.

TOOTH, H. H.: Some observations on the growth and survival period of intracranial tumors. Brain 35, 61–108, 1912.

TORKILDSEN, A.: Tumors of the glioma group. Acta psychiatr. neurol. K'hvn. 10, 163–196, 1935.

TORKILDSEN, A.: Ein Beitrag zur Klinik der Frontalhirntumoren. Zbl. Neurochir. 2, 291–301, 1937.

TROLAND, C. E. et al.: Ependymoma: A critical re-evaluation of classification with report of cases. J. Neuropath. 10, 295, 1951.

TROLAND, C. E., P. F. SAHYOUN and F. B. MANDEVILLE: Primary mesenchymal tumors of the brain, so-called reticulum cell sarcoma. Report of five cases. J. Neuropath. 7, 322–334, 1950.

TROWBRIDGE, W. V. and J. D. FRENCH: Disseminated oligodendroglioma. J. Neurosurg. 9, 643–648, 1952.

TSCHERNYSCHEFF, A., M. KOPYLOW und K. TERIAN: Über einen Fall von Plexus-Chorioideus-Psammom im rechten Seitenventrikel. Zschr. Neurol. 129, 713–723, 1930.

TURNER, O. A. and J. W. KERNOHAN: Malignant meningeoma, a clinical and pathologic study. Surg. Gynec. Obstetr. 11, 81–100, 1944.

TURNER, O. A. and J. W. KERNOHAN: Vascular malformations and vascular tumors involving the spinal cord. Amer. Assoc. Neuropath. 1941.

TURNER, O. A. and M. A. SIMON: Malignant papilloma of the choroid plexus. Amer. J. Cancer 30, 289, 1937.

UDVARHELYI, J. B.: Über einen riesigen Tumor des Septum pellucidum mit ungewöhnlich kurzer Vorgeschichte. Zbl. Neurochir. 14, 293–297, 1954.

UDVARHELYI, G. B., W. WALTER und W. SCHIEFER: Die Gefäßstruktur des Glioblastoma-multiforme in angiographischer und histologischer Darstellung. Acta Neurochir. Wien 4, 109–127, 1955.

UIHLEIN, A., E. M. GATES and R. G. FISHER: Meningeal meningiomatosis. Report of case. J. Neurosurg. 6, 81–89, 1949.

URBAN, H.: Ein Beitrag zur Kenntnis der Chorioidal-Plexustumoren, Ependymome und Neuroepitheliome. Frankf. Z. Path. 44, 277, 1932.

URBAN, H.: Zur Klinik und Pathologie der Angioblastome im Zentralnervensystem. Zschr. Neurol. 155, 798, 1936.

URBANEK, K.: Zur Kenntnis der gutartigen Melanome des Gehirns. Zschr. Neurol. **175**, 459—475, 1943.

VERAGUTH: Über die Beziehungen zwischen Trauma und einigen Nervenkrankheiten. Dtsch. Z. Nervenhk. **124**, 123—129, 1932; Schweiz. Arch. Neurol. **29**, 153, 1932.

VERBIEST, H.: Die Epidermoide des Rückenmarkes. Analyse eines Falles, zugleich Beitrag zur Frage der Entstehung der aseptischen Meningitis nach Epidermoidoperationen. Zbl. Neurochir. **4**, 129—141, 1939.

VERBIEST, H.: Expériences neurochirurgicales dans l'atrophie optique héréditaire. Rev. neurol. **80**, 657—676, 1948.

VERBIEST, H. und J. ZELDENRUST: Dermoidzyste der Zyst. cerebri magna. Nervenarzt **11**, 366—369, 1938.

VERBRUGGHEN, A.: Paragasserion tumours. J. Neurosurg. **9**, 451—460, 1952.

VERHOEFF, F. H.: Primary intraneural tumors of optic nerve. Arch. Ophth. **51**, 120—140, 1922.

VERHOEFF, F. H.: Tumors of the optic nerve. PENFIELDs Cytology and cellular pathology, Vol. 3, p. 1029. Hoeber 1932.

VEROCAY, J.: Multiple Geschwülste und Systemerkrankungen am nervösen Apparat. CHIARI-Festschrift, Wien u. Leipzig 1908.

VEROCAY, J.: Zur Kenntnis der Neurofibrome. Festschrift für Chiari 1908. 13. Tagg. d. dtsch. Ges. f. Path. 1909; Beitr. path. Anat. **48**, 1910.

VINCENT, C. et al.: Papillomes du 4 ventricule etc. Rev. neurol. **1931**, I, 811.

VINCENT, C., P. PUECH et M. DAVID: Hémangioblastome cérébral. Rev. neurol. **1930**, I.

VINCENT, C., P. PUECH et M. DAVID: A propos de 7 cas d'arachnoidite optochiasmatique. Rev. neurol. 1931.

VINCENT, C. et P. RAPPOPORT: Contribution à l'étude des pinéalomes. Rev. neurol. **40**, 1933.

VIRCHOW, R.: Zur Entwicklungsgeschichte des Krebses usw. Virchows Arch. **1**, 94, 1847.

VIRCHOW, R.: Das wahre Neurom. Virchows Arch. **13**, 1858.

VIRCHOW, R.: Die krankhaften Geschwülste. Hirschwald, Berlin 1863/1865.

VIRCHOW, R.: Das Psammom. Virchows Arch. **160**, 32, 1900.

VOLLAND, K.: Über traumatische Gliomentstehung. Münch. med. Wschr. **37**, 1544—1546, 1925.

VOLLAND, W.: Über multiple Chondrome der Dura mater spinalis. Zbl. Path. **69**, 162, 1938.

VONDERAHE, A. R. and N. R. ABRAMS: Ependymoma of third ventricle. Arch. Ophth. **12**, 693—698, 1934.

VONDERAHE, A. R. and W. T. NIEMER: Intracranial lipoma. J. Neuropath. **3**, 344—354, 1944.

VONWILLER, P.: Über das Epithel und die Geschwülste der Hirnkammern. Virchows Arch. **204**, 230, 1911.

VORIS, H. C. and A. W. ADSON: Tumors of corpus callosum. Arch. Neurol. Psychiat, **34**, 965, 1935.

VOSSKÜHLER, P.: Ein weiterer Beitrag zur Ausbreitungsweise der Hypophysenadenome. Zschr. Neurol. **169**, 444—451, 1940.

WÄTJEN, J.: Ein Ganglioglioneurom des Zentralnervensystems. Virchows Arch. **277**, 441—465, 1930.

WAGENEN, W. P. VAN: Tuberculoma of the brain: its incidence among intracranial tumors and its surgical aspects. Arch. Neurol. Psychiat. **17**, 57—91, 1927.

WAGENEN, W. P. VAN: Papillomas of the chorioid plexus. Arch. Surg. **20**, 199—231, 1930.

WAGENEN, W. P. VAN: Verified brain tumours: end results of 149 cases 8 years after operation. J. A. M. A. **102**, 1454—1458, 1934.

WAGENEN, W. P. VAN and R. B. AIRD: Dilatations of the cavity of the septum pellucidum and Cavum vergae. Amer. J. Cancer **20**, 539—557, 1934.

WAGGONER, R. W. and K. LÖWENBERG: Clinico-pathologic study of astrocytomas. Arch. Neurol. Phychiat. **38**, 1208—1223, 1937.

WAGNER, W. und H. COSACK: Hirnzysticerkose. Zschr. Neurol. **156**, 660, 1936.

WALKER, A. EARL: Astrocytosis arachnoideae cerebelli. Arch. Path. **45**, 520, 1941.

WALKER, A. EARL: A history of Neurological Surgery. The Williams & Wilkins Co., Baltimore 1951.

WALKER, A. EARL et C. E. ALLÈGRE: Histopathologie et pathogénie des anévrysmes artériels cérébraux. Rev. neurol. **89**, 477—490, 1953.

WALKER, A. EARL and P. C. BUCY: Congenital dermal sinuses: a source of spinal meningeal infection and subdural abscesses. Brain **57**, 401—421, 1934.

WALKER, A. EARL, H. C. JOHNSON and K. M. BROWNE: Hemangiomas of the fourth ventricle. J. Neuropath. 11, 103–115, 1952.

WALKER, J. C. and G. HORRAX: Papilloma of the choroid plexus. J. Neurosurg. 4, 387–391, 1947.

WALTER, W.: Über die sogenannten Zylindrome an der Hirnbasis. Zbl. Path. 93, 422, 1955.

WALTER, W.: Zur Wirkung der Röntgenstrahlen auf das Hirn. Zbl. Neurochir. 14, 297–301, 1954.

WALTHER, H.-E.: Krebs-Metastasen. B. Schwab, édit., Bâle 1948.

WEBER, E.: Über den Bau der Meningeome. Zschr. Neurol. 161, 211–214, 1938.

WEBER, E.: Die Teratome und Teratoide des Zentralnervensystems. Zbl. Neurochir. 4, 47–57, 1939.

WEHRLI, G. A.: Zur Gliom- und Rosettenfrage. Graefes Arch. Augenhk. 71, 1909.

WEIGERT, C.: Zur Lehre von den Tumoren der Hirnanhänge. Virchows Arch. 65, 212–219, 1875.

WEIL, A.: Experimental production of tumors in the brains of white rat. Arch. Path. 26, 777–790, 1938.

WEIL, A. and B. BLUMKLOTZ: Experimental intracranial epithelial cysts. J. Neuropath. 2, 34–44, 1943.

WEIL, A. and M. P. ROSENBLUM: Astrocytoma of fifteen years duration. A case report. J. Neuropath. 11, 409–420, 1952.

WEIMANN, W.: Tuberkulose, Aktinomykose, Hefeinfektionen. Handb. d. Geisteskrankh., Bd. XI/VII: Die Anatomie der Psychosen, S. 130–156. Springer, Berlin 1930.

WEINBERGER, L. M. and F. GRANT: Precocious puberty and tumors of the hypothalamus. Arch. int. Med. 67, 762, 1941.

WEISS, P.: Über einen Kombinationstumor des Gehirns. Frankf. Z. Path. 44, 1932.

WENZEL, J. C.: Über die schwammigen Auswüchse auf der äußeren Hirnhaut. Mainz 1811.

WERNER, I.: Kyste épidermique intra-rachidien. Nord. Med. 41, 815-817, 1949.

WERNER, T.: Ein Pinealom mit diffuser Metastasierung in die Meningen. Zbl. Neurochir. 4, 155–160, 1939.

WERTHEIMER, P., G. ALLÈGRE et A. GARDE: Les tumeurs épendymaires de la moelle et du filum terminale. Rev. neurol. 82, 153–162, 1950.

WETTLER, H.: Das intrakranielle Epidermoid. Mschr. Psychiatr. 115, 233–276, 1948.

WILKE, G.: Zur Angioarchitektonik der gliomatösen Hirntumoren. Arch. Psychiat. 116, 4, 1943.

WILKE, G.: Über primäre Reticuloendotheliosen des Gehirns. Dtsch. Z. Nervenhk. 164, 332–380, 1950.

WILKE, G.: Über Rethotelsarkome des Gehirns. Verh. Dtsch. Ges. Path. Hannover 1951. Stuttgart: Piscator-Verlag 1952, S. 178.

WILKE, G.: Granulomatous encephalitis, with reference to known and unknown aetiologies. Excerpta Med. Neurol. and Psychiat. 8, 824, 1955.

WILLIS, R. A.: Pathology of tumours. Butterworths and Co., London 1953.

WNKELMAN, N. W. jr., C. CASSEL and B. SCHLESINGER: Intracranial tumors with extracranial metastases. J. Neuropath. 11, 149–168, 1952.

WINKLER: Sarkome. Erg. allg. Path. 23, 22, 1930.

WINTERSTEINER, H.: Das Neuroepithelioma retinae. Deuticke 1897.

WISLOCKI, G. B. and T. J. PUTNAM: Note on the anatomy of the area postrema. Anat. Rec. 27, 151–156, 1924.

WITT, J. A., C. S. MACCARTY and F. R. KEATING: Craniopharyngioma (pituitary adamantinoma) in patients more than 60 years of age. J. Neurosurg. 12, 354–360, 1955.

WITTERMANN, E.: Hypophysengangstumoren und vegetative Zentren des Zwischenhirns. Nervenarzt, 9 441–516, 1936.

WOHLWILL, FR.: Über gleichzeitiges Vorkommen von Hirngliomen und Sarkomen. Mitt. aus der Hamburger Staatskrankenanstalt 1910.

WOHLWILL, FR.: Ein Fall von Angiomatosis des Zentralnervensystems (Lindausche Erkrankung). Zbl. Neurol. 46, 456, 1927.

WOHLWILL, FR.: Zur pathologischen Anatomie der malignen medianen Kleinhirntumoren der Kinder. Zschr. Neurol. 128, 587–614, 1930.

WOLF, A. and D. COWEN: Angioblastic meningiomas. Bull. Neurol. Inst. New York 5, 485–503, 1936.

WOLF, A. and F. ECHLIN: Osteochondrosarcoma of the falx. Bull. Neurol. Inst. New York 5, 515–525, 1936.

WOLF, A. and B. F. MORTON: Ganglion cell tumors of the central nervous system. Bull. Neurol. Inst. New York **6**, 453–488, 1937.

WOLF, A. and S. T. ORTON: Intranuclear inclusions in brain tumors. Bull. Neurol. Inst. New York **3**, 113–123, 1933.

WOLF, N.: Gliom und Kriegsverletzung. Nervenarzt **22**, 430/431, 1951.

WOLF, N.: Kriegsverletzung des Gehirns und Hirntumorenentwicklung. Z. Unfallmed. u. Berufskrankh. **44**, 279–284, 1951.

WOLMAN, L.: The origin of the fibrous tissue in meningiomata. J. Neuropath. **12**, 194–200, 1953.

WOLLSTEIN, M. and F. H. BARTLETT: Brain tumors in young children. Amer. J. Dis. Child. **25**, 257–283, 1923.

WOLTMAN, H. W.: Malignant tumors of the nasopharynx. Arch. Neurol. Psychiat. **8**, 414–429, 1922.

WOLTMAN, H. W., J. W. KERNOHAN and A. W. ADSON: Gliomas of the cerebellopontine angle. Proc. Staff Meet. Mayo-Clinic **24**, 77–82, 1949.

WOLTMAN, H. W., J. W. KERNOHAN, A. W. ADSON and W. McK. CRAIG: Intramedullary tumors of spinal cord and gliomas of intradural portion of filum terminale: Fate of patients who have these tumors. Arch. Neurol. Psychiat. **65**, 378–393, 1951.

WOOLSEY, R. D.: Hemangioblastoma of cerebellum with polycythemia. J. Neurosurg. **8**, 447–449, 1951.

WRIGHT, J. H.: Neurocytoma or neuroblastoma, a kind of tumor not generally recognized. J. exper. Med. **12**, 556–560, 1910.

WYCIS, H. T.: Oligodendroglioma of the cerebellum. Arch. Neurol. Psychiat. **59**, 404, 1948.

YAKOVLEV, P. I. and R. H. GUTHRIE: Congenital ectodermoses (neurocutaneous syndromes) in epileptic patients. Arch. Neurol. Psychiat. **26**, 244, 1931.

YENERMAN, M.: Histological and topographical study of gliomas in Turkey. Excerpta med. Neurol. Psychiat. **8**, 797, 1955.

YUHL, E. T. and C. W. RAND: Tuberculous opticochiasmatic arachnoiditis. J. Neurosurg. **8**, 441–447, 1951.

ZAAIJER, J. H.: Über die Behandlung von metastatischen Tumoren. Zbl. Neurochir. **3**, 7–12, 1938.

ZALKA, E. v.: Beitrag zur Pathohistologie des menschlichen Plexus chorioideus. Virchows Arch. **267**, 379–412, 1928.

ZAMORA, M. M.: Patogenia de las lesiones tuberculosas del sistema nervoso. Anais do IV. Congr. Sul-Americano de Neuro-Cirurgia, Porto Alegre, Bras., Mai 1951, S. 67–76.

ZANDER, E.: 6 Fälle von Papillomen des Plexus chorioideus. Mschr. Psychiatr. **118**, 321 –363, 1949.

ZEHNDER, M.: Subarachnoidalzysten des Gehirns. Zbl. Neurochir. **3**, 100–112, 1938.

ZEITLHOFER, J. und H. KRAUS: Über die extrakranielle Metastasierung der Gliome. Zbl. Neurochir. **12**, 347–357, 1952.

ZEITLIN, H.: Adamantinomas of the hypophysial stalk. Amer. J. Cancer **23**, 729–740, 1935.

ZEITLIN, H.: Tumors in the region of the pineal body. Report of 3 cases. Arch. Neurol. Psychiat. **34**, 567, 1935.

ZEITLIN, H.: Hemangioblastomas of the meninges and their relation to Lindau disease. J. Neuropath. **1**, 14–23, 1942.

ZEITLIN, H. and LEVINSON: Intracranial chordoma. Arch. Path. **45**, 984, 1941.

ZEMAN, W.: Zur Frage der Röntgenstrahlenwirkung am tumorkranken Gehirn. Arch. Psychiatr. **182**, 713–730, 1949.

ZEMAN, W.: Die Toleranzdosis des Hirngewebes bei der Röntgentiefenbestrahlung. Strahlentherapie **81**, 549–556, 1950.

ZIMMERMANN, H. M.: Experimental brain tumours. II. Intern. Congr. of Neuropathology, London 1955.

ZIMMERMANN, H. M.: The nature of gliomas as revealed by animal experimentation. Amer. J. Path. **31**, 1–30, 1955.

ZIMMERMANN, H. M. and H. ARNOLD: Experimental brain tumors I. Tumors produced with methylcholanthrene. Cancer Res. **1**, 919–938, 1941.

ZIMMERMANN, H. M. and H. ARNOLD: Brain tumors produced with benzpyren. J. Neuropath. **1**, 123, 1942. — Amer. J. Path. **19**, 939–955, 1943.

ZONDEK, B.: Hypophyseal tumors induced by oestrogen hormone. Amer. J. Cancer **36**, 555, 1949.

ZSCHAU, H.: Beitrag zur Kenntnis der Cauda equina. Frankf. Z. Path. 38, 400–438, 1929.

ZÜLCH, K. J.: Zur Histopathologie der Großhirngliome in den ersten beiden Lebensjahrzehnten. Zschr. Neurol. 158, 369–374, 1937.

ZÜLCH, K. J.: Zur histologischen Schnelldiagnose bei der Operation von Hirngeschwülsten. Arch. klin. Chir. 189, 492–493, 1937.

ZÜLCH, K. J.: Die Hirngeschwülste des Jugendalters. Zschr. Neurol. 161, 183–188, 1938.

ZÜLCH, K. J.: Die Gefäßversorgung der Gliome. Zschr. Neurol. 167, 585–592, 1939.

ZÜLCH, K. J.: Über die geschichtliche Entwicklung und den heutigen Stand der Klassifikation der Hirngeschwülste. Zbl. Neurochir. 4, 251–272, 325–331, 1939.

ZÜLCH, K. J.: Über das sog. Kleinhirnastrocytom. Virchows Arch. 307, 222–252, 1940.

ZÜLCH, K. J.: Hirngeschwülste im Jugendalter. Zbl. Neurochir. 5, 238–274, 1940.

ZÜLCH, K. J.: Das Medulloblastom. Arch. Psychiatr. 112, 343–367, 1940.

ZÜLCH, K. J.: Die Pathologie der Hirngeschwülste (insbesondere der Gliome) und ihre Bedeutung für die Klinik. Wien. klin. Wschr. 53, 498, 1940.

ZÜLCH, K. J.: Über die morphologischen Folgen der Anwendung elektrischen Stromes zum Schneiden und Koagulieren des Hirn- und Geschwulstgewebes. Dtsch. Z. Nervenhk. 151, 141–145, 1940.

ZÜLCH, K. J.: Das Oligodendrogliom. Zschr. Neurol. 172, 407–482, 1941.

ZÜLCH, K. J.: Ein Medulloblastom mit glatten Muskelfasern. Arch. Psychiat. 114, 349–352, 1941.

ZÜLCH, K. J.: Hirnödem und Hirnschwellung. Virchows Arch. 310, 1–58, 1943.

ZÜLCH, K. J.: Pathologische Anatomie und Biologie der intrakraniellen Geschwülste. In: KIRSCHNER-NORDMANN „Die Chirurgie“, Bd. III, S. 665, 1948.

ZÜLCH, K. J.: Sobre a significacão clinica de uma classificacão apropriada dos tumores encefalicos. Arqu. Neuro-Psiquiatr. (S. Paulo, Brasil) 7, 113–125, 1949.

ZÜLCH, K. J.: Häufigkeit, Vorzugssitz und Erkrankungsalter bei Hirngeschwülsten. Zbl. Neurochir. 9, 115–128, 1949.

ZÜLCH, K. J.: Zur Pathologie der äußeren Liquorräume. Zbl. Neurochir. 10, 25–38, 1950.

ZÜLCH, K. J.: Vegetative und psychische Symptome bei umschriebenen traumatischen Zwischenhirnschädigungen. Zbl. Neurochir. 10, 73–97, 1950.

ZÜLCH, K. J.: Über die „unklassifizierten“ Hirngeschwülste. Acta Neurochir. 1, 283–299, 1950.

ZÜLCH, K. J.: Fortschritte auf dem Gebiet der Morphologie und Biologie der Hirngeschwülste unter besonderer Darstellung der Klassifikation. Fortschr. Neurol. Psychiatr. 18, 513–538, 1950.

ZÜLCH, K. J.: Diskussionsbemerkungen zu den Frontallappengeschwülsten. Zbl. Neurochir. 11, 286–287, 1951.

ZÜLCH, K. J.: Vorzugssitz, Erkrankungsalter und Geschlechtsbevorzugung bei Hirngeschwülsten als bisher ungeklärte Formen der Pathoklise. Dtsch. Z. Nervenhk. 166, 91–102, 1951.

ZÜLCH, K. J.: Schema zur Erleichterung der Klassifikation der neuroepithelialen Geschwülste. Acta Neurochir. 3, 104–110, 1952.

ZÜLCH, K. J.: Estado actual de la classificacion de los tumores cerebrales. Folia clinica internacional 2, 1952.

ZÜLCH, K. J.: Über die primären Hirnsarkome. Arch. Int. Stu. Neur. Firenze 2, 1–35, 1953.

ZÜLCH, K. J.: Hirngeschwülste als Schädigungsfolge. Ärztl. Forschg. 7, I/535–543, 1953.

ZÜLCH, K. J.: Hirnschwellung und Hirnödem. Dtsch. Z. Nervenhk. 170, 179–208, 1953.

ZÜLCH, K. J.: Betrachtungen über die Entstehung der frühkindlichen Hirnschäden auf Grund der klinischen und morphologischen Befunde. Arch. Kinderhk. 149, 1–27, 1954.

ZÜLCH, K. J.: Mikroskopischer Farbatlas der Hirngeschwülste. (Leitz-Wetzlar, Agfa-Leverkusen) 1955.

ZÜLCH, K. J.: Biologie und Pathologie der Hirngeschwülste. Im Handbuch der Neurochirurgie. III. Bd.: Pathologie, Anatomie der raumbeengenden intrakraniellen Prozesse. 702 S., Springer 1956.

ZÜLCH, K. J.: La génèse des tumeurs cérébrales. La malignité des tumeurs de l'encéphale et ses problèmes. Vorträge, gehalten im Curso de Tumores Intracraniales der Universität Santander (Spanien) August 1955. — Ref. Zbl. Neurochir. 16, 52–54, 1956.

ZÜLCH, K. J.: Problems in the diagnosis of oligodendrogliomas. Excerpta Med., Neur., Psych., 8, 816, 1955. Ref. Zbl. Neurochir. 16, 46–48, 1956.

ZÜLCH, K. J. siehe W. F. BORCK: Über die Erkrankungshäufigkeit der Geschlechter an Hirngeschwülsten. Zbl. Neurochir. **11**, 333–350, 1951.

ZÜLCH, K. J. und W. F. BORCK: Tafeln über die relative Häufigkeit der Hirngeschwülste in verschiedenen Altersklassen. Zbl. Neurochir. **12**, 93–97, 1952.

ZÜLCH, K. J. siehe G. KRAUSE: Über die Häufigkeit der Hirntumorarten in den verschiedenen Regionen. Zbl. Neurochir. **11**, 221–230, 1951.

ZÜLCH, K. J. und F. PINTO: Zur Klassifikation polymorpher Gliome. Zbl. Neurochir. **13**, 27–40, 1953.

ZÜLCH, K. J., F. POMPEU und F. PINTO: Über die Metastasierung der Meningeome. Zbl. Neurochir. **14**, 253–260, 1954.

ZÜLCH, K. J. mit D. RIESSNER: Über die Formveränderungen des Hirns (Massenverschiebungen, Zisternenverquellungen bei raumbeengenden Prozessen). Dtsch. Z. Chir. **253**, 1–61, 1939.

ZÜLCH, K. J. und E. E. SCHMID: Über das Ependymom der Seitenkammern am Foramen Monroi. Arch. Psychiatr. **193**, 214–228, 1955.

ZÜLCH, K. J. und E. E. SCHMID: Eigenartige intermittierende Einklemmungsanfälle beim Angioblastom ohne Zeichen des Hirndrucks. Zbl. Neurochir. 1956. (Im Druck.)

ZÜLCH, K. J. siehe D. RIESSNER: Über die Formveränderungen des Hirns (Massenverschiebungen, Zisternenverquellungen bei raumbeengenden Prozessen). Dtsch. Z. Chir. **253**, 1–61, 1939.

ZÜLCH, K. J. siehe A. STENDER: Über die Ventrikeltumoren bei tuberöser Sklerose. Zschr. Neurol. **176**, 556–578, 1943.

ZÜLCH, K. J. siehe W. TÖNNIS: Das Ependymom der Großhirnhemisphären im Jugendalter. Zbl. Neurochir. **2**, 141–164, 1937.

ZÜLCH, K. J. siehe W. TÖNNIS: Intrakranielle Ganglienzellgeschwülste (mit ausführlicher Beschreibung einer einheitlichen Gruppe im Großhirn). Zbl. Neurochir. **4**, 273–307, 1939.

ZÜLCH, K. J. siehe L. TELTSCHAROW: Das Astrozytom des Großhirns vom pathologisch-anatomischen Standpunkt aus. Arch. Psychiatr. **179**, 691–720, 1948.

INDEX